CONDITIONING TO THE CORE

Greg Brittenham

Daniel Taylor

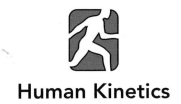

Human Kinetics

Library of Congress Cataloging-in-Publication Data

Brittenham, Greg.
  Conditioning to the core / Greg Brittenham, Daniel Taylor.
    pages cm
  1. Exercise--Handbooks, manuals, etc. 2. Abdominal exercises. 3. Back exercises. I. Taylor, Daniel, 1979- II. Title.
  GV508.B755 2014
  613.7'1--dc23

                        2014003256

ISBN: 978-1-4504-1969-7 (print)

Developmental Editors: Laura E. Podeschi and Julie Marx Goodreau; **Assistant Editor:** Tyler M. Wolpert; **Copyeditor:** John Wentworth; **Graphic Designer:** Fred Starbird; **Cover Designer:** Keith Blomberg; **Photograph (cover):** Larry C. Lawson/Icon SMI; **Photographs (interior):** Neil Bernstein, unless otherwise noted; **Photo Asset Manager:** Laura Fitch; **Visual Production Assistant:** Joyce Brumfield; **Photo Production Manager:** Jason Allen; **Art Manager:** Kelly Hendren; **Associate Art Manager:** Alan L. Wilborn; **Illustrations:** © Human Kinetics, unless otherwise noted; **Printer:** Premier Print Group

We thank Wake Forest University for assistance in providing the location for the photo shoot for this book.

Human Kinetics books are available at special discounts for bulk purchase. Special editions or book excerpts can also be created to specification. For details, contact the Special Sales Manager at Human Kinetics.

Printed in the United States of America   10 9 8 7 6 5 4 3

Human Kinetics
P.O. Box 5076
Champaign, IL 61825-5076
Website: www.HumanKinetics.com

In the United States, email info@hkusa.com or call 800-747-4457.
In Canada, email info@hkcanada.com.
In the United Kingdom/Europe, email hk@hkeurope.com.

For information about Human Kinetics' coverage in other areas of the world,
please visit our website: **www.HumanKinetics.com**   E5582

Tell us what you think!
Human Kinetics would love to hear what we
can do to improve the customer experience.
Use this QR code to take our brief survey.

For Dad. Well into his sixth decade of training athletes and still a pioneer in the field of sport performance, Dad's unwavering passion to help people is matched only by his inspiring personal convictions and thirst for learning. He continues to amaze me with his creativity, kindness, and one singularly focused agenda: to do good in this world. Dad, you never gave up on me even after the repeated failures of my QI tests.

Greg Brittenham

For my beautiful wife, Erin, who I know will always meet me where the flame turns blue.

Daniel Taylor

Contents

Acknowledgments

It would be impossible to express my appreciation to all the decent people in my life who, through their example, inspired me to choose the path less traveled. These people lack arrogance and self-absorbed duplicity; their sincerity and creative influence have helped to mold my personal philosophy. These pages may not have all the answers, but at least it is an honest attempt at inspiring the reader's own creativity.

In so lacking the necessary basal ganglia to adhere to any sort of logical compositional constructs, most of the acknowledgments that follow make about as much sense as George W. Bush's "strategery" toward fiscal responsibility. You never know who might want to include me in their will. Therefore, I'd like to acknowledge these people:

Luann, my wife, you're a real mensch whose constant stream of positive support is equaled only by your naïveté toward sarcasm. Thank you for your trust and unwavering confidence that I could achieve anything that you put your mind to.

Max and Rachel, your father, being one neuron short of a synapse, fell out of the family tree and hit every branch on the way down, landing in the gene pool while the lifeguard was adding chlorine. Nevertheless, you both emerged from the primordial ooze with integrity, work ethic, and moral certitude. Kids, you are a constant source of joy and inspiration. You *will* change the world.

Steve Brittenham, you are a remarkable brother, father, husband, and coach. I aspire to your vast accomplishments. You always said that anyone with half a brain could write an abdominal book. Well, here it is.

Dan Furlong, you are a fantastic teacher, a phenomenal parent, and unquestionably the best person I know. My friend the phoenix, you continually rise from the flames. Your collection of pink slips from the Knicks could wallpaper a . . . umm . . . sorry . . . lost my train of thought. Was thinking about my deck.

Jean Smith, you taught me that ambiguity was something entirely different. Ron Smith, you taught me to love all animals. Especially barbecued with a less-than-subtle chipotle pepper, cilantro, oregano, cumin, and orange peel rub and a side of creamed peas and potatoes.

Lauren Huff, who is excited about her recent discovery of a remedy for her insomnia in that, every time she starts to read one of my books, she falls asleep. Lyle Huff, host of the wildly entertaining and informative *Safety Show* on KHNS Public Radio in Haines, Alaska: After a recent inspection of my camping skills, you concluded that it would take me only one match to burn down a forest but an entire box to start a campfire.

Jeff Bzdelik, when you called and said you needed a player development coach in the worst way, I said, "I'm your man." Since my arrival at Wake, I finally feel a sense of family in which our collective efforts are not wasted on pretense but truly serve a higher purpose. I embrace denunciation of player pampering and wholeheartedly welcome your belief in hard work and focused training.

Jeff Nix, you taught me that to err is human, and to blame it on the players shows coaching potential. Nietzsche said, "To live is to suffer; to survive is to find some meaning in the suffering." If wisdom were the consequential result from circumstances of difficulty, then I must be the smartest guy in the world. You believed when others refused to. For that I am eternally grateful.

Mary Ann Justice, without you I would most certainly miss mandatory meetings, required fees, and compulsory appointments. I've had a bad memory for as long as I can remember. People pay big money for the psychotherapy services that you provide for free. Enough of me talking about me. Why don't *you* talk about me for a while?

The sport performance staff at Wake Forest University: knowledgeable, ethical, high-character, selfless, and enthusiastic colleagues. Your genuine concern for your charges is refreshingly unique. It's amazing what can be accomplished from a singularly-focused agenda.

To our models, Abbe Brooks, Erin Brooks, Brad Beauregard, Will Murphy, Zak Butler, and Max Brittenham, your photos radiate infectious smiles, positive dispositions, competitive spirits, concentration, and athleticism. Dan and I are honored that each of you have become the focus of the book, and we are convinced that the bar has been raised extremely high for the readers. And of course, to Randolph Childress, 1995 ACC Tournament MVP, ACC Athlete of the Year, NCAA All-American, NBA first-round draft pick, a wonderful family, and now this book. I can only assume that your wildest dreams have now been completely fulfilled. Thanks to everyone for your participation.

To the Winston-Salem University Parkway Starbucks morning crew, who kept me sufficiently caffeinated during the writing of this book. My heart attack while sitting in the big comfy chair in front of the fireplace in the quiet room did not deter me from returning, four days later, to your wonderful establishment to delight in your friendly service and exceptional fair-trade product while trying to finish chapter 8 prior to the publisher's deadline. . . thrombosis notwithstanding. Another stream of consciousness sentence. Thank you, James Joyce.

To Barry Slotnick of Varisport, who provided support, encouragement, friendship, and the best slideboard on the planet.

To Nike for providing the shoes and apparel that make the content look credible and further support the illusion that I am qualified to have anything to do with writing a book.

Pat Riley, in the early '90s, you established my career by believing in a radically unique training methodology.

All the coaches, mentors, athletes, and staff (too numerous to mention all) who made working with the Knicks during the '90s exciting, successful, rewarding, educational, and the greatest experience of my life: Jeff Van Gundy, Allan Houston, Patrick Ewing, Don Chaney, Doc Rivers, Mark Jackson, Herb Williams, Larry Johnson, Dr. Jack Ramsey, Mike Breen, Mike Martinez, Jonathan Supranowitz, Matt Harding, Mike Smith, John Donahue, Lenny Wilkins. And special thanks for the truthfulness and authenticity of Mike Saunders, Said Hamdan, Dr. Norman Scott, Dr. Peter Bruno, and Dr. Fred Kushner, who had no other personal agenda but to help the team move closer to our collective goal of winning a championship.

Greg Brittenham

E rin—girlfriend, fiancée, best friend, wife, companion, director of household operations, and now mother to our children—you have always been and will always be everything to me. Your love, support, and unmitigated faith in me are at times humbling, and I consider myself fortunate to be able to forever call you Mrs. T.

Lorelai and Jackson, my twins, you were born during the inception of this book, and this project has grown as you have. In two short years you have redefined for me what being a man and a father are all about. In you I finally understand love in its purest form, and seeing the wonders of the world through your virgin eyes is an ongoing, delightful journey. More than anything else, you have taught me that nothing in life is more important than your mother's face, Mickey Mouse, and a new pair of wellies.

Thanking my parents in the acknowledgments page of this book can only go a short way in repaying them for everything they have done for me. If I end up being half as good a parent as you have been to me, then my life as a father will have been a success. Mum, you gave me

wings and told me I could fly; Dad, you stressed the importance of first learning how to use them before I left the ground. These tools combined with my brother's unabashed love, respect, and praise for the man I have become have made me able to soar to heights that even I would never have thought possible.

Greg Brittenham, thank you not only for inviting me to work with you on this project also but for extending me the hand of friendship and for sharing with me many, many years of experience. The most important lesson that you have taught me is that even though we should perform serious work, we must always remember to laugh a lot while doing it.

A few years ago I decided that when I grow up I want to be Dr. Jeremy Sheppard, the sport science manager and head of strength and conditioning for Surf Australia. A native Canadian who works with the best surfers in Australia! Jeremy, you are the best strength coach I have ever met and, more important, a gracious friend. Given the distance between us and the limited time we spend together, I am always grateful for your friendship and shared knowledge.

I would be incredibly remiss in not thanking Siena College as an institution and a staff for supporting me unquestionably and for allowing me to grow as a professional. Specifically I want to thank the hundreds of athletes who have come through the doors of my weight room and trusted my decisions and guidance every step of their journey. Particular thanks go to Kenny Hasbrouck. At the lowest point in your fledgling pro career, you put your future in my hands; in doing so, you afforded me one of the most rewarding experiences of my professional life.

We will forever be grateful to the gifted hands of our editors, Laura Podeschi and Julie Marx Goodreau, along with the sage wisdom of VP Ted Miller for turning the frustrated ramblings of a strength coach into something resembling elegant prose. You epitomize professionalism and guided me through an industry I know very little about. I thank you for bringing creativity, direction, and levity to my experience with this project.

Thanks to every member of the Human Kinetics staff we have worked with on various aspects of this book over the last few years. You are all incredible at what you do, and I thank you for making a summertime phone conversation with Greg turn into a beautiful reality.

Special thanks to Sally Herrick, Jerri Wassenaar, Christina De Lella, Linda Bartlett, and the whole O'Hara family for serving as guinea pigs, friends, and confidants over more years than I can remember. To our amazing models, Erin, Max, Will, Zak, Abbe, Randolph, and Brad. Your enthusiasm and commitment to this project show through in every picture.

Coach Reeve and the strength and conditioning staff at Wake Forest, thanks for letting us take over your weight room for a crazy weekend.

As a big believer in the fact that as a young professional I stand on the shoulders of giants (Greg's father Dean among them), with grave sincerity I thank many of the often nameless and faceless professionals whose ideas, philosophies, and victories echo throughout my work. You have given me a profession I love and a job I marvel over every single day.

Daniel Taylor

Introduction
Unleashing Your Core Potential

A 95 mile per hour fastball, a slam dunk over a defender: Both of these actions provide a quintessential moment in their respective sport. Honing these abilities is critical for the serious participant who strives to maximize performance potential; a myriad of "throw harder, jump higher, and run faster" training programs are incorporated with this very objective in mind. The truth of the matter is, though, that instead of looking to the outside for extrinsic activities that may help with this development, one should look within. A functionally trained core region will enhance athletic efficiency and better transfer power throughout the various links in the body, which can lead to a triple-digit mile per hour fastball or help you evolve from a perennial rim toucher to a full-blown slam dunker.

How, then, does the core play such an important role in all of this, when your legs appear to drive your movement and the dexterity of your arms is displayed in all facets of life? Because *all force generated by upper- and lower-body musculature originates in, is stabilized by, or is transferred through the trunk and low torso.* This has huge fitness and athletic ramifications, especially when you look at the core from a performance standpoint. If we strengthen the core—the transfer of energy—the efficiency of our actions and next-level performance variables will most certainly increase while, simultaneously, the risk of injury will decrease.

The core should be trained in the same way it was originally developed, following this sequence: Stability precedes strength, and strength comes before power. An easy way to visualize this training is to think about a newborn baby. Initially, the child has no core control. The first big event for new parents is the predictable process whereby the newborn begins to stabilize the core. This in turn leads to heightened total body control, which can then facilitate rolling over. The developmental process of moving from the realm of primitive and postural reflexive actions to the phase of rudimentary movement patterns is of utmost importance. If this transference does not take place or is delayed for some reason, further development will be inhibited. So much of that last statement is true with regards to the successful implementation of and exercise regimen as well. Plateaus are the athlete's nemesis.

Now that the baby can roll over, she is in a position to draw her limbs under their mass, and as the muscles become more potent, the crawl is soon to follow. This is a display of strength; for a crawl to be effective and synchronized, the core must be strong enough to not only stabilize the pelvis and spine but also to pass the aforementioned forces to the limbs to create movement. Lastly are the epic first wobbly steps. While this may not be as impressive as a fully-fledged run, the ability to control the core in a vertical fashion while lifting limbs and balancing is the beginning of true core power.

The technical term for this process is proximal-to-distal development. Motor development, or movement skill, begins with the larger and slower muscles of the core (the proximal muscles) early in a child's life. As a healthy child matures, development moves gradually away from gross motor patterns associated with the center of mass and out to the smaller muscles of the extremities (the distal muscles), which are responsible for fine motor skills. Whether you perform a fine motor skill, such as throwing darts, or a gross motor pattern, such as rowing a skull, you must have a strong core to ensure safe, efficient, and effective function.

Each chapter of this book will build on the one before, allowing you to understand the system we use and teaching you that all core work is essentially a series of functional progressions. All of the exercises are color-coded (blue for stabilization, red for strength, green for power), helping to aid in your understanding of which area of the core is being targeted. Along with photographs and descriptions, the exercises will demonstrate how to either progress or regress depending on your level of ability.

Finally, we will outline a number of tests that will allow you to determine a starting point for your training. These tests will also help you to organize and periodically monitor an intelligent progression so you do not advance too quickly through a phase or restrict yourself from jumping to the next phase when you should. While these tests will illuminate areas of weakness and assist you in identifying asymmetries with your core's dynamic functionality, fear not, for they will also identify your core strengths. Our goal is to continue to reinforce your established core strengths while gradually balancing out the asymmetries and greatly lessening and hopefully eventually eliminating your core weaknesses. Combined with these tests are sample workouts of each level of core training, which enable you to see how everything comes together in a seamless, time-efficient workout.

The information in this book is essential to building a strong core program that should be highlighted and focused on as much as any part of your training. With that being said, to reach your full athletic potential other areas of training, such as mobility, strength, and agility, must also be attended to. With that in mind, the workouts presented in later chapters should only take between 15-20 minutes, allowing more time to have a full, comprehensive training session.

Ultimately, no matter your present level of fitness or athleticism, this book will lay the foundation on which you can unleash your physical potential to the fullest.

CORE BENEFITS

Sport and athletic performance has gripped the country with such a fervor that sports enthusiasts can now find TV channels dedicated to sporting events 24 hours a day. Not only is participation in physical activity and sport on the rise, but sports lovers looking to escape into the world of observation are at unprecedented levels. You need look no further than the Olympics, the World Series, the World Cup, and the king of all American sports viewership, the NFL's Super Bowl, to recognize that sport is a multibillion-dollar business. Our infatuation with sport has become a part of the national psyche as much as apple pie and hot dogs.

This hyperfocus has created a ripple effect. Never before have we lived at a stage of athletic advancement when so much is at stake—be it a full scholarship to the institution of your dreams or bragging rights in your backyard—which means athletes are constantly looking for ways to gain an edge over the competition. Also, more than ever before, we are engaged at a time when rules prevent pushing the boundaries of fair play within competition. Thus it is the flesh-and-blood vehicles that now drive our sports—our bodies—and these vehicles have boundless room for improvement and advancement. In this area, the possibilities are only just being discovered by science, and they seem to change every generation. What was true then is false now, and what was once thought physically impossible by our grandfathers is now seen on television on weekend afternoons. As gene pools mix and sport taps into a growing global marketplace, exploding the limits of popularity and participation, physical capacities will be stretched even further.

A NEVER-CHANGING TRUTH

One truth that has never changed, and is not likely to, is that the core of the body is the anchor to almost all success—be it as epic as an Olympic gold medal or as discretely effectual as a full recovery following back surgery. The core's importance, in its many delineated manifestations, has been a known entity since antiquity, when warriors were taught to maintain balance with resistance in the form of rocks in their hands. With the changing of generations, more and more information regarding the core has come to light, but as frequently occurs, information can be fragmented or watered down.

Many disciplines that work with the body have developed, but this does not always lead to greater overall knowledge. Chiropractors tend to know a lot about the spine but typically not much about progressive overload. Strength professionals know about progressive overload but usually not as much about quality of movement and preventive exercise. Most physiotherapists intimately understand quality of movement but sometimes avoid pushing global strength and spend too much time on isolated or regional development. Doctors and athletic trainers can excel at healing the body but might lack understanding of the full process of athletic development, even at the elite level, where resources abound.

The combined knowledge of these practitioners could equip an army of athletes, and the most successful teams have a symbiotic relationship among members of such a support staff. More often than not, however, each specialist has a reluctant attitude toward collaboration and avoids any cross-pollination of knowledge. Sadly, this leads to many schools of thought; though they all have the same fundamental message—the need for core development—we are left in a confusing maze of how to get to it.

The beauty of this book is that it ties information together and creates one map for the reader, using the most credible and scientifically backed information pertaining to training the core. This same information is available to all practitioners who work with the body, but here we channel it into one voice for clarity and with distinct purpose.

To achieve this, we start at the beginning by dissecting and reexamining the benefits of the core, updating outdated information, and eradicating falsehoods and jargon. We thus arm you with the knowledge of how you need to train, why you need to train this way, and the benefits you will reap—and the pitfalls you will avoid—by doing so.

The process of selecting a training protocol specific to the needs of each individual can be a brilliant journey of self-discovery, but it can also be an intimidating maze full of strange terminology, inconsistent advice, and bewildering compromises. In this book we will guide you through the process; along the way you might discover a little bit about yourself and which of your needs, desires, and goals are most important to you.

INTRODUCING THE CORE

Our discussion begins in chapter 1, in which we retell the tale of the core in sports, providing a deeper understanding of the forces moving within and illuminating the truly remarkable nature of heightened athletic performance. Discussions of force are thrown around by many when describing explosive feats or impressive individuals, but these merely paint a larger picture—the details of which are within the core.

For you to be an educated consumer, or simply a conscientious user, you must understand that if you do not know what you are dealing with, you have little hope of improving it.

From a synergistic perspective, we next examine anatomical features, including the primary muscles associated with core performance. Our approach is to lay the groundwork of basic anatomy and then assemble a comprehensive understanding of the amazing integrated functionality of the human body and the core's role in tying it all together. To this end, chapter 2 presents a discussion of the muscles in classic isolation and, ultimately, the mechanics behind their unified responsibilities in the seeming fluidity of human movement.

We have established that the stakes are at an all-time high within the sporting spectrum, so it is prudent to explain in detail in chapter 3 how a well-developed core can help immeasurably in reducing your chance of injury and creating resiliency from within. Athletes will always be susceptible to injury, but considering the vast number of noncontact, preventable injuries occurring daily, strength and conditioning professionals must search as many avenues as possible to bring the injury numbers down. Core training should be the number-one priority in any comprehensive, periodized, annual training plan.

With a need to broaden the horizon of core training and forge an understanding of all the core properties, we endeavor to explain the core's role in power production and control. In chapter 4 we provide a detailed explanation of what power is, how it relates to strength, and why harnessing power through the core is vital to athletic achievement. Our ultimate aim is to leave you with an underlying appreciation of the seamless nature of all core qualities and an understanding that each one underpins the other and none stands alone.

Finally, in chapter 5, we set the stage for the drills in parts II through IV by explaining some of the nuances of exercise selection, outlining the specific benefits of the drills to come, and providing training guidelines to incorporate into your program.

Key Sports Performance Factor

Throughout *Conditioning to the Core*, it is our intention to rigorously analyze the key elements of the core, providing as much detailed information as possible. In doing so, we will be delving into applicable aspects of human anatomy, medically relevant injury prevention, and physics-riddled force and power production. These discussions are critical to a complete understanding of the core.

That said, in this first chapter we begin our discussion at the end and examine the final product, the fruits of your labors—that being high-quality core training's ultimate impact on sport and why it is such a key factor to performance. We begin here because much of what we present in later chapters is more theoretical and deals with factors and components that cannot be seen. In this chapter we operate on a more visceral level, discussing matters we can see and feel.

THE MULTIFUNCTIONAL CORE

Everyone in our field has heard the story of Milo of Croton, the father of progressive overload training, who woke up each morning, downed a macrobiotic mung bean protein shake, headed to the coliseum, hoisted a newborn calf onto his shoulders, and performed squat thrusts in his loin cloth. Each day, as the calf grew, Milo's strength subsequently had to adapt to the bovine's cumulative weight gain to the point at which Milo, with a full-grown ox across his shoulders, could execute a perfect petit jeté while leading a conga line at the Fred Persky Dance Studio.

Throughout history, artist renderings and Greek sculptures of Milo show a man with an absurdly remarkable set of abs with more musculature than can possibly exist. His core stabilization capability must have been spectacular, quite possibly second only to the marble statues themselves. Until recent years, the goal of core training was to acquire a similarly great set of abs, more for appearance than for functionality. The importance of the core had yet to be fully appreciated by coaches, physiotherapists, and athletes alike.

All movement originates, couples through, or is stabilized by what we will broadly refer to as the core. Effective stabilization of the osteoarticular system is necessary prior to the initiation of movement. Postural control is the precursor to effective mobilization. Without spinal stabilization, copious difficulties, including poor posture, will appear, leading to diminished movement efficiency. Other compensation issues that can occur as a result of poor spinal control include, but are not limited to, reciprocal inhibition, synergistic muscle dominance, and the inhibition of the arthrokinetic reflex. Enigmatically, intended functional movement can in fact create deleterious scenarios, and the deep stabilizers are the protective mechanism in the avoidance of the above-mentioned problematic compensation. Without this stabilizing mechanism, the possibility of the pain–injury cycle is heightened. Greater stress, typically in the form of microtrauma, will be placed on the contractile and noncontractile tissue of the muscle, leading to further compensation issues and biomechanical changes.

Thus developmentally, consistent with the Milo legend, there should be a progression in which deep-stabilizer sequencing precedes and provides the foundation for continual development of the mobilizers. Unfortunately, today's YouTube methodology is to focus on excessive amounts of the prime movers—whether with machines that intentionally disregard the deep stabilizers or by performing thousands of crunches in front of a mirror, which does little toward laying the groundwork for further functional core development.

Our task is to maximize foundational control of the trunk and torso during dynamic movement. With further development of the inner stabilizing musculature and its effective support of the articular vertebrae, the outer mobilizers are discharged of any significant postural stabilization responsibility and are thus left to function as intended, commanding strength, power, and efficiency of movement—the ultimate goal of all serious athletes.

THE CORE AS A BRIDGE

Much of the appeal of sport is the display of athletic performance and the unpredictable outcomes of competition. Yet, when a coach develops a conditioning program and asks athletes to train within the parameters of that program, there needs to be some assurance that the outcome will yield a high probability of success; everyone involved wants to be certain that the time and energy invested will pay off. Such certitude is achievable only if the program is based on universal principles.

Biomechanical analysis of a range of athletic movements confirms that all such movement relies on Newton's third law of motion. In its elegant precision, the law states that "for every action, there is an equal and opposite reaction." A clear example of this law comes into play when an athlete applies a certain amount of force into the ground (for instance, a sprinter pushing down through the balls of the feet during the first part of a race). The ground is an immovable object in that we cannot actually push the earth away from us. Thus the "equal and opposite reaction" occurs, sending the force back through the body, and for our purposes, back through the core, such as occurs when a sprinter pushes off the ground to propel the body forward. This is known as ground reaction force (figure 1.1).

As these forces are created, they must be distributed with appropriate specificity around the body to allow for efficient movement with dynamic precision and controlled energy. This force summation is expressed in different ways; in the case of a gymnast performing on the parallel bars, where there is no foot contact, force summation is identified from the top down;

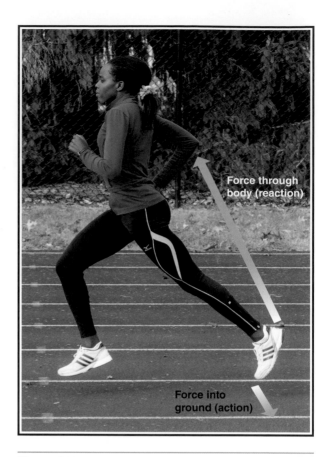

Force through body (reaction)

Force into ground (action)

Figure 1.1 Ground reaction force.

conversely, for a sprinter, the force travels from the ground up.

Throughout this book we will refer to motor development within the progressive context of proximal to distal functioning. In other words, in the early stages of development, specifically the primitive and postural reflexive stage, all movement begins close to the midline of the body—basically, from the center of mass (proximal) to the outer extremities (distal). A "motor unit" is a motor neuron and all of the muscle fibers that it innervates. When a neuron fires, all corresponding fibers contract simultaneously and maximally. In terms of force summation, the order of muscle involvement follows the same general rule. The smaller muscles located near the center of the mass initiate the movement, followed by the larger and stronger muscles of the extremities, which are more involved with accuracy, control, and coordination. The maximum amount of force employed is the aggregate total of the individual muscles involved. For less than maximal force production, the number of motor neurons would be less. Less muscle involvement equals less force; more muscle involvement equals more force.

For an example, let's consider the baseball pitch. The muscles recruited during the movement are the core, hips, legs, chest, deltoid, arm, wrist, and hand, roughly in that order. To maximize force potentiation, precise synchronization and accurate involvement from the deep stabilizers to the mobilizers to fine motor skills define the summation of forces, thus allowing for a 100-mile-per-hour throw with pinpoint accuracy.

To allow the energy recognized by Newton's third law to be channeled through the body, a bridge must be used to enhance the transfer of force from the lower limbs to the upper limbs, and vice versa.

The midsection of the body, or proximal core, is that bridge. The beauty of training the core as an osteoarticulating stabilizer concurrent with active mobilizing properties is that, when speaking in terms of functionality, all modalities of training benefit from the core's aforementioned attributes. Thus such exercises as the power clean, box jump, front squat, and flamingo cable fly will *all* benefit from and contribute to total body strength and power development.

It is extremely short sighted to presume that one modality of training always holds a superior advantage over another. The ultimate goal of any program is to maximize potential, and there are many roads on the map to reach that destination. Identifying individual strengths and weaknesses is of critical importance in determining which modality is best suited for a particular athlete. A strength jumper would benefit from an elastic program, and an elastic jumper would profit from a strength program. Regardless, whether you are doing a deep squat or a step-up curl alternate-arm shoulder press, the movement originates at the core, and as such there can be no wrong approach as long as the program is safe, progressive, specific to your needs, time efficient, and measurably productive. Perform the Olympic lifts, incorporate corrective therapies, be creative with functional modalities—the point is to stop isolating individual muscles and instead train globally, the way our bodies were designed to perform. When the focus of training is on one singular area of the body while marginalizing other areas, the results can be methodological flaws and ineffective performance.

The influence of an efficiently functioning core on sport performance has been well documented. On the other hand, a poorly functioning core does little to stabilize the spine or serve as the force-transfer conduit. This can result in inconsistent, extraneous movements, which in turn cause negative energy leaks. These leaks are displayed in inefficient actions, which cause poor athletic output and, if left unchecked, can certainly lead to a physiological or mechanical breakdown, often resulting in a pain–injury cycle. This tends to happen when a force is traveling to or through an area that is not well equipped to cope with the force. For example, after thousands of serves, forehands, and backhands, a tennis player might develop a chronic injury in the lower back, shoulder, or elbow. The primary cause of this compensation issue is the repetitive, powerful motion of the swing through the shoulder—with an implement in the hand, no less.

A rigid or well-conditioned core allows for a seamless transfer of force, enabling athletes to perform in a highly efficient, powerful, precise, and physically stress-free way. We will look to further explain the core's role in all athletic movements by presenting various examples from different sports; remember, however, that the core is all-inclusive to every unique body and unique action.

Ground Reaction Forces at Work

Walking, running, and jumping are easy ways to visualize ground reaction forces at work. These movement patterns occur primarily within the sagittal plane. Most sports are multifaceted when it comes to movement, and the need for Newtonian physics must be expressed in consideration of all planes. Change of direction, force production, force reduction, and dynamic stabilization all occur in the blink of an eye. We are not trying to write a physics textbook, but it must be understood that ground reaction forces change in magnitude, direction, and point of application during the time that an athlete is in contact with a surface.

Running and Cutting

In an all-out event such as the Olympic 100-meter dash, it is easy to see the core working optimally. If you examine a still photograph of one of these Olympic champions (Yuliya Nesterenko being a flawless example—see figure 1.2), you will notice a powerful leg cycle combined with an equally commanding and perfectly synchronized arm action. Between the two, you see an upright solid column that allows the limbs to work together to efficiently transfer energy, resulting in gold-medal speed. Upon closer examination of the photo of Nesterenko, you can actually see

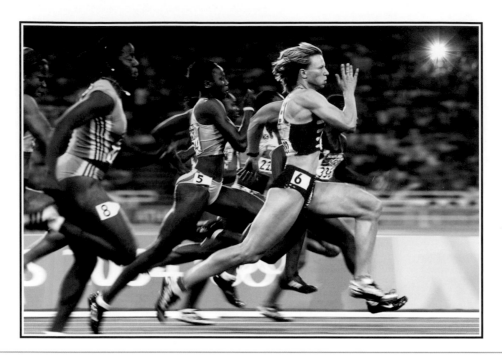

Figure 1.2 Yuliya Nesterenko won the women's 100 meters in the 2004 Summer Olympics by maintaining proper mechanics and total core control.

the core actively restraining the rotation of the hips to reduce unwanted extraneous movement.

At the point of ground contact and the subsequent drive into the next stride, the efficient sprinter is very close to a straight line through the body—you could lay down a ruler and connect the points of the ear, shoulder, hip, knee, and ankle. When observed from the front, as if the athlete were running at the camera, you would see very little unnecessary twisting or bobbing.

If the goal is to sprint straight ahead, then all energy should be channeled in the direction of that goal. Unfortunately, most of the other runners in the photo have speed-reducing body-alignment issues or extraneous motions such as twisting, rotating, low knee lift, cross-body arm action, incorrectly phased plantar flexion, or kyphotic posture. Nesterenko won that race because she maintained proper mechanics for the duration, while the other sprinters broke down because of a lack of total core control.

The effect holds equally true for athletes of any sport. For example, every hard foot plant that a running back makes, which is intended to change direction quickly, will be enhanced by a strong core controlling his body as the force travels up through his hips. This essential control, which originates in the core, enables the running back to leave the abdominally challenged defensive back in his dust.

Hitting

The benefits of a highly trained core do not stop at running and cutting. Yes, a sprinter wants to eliminate extraneous movements such as twisting and bobbing, but in other sports, such as tennis, actions such as twisting and bobbing are not extraneous and are critical to success. A solid core section is fundamental in sports that emphasize rotational movement. Hip separation and powerful rotations are key for those swinging an implement in sports such as baseball, cricket, golf, tennis, or throwing the disc. Here, the force from the ground is transferred from a more linear pattern to a strong rotary pattern, resulting in the object traveling at great speed, sometimes for incredible distance, and in many cases with extreme precision.

As we will discuss in chapter 2, successful sport performance, with a powerful rotational component, is not the net result of strong oblique musculature as is often thought. Rather, it is the result of a core-controlled mechanical process whereby after the initial hip-torso separation the whole of the core unit rotates in one quick and controlled motion. As with most athletic movements, this involves using the pelvic girdle as the driver but also requires the whole torso to be synchronized and well conditioned from a stability, strength, and power perspective, in addition to maintaining heightened motor control.

Jumping

Athletes in sports that require frequent jumping, such as volleyball, also benefit from a well-crafted core routine. Though these athletes must be quick and agile, they must also be able to accelerate into the air. Great leapers are often by-products of genetics and excellent mechanics, but an effective bridge between the upper and lower body that allows power from the legs to create tremendous upward force can be attained by nearly anyone to varying degrees. The ability to use horizontal velocity, as with an approach or penultimate step, and transfer that energy to vertical lift is the single-most identifying characteristic of great leapers.

Note that sport-specific training involves training the energy systems, the strength and power foundations, and the movement mechanics required of your particular sport (and, whenever possible, for your particular position within that sport). Unfortunately, many training protocols fail to apply the principles of sport-specific training. For instance, though it is rare in sport for an athlete to simply stand and jump, the typical protocol for training rarely involves an approach step (a horizontal velocity component), and testing the vertical jump is typically from a standing (non-displacement), stationary position.

Energy is generated by movement. If this energy can be quickly and efficiently transferred to a different purpose, such as taking a couple of steps prior to jumping, then the resultant action, such as dunking a basketball, might be explosive enough to earn a top 10 showing on ESPN's *SportsCenter*. But optimal energy transfer cannot occur without a well-conditioned bridge. A great thing is that by harnessing your core strength you will increase your vertical leap, even without the benefit of a jump-training program. But imagine if you did both!

Striking

Finally, an often overlooked aspect of core training is demonstrated by athletes in striking sports. In boxing, for example, a well-conditioned core not only allows competitors to withstand an opponent's blows to the midsection but also enables them to punch more effectively. Throwing punches is all about rotational power in the core. A single hard jab is not nearly as effective as combinations of punches thrown repeatedly from a strong foundation.

Stability, strength, and power in the core allow the boxer to create force quickly through the ground and to immediately repeat the action from a variety of angles. Very few, if any, boxers have been successful without a stable, strong, and powerful core. Earlier in the chapter we discussed the summation of forces. Never is the aggregate sum of forces more important than when fighting for your life in the ring.

Groundless Forces

In some sports, using ground force reaction is impossible, so another means of force generation and transfer must be used. Surfing and swimming are two examples. In swimming, other than the initial pushoff from the blocks or pool wall, there are no opportunities for grounding. Instead, swimmers move through water by creating propulsion and minimizing the effects of drag forces on the body.

Propulsion is the by-product of the limbs pushing backward into the water to allow forward movement. Water is not solid, so energy generated is not transferred solely to forward movement but is also disbursed into the water. As is true for land athletes, aquatic athletes want to be as efficient as possible; every potential advantage to maximize efficiency must be exploited.

Swimmers speak in terms of *propulsive efficiency*. For elite swimmers, 80 percent of energy goes into moving the body forward, and the remaining 20 percent simply moves the water around them. Elite competitive swimmers can reach this 80 percent in two ways. First, through endless hours in the pool, they have learned to maximize perfectly efficient technique. Second, and of equal importance, they have conditioned their core to be unyielding in keeping unproductive, wasted energy in check. Possibly more so with swimming than any other sport, extraneous movement will deter from the intended goal of forward propulsion. It should be conceptualized that the forces are created and controlled from within, and core training for swimming should reflect that. (The rolling exercises outlined in chapter 7 are an excellent place to start.) Swimmers should see themselves as torpedoes, with control coming from within and propulsive forces pushing behind a solid cylindrical shaft that allows them to move through water at astounding speeds.

Another interesting example to make this point is the sport of surfing. Surfers take a different

In-Season Training and Performance

Back in the 1960s, my father, Dean Brittenham, a pioneer in the field of performance-enhancement training, spoke to his charges at the University of Nebraska about the importance of dynamic control and abdominal stabilization. I recall watching him work with his athletes, having them carry cinder blocks while performing twisting lunge walks up a grassy hill or twist-tossing leather medicine balls to each other while standing in the sand of a long-jump pit. I remember his long-jumpers locking their arms around the ladder in the pool and executing knee drives and straight-leg raises against the resistance of water. Little, if any, time was spent in a weight room using free weights (there were no machines back then) to train the efficiency of the core. Dad understood that common sense dictates training the core specific to its function. You don't throw darts to improve your golf putt.

I share my Dad's training philosophy and have practiced his teaching every day of my life. One constantly needs to adapt to the personnel, environment, available equipment, and the goals and objectives of the team in order to have an effective influence season after season. While no two teams, athletes, or schedules are exactly alike, there are some constants in regard to intensity, frequency, and duration of training that, when intelligently manipulated, can result in further growth and development, even during the season. Neither of us has ever been of the mindset that in-season training is a time of maintenance. To be sure, just the opposite is our philosophy. In-season training, while modified in its intensity and often in its frequency, can still be challenging enough to demand positive physical adaptation. Imagine becoming a stronger, more powerful, and better conditioned athlete as the season progresses, while your opponent is either maintaining or even experiencing diminishing strength and conditioning levels because of in-season interrupted training.

All too often, teams mistakenly incorporate a maintenance program during the in-season. The misguided rationale is a fear of overworking the players that could result in poor performance. But my experience has been quite the opposite. During the competitive season, my players work at or close to their off-season training intensity. Each athlete's strength, power, endurance, and confidence improves and is noticeably superior to that of opponents. For example, in the

concluding stages of each season during the 1990s, the Knicks showed improved athleticism, strength, and conditioning. This was demonstrated in three ways:

- Statistical improvements in all facets of the game at the end of the season when compared to the start of the season
- Empirically via a noticeable dominance over the opponent
- An increased winning percentage at the end of the season and during the playoffs every year of the decade

The NBA season is an eight-month marathon. A team can ill afford to pander to the pampering fancies of the spoiled player. Recovery techniques are certainly not ignored, and more often than not, they hold high priority, especially for athletes playing significant minutes. Because of the hectic in-season schedule, duration and frequency of training are unavoidably altered; however, the intensity of the remaining in-season training sessions must stay high throughout in order to realize continual positive adaptation to the exercise stress imposed. Successful teams such as the 1990s Knicks embrace this in-season training philosophy, which can be summed up by the following statement: The athlete should train *through* the competitive season, not *to* the competitive season.

Unfortunately, the tough teams and players of the '90s era who sported a philosophy of robust self-reliance have given way to protocols of delicate dependence. Low-intensity or, more accurately, *no*-intensity methodologies, such as manual therapy, have become an all-too-common system for the preparation of high-level performance. From a developmental perspective, motor reeducation is a cognitive reliant process. In other words, learning new motor patterns (or relearning lost motor patterns as a result of inactivity after injury) is a process requiring conscious appreciation on the part of the athlete—*not* the coach or therapist imposing his or her own personal awareness on the athlete. One of the great deceptions of manual therapy is that the athlete will enhance an existing movement skill or even learn a completely new motor pattern as a result of the passive therapy. The notion that a coach manually moving an athlete's arm through a range of motion or a therapist digging an elbow painfully deep into a player's IT band will somehow improve movement efficiency, accuracy, or effectiveness is complete nonsense. The only way an athlete can learn a new movement pattern is through actively participating in the process both physically and cognitively.

Again, I refer back to the Knicks of the 1990s. Those teams had a reputation for a high-energy, strong, and physical style of play from the start of the game to the end of the second overtime. In fact, the '90s Knicks were stronger and better conditioned at the end of the season heading into the playoffs than they were at training camp. This was largely because of a coaching philosophy that embraced high-intensity, multiset strength training, and a continued high-level conditioning straight through the season. Recovery days were more than adequate, with each player being closely monitored and appropriate rest-and-regeneration techniques being applied on an individual, as-needed basis. As a result of the strength and toughness of these Knicks teams, the NBA saw fit to change the rules to reflect the new physicality of play. It was during this time that NBA referees began a regimented training program of their own to ensure a standard of fitness necessary to run with the evolving contemporary NBA player.

path. Their sport is also aquatically based and puts them at the mercy of the elements, but between the water and the surfer is a board, which can be used in somewhat the same way as land athletes use the ground. However, because the board rests on top of an ever-moving liquid, it is highly unstable.

Research shows that what separates good surfers from beginners is the ability to maintain board stability no matter what waves lie beneath. This creates a relatively secure platform to work from, thereby allowing Newton's third law to take hold. Maintaining an elevated level of stabilization is the art and skill of surfing, and it is tied directly to a stable core. In a constantly changing environment, excellent core strength will brace the body no matter what direction or velocity external forces are coming from. This allows the surfer to maintain balance and increase control over the environment. Conversely, an inefficient core allows unstable forces to overwhelm the physiological system and ultimately throw the surfer from the board.

THE BODY'S CENTER OF GRAVITY

The body's center of gravity (or, more generally, center of mass) is the location within the body where all the particles of the body are evenly distributed. It is also the balancing point of the body. An individual's center of gravity is located within the core. In a standing, rested state, the center of gravity is typically about two inches (five centimeters) below the navel.

Sporting movements tend to alter the location of the center of gravity. The high jump is a perfect example. Before the 1968 Olympics, when Dick Fosbury displayed his new back-first technique (coined the Fosbury Flop) to the tune of a gold medal and a new Olympic record, most athletes were roll-jumping or scissor-kicking over the bar. By the 1972 Munich Olympics, 28 out of 40 competitors were using the back-first technique to high degrees of success. What makes the flop so successful is that it lowers the center of gravity, leading to a vast change in speed and projection angle, which improves the outcome.

The importance of influencing the body's center of gravity is common in sport. In evasive sports such as football and rugby, we try to move our center of gravity around an opponent; in basketball or netball, we change the position of our legs up under our bodies to offset the downward pull of gravity as we attempt to make a shot under pressure. The ability to execute an athletic movement of any kind requires the need for a rapid change in the location of the center of gravity. Those who exhibit a high degree of control in the body's center of mass are commonly called gifted or natural athletes. They seem to possess an ability to change direction without a concomitant sacrifice in speed—an ability we call agility. This change of direction might be from left to right around a tackler, from the floor to the rim for a fast-break alley-oop, or from a backpedaling overhead smash to charging the net for a match-winning drop shot.

To be successful in executing such movements, athletes must be physically able to control the change of direction rather than allowing the change to control them. The difference is as fundamental as one of us falling on the ice as opposed to a conditioned skater quickly leaning to change direction. Those who can control their core have control over their center of power. Mastery of the core is the single-most manageable athletic attribute and is critically important to athletic prowess.

The specific requisite necessary to play at a high intensity is determined by the level of your physical base. If your physical base is poorly developed or decreases because of extended inactivity, your physical performance will decline. Obviously, to maximize your performance potential, you must train not only your sport-specific skills but also the physical base that supports those skills.

A great deal goes into making an athlete a top performer. Some determinants are beyond our control. Genetics play a major role in affecting height, body type, limb length, muscle fiber type, and so on, whereas geography and culture often determine our sport of choice and nature of participation. However, one thing remains constant and is within our control: our ability to intelligently prepare our bodies for high-level performance. We might not be training for the Olympics or the NBA Finals, but we certainly can train to be better than we are right now. We must never be satisfied with mediocrity. We must reach for that which is beyond our grasp. If you make training the core the centerpiece of your conditioning program, you can make those crazy sports clichés come true. Preparation is what you make it.

Anatomical Lynchpin

Our aim in this chapter is to look at core anatomy in a way that truly illustrates its purpose. We begin by discussing muscles in the classical, detached way. Our primary intention, however, is to show what happens to these muscles during integrated movement, which is the essence of athletic grandeur.

TRAINING THE CORE GLOBALLY: A NONTRADITIONAL APPROACH

Conventional core development has moved across the entire training spectrum, from muscle isolation modalities of the 1980s to global movement patterns of the late 1990s and early 2000s. Unfortunately, in recent years, there has been a strong push back to the archaic muscle isolation movements of the past, the thinking being that weaknesses in one or more individual muscles within the kinetic chain will lead to dysfunctional and asynchronous movement patterns that can in turn lead to poor performance or a "weak link" injury. This push has triggered an epidemic of muscle isolation training, in which entire training sessions are devoted to the one delinquent muscle within the chain at the expense of all others (for example, crunches for the rectus abdominis, or clam raises for the gluteus medius).

Following an isolationist approach to core training is, unfortunately, "fool's gold." Although the area of focus might improve in aesthetic appearance or muscle tone, this alone is worthless in the pursuit of heightened athleticism. Motor development is the process of developing movement patterns and fine motor skills throughout one's life. Embracing the broader perspective of the movement paradigm, specific muscle isolation, including first-stage motor development reflexes (such as palmar grasp or asymmetrical tonic neck reflex), must unquestionably be inhibited prior to continued advancement to subsequent stages of motor development, such as the second-stage, rudimentary movement patterns (rolling over, sitting up, and eventually walking).

Developmentally, purposeful muscle isolation should have been inhibited during the first stage of motor development. For example, an infant lying supine with one arm extended in the direction that his or her head is facing characterizes asymmetrical tonic neck reflex. If the child turns his or her head in the opposite direction, the opposite arm will extend in that direction. If the child does not learn how to inhibit this postural reflex, further development in complex multimuscular movement patterns cannot take place. Thus if the infant does not learn how to tuck the extended arm tight to the body, he or she will not be able to roll over, which is the impetus for crawling, which leads to sitting up, which triggers standing, cruising, walking, running and so on.

Muscle isolation and its eventual yielding from the first stage promotes further development within the second stage. As mentioned, simple movement patterns during the second stage must give way to more complex patterns during the third stage (fundamental movement patterns), and these movement patterns are eventually applied during the final stage of development: sport skill patterns. Thus athletes and trainers with a penchant for muscle isolation training or singular muscle contraction regimens rather than complex global movement patterns are in actuality moving backward in their motor development.

So why has muscle isolation become a popular training modality? Curiously, it appears that today's strength coaches, physiotherapists, and personal trainers see isolation training as a simple yet trendy and marketable methodology that is relatively easy to administer. For example, suppose your gluteus medius is underperforming. A well-intentioned coach, articulating this current training idiom, might say that this particular muscle is "not firing" and proceed to design a program to address the culprit specifically.

Unless a neurodegenerative disease is affecting an athlete, it is physiologically impossible for a muscle not to fire (i.e., activate). Try this simple test: First, stand up; second, take a lateral step to the side. Your gluteus medius just "fired," and so did your other deep stabilizing and outer mobilizing musculature and joint stabilizers and mobilizers along the kinetic chain. How do you know that your gluteus medius was involved in that lateral step? Because if the gluteal muscles had not been active during the foot strike, you would have collapsed to the floor. Are you still standing? Good! Gluteus medius fired.

Muscle isolation training is so far removed from ground-based athletic performance that athletes are in fact detraining other important systems, and spending precious time doing it— time that could be far more productive practicing the skills of their sport or improving on their less developed athletic traits. There are infinite combinations of movement patterns that involve the gluteus medius within the framework of the third and fourth stages of motor development (fundamental movement patterns and sport skill application, respectively). So, you tell me—would you rather perform isolated movements, or train specific to the needs of your sport, position, or activity? In other words, would you rather lie on the floor and isolate your psoas with a straight-leg raise or sprint up a hill to dynamically incorporate the psoas along with all the other kinetic chain musculature and their corresponding patterns that will be involved with all athletic movements? You say sprint up a hill? Good! Because that is what this book is all about: integrated core development.

The nontraditional approach we intend for you to take involves training the core globally and avoiding programs that focus on muscle isolation—with the possible exception of specific and unique needs such as injury rehabilitation.

Throughout the book, we reinforce the concept of inclusive musculature training from a performance-based perspective. Michael Jordan, regardless of his superior basketball skills and heightened athleticism, could not have won six championships without the cooperative assistance of the rest of the Chicago Bulls. Likewise, regardless of the function at hand—stability or mobility—isolating muscles makes no sense within the integrated world of motor control. The Bulls would never practice with just Michael Jordan; they would practice with the entire team. Likewise, you wouldn't train just one muscle if the entirety of the system is required to perform maximally.

DEFINING THE CORE

Although coaches, athletes, academicians, scientists, doctors, and personal trainers might differ in their definitions of what constitutes the core, they tend to argue only about the musculature of the core's periphery—there is no contention regarding the heart of the core. The myofascial center and the muscles that attach to and around the lumbar spine and pelvic girdle region are considered to be the core's foundation, and together are referred to as the lumbo-pelvic hip complex (LPHC.)

The LPHC is an integral part of a series of links that create our strong, self-repairing framework. This sequence of links is encompassed by the systems next discussed.

The Fascial System

The fascial system is a paper-thin web that subcutaneously covers the body. Structurally, this system contains tightly packed bundles of fibers made from collagen. Although the fascia may not be specifically addressed in this text, it plays a major role and through its vast area of coverage creates important links across the body.

The Neural System

The neural, or nervous, system is the control system within all of us. It coordinates all of our actions by transmitting signals among and throughout the various systems of the body. The neural system consists of the central nervous system (CNS), comprised of the brain and spinal cord, and the peripheral nervous system (PNS), which is made up of cranial nerves, spinal nerves, and sensory receptors that create a web of long fibers connecting the CNS to the rest of the body.

The Articular System

The articular system is comprised of the many joints of the body, which number around 230. These joints link the skeleton and enable or restrain movement. Because this is an active system, with all joints linked, the movement of one directly affects the motion of others. This is an important consideration that dictates our suggested training philosophy.

The Muscular System

The body's actions may well be controlled by the brain and the nerves, but for movement to occur the body must have a mechanism that the neural system commands in order to move the skeletal framework. This mechanism is the muscular system, which is comprised of muscles that generate internal tension. With signals from the central nervous system, these muscles manipulate the bones of our bodies through their ligamentous and tendinous attachments to produce movement. As we will see, the muscular system provides both locomotion and stabilization for the body.

The Skeletal System

All of the aforementioned systems are hung from, connected to, woven around, or covering the skeletal system, which is the framework for the body's structure and movement. The skeletal system plays a fundamental role in determining body size and shape. This system includes two areas: the axial skeleton (comprised of the skull, vertebral column, and rib cage) and the appendicular skeleton (consisting of the pectoral and pelvic girdles and upper and lower limbs).

Working together, these systematic links are known as the kinetic chain. Whether turning a double-play or cleaning leaves out of the gutter, a multifactorial collaborative effort from each link of the kinetic chain ensures consistent reliability and quality of movement, regardless of the skill complexity. Any imbalance within this chain leads to decreased level of performance and increased risk of injury.

For the kinetic chain to work optimally, a high level of postural control is required. Poor posture has detrimental effects on physical capacity and impairs the force-transfer abilities so highly touted in chapter 1. A functionally stable and controlled LPHC is undoubtedly the anchor of good posture.

Sitting atop the LPHC is the thoracic area of the body, which transitions into the shoulder girdle and arms. Almost every sport relies heavily on the thoracic region, and thus the stability, strength, and power of this area must be addressed. Understanding the core in this way identifies additional regions and musculature, as the core was traditionally thought of as simply the abs and lower back. But if we disregard the head (which is the control center for everything discussed to this point) and the upper and lower limbs (which we have established to be extensions of core activity), we are essentially left with the torso and gluteal complex.

Let's present a new working definition of the core. Think of the core region as a staging area. Whether stabilizing, transferring a force, or coordinating upper- and lower-extremity movements, the core is capable of every type of muscle contraction. These contractions may be fast concentric (in which the muscle rapidly shortens and its origin and insertion point move closer together), slow eccentric (in which the muscle lengthens in a controlled manner and its origin and insertion move apart), fast (or rapid eccentric, which is what agility is all about), static isometric (in which the muscle is placed under tension but there is no perceivable change in length), or any number of combinations. A finely tuned core allows for unconnected movements among zones of the body. For example, efficiently stabilizing one area while mobilizing another can result in a world-record performance. Conversely, the inability to disjoin body parts can lead to poor mechanical performance and possibly to injury.

INTEGRATED CORE ANATOMY

The musculature of the core can be likened to a cylinder (figure 2.1). Conceptually, the cylinder acts like a woven basket, in which structural integrity comes from the overlapping weave. If you twisted the basket, one side would tighten and one side would resist, but the structure would remain intact. The same is true if the basket is compressed or lengthened. All parts work together for the benefit of the whole. This is much like the core section of the body—it is a strong, durable, and functional unit. If you take nothing from this chapter but the idea to train the core with this cylinder in mind, you are at least on the right track.

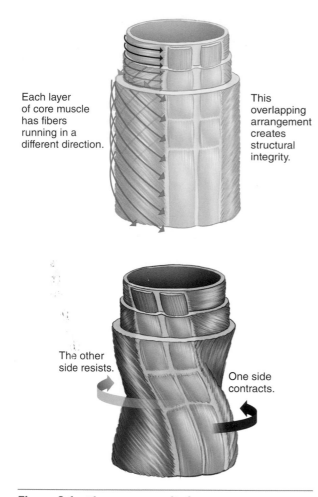

Each layer of core muscle has fibers running in a different direction.

This overlapping arrangement creates structural integrity.

The other side resists.

One side contracts.

Figure 2.1 The core as a cylinder.

Over the years, our functional experience suggests a reclassification of the core musculature into two functionally integrated groups: the deep stabilizers and the outer mobilizers. The deep stabilizers make up the core's foundation, and the outer mobilizers comprise the core's precise multifunctional athletic musculature. Categorizing the core in this way allows for a useful and integrative understanding of the relation of the two groups.

Adhering to the concept of proximal to distal progression with regard to motor development and the eventual efficiency of movement (both precision and endurance), the deep stabilizers are recognized primarily as the proximal myofascial nucleus. This musculature must be engaged first to provide joint support prior to the execution of complex movement patterns by the distal complex, or outer mobilizers. These movement patterns are either stabilized *by* or activated *through* the deep stabilizers and outer mobilizers via fine neural control and articular coupling.

Deep Stabilizers

Deep stabilizer musculature is the core's foundation and, sequentially, must be recruited first to facilitate subsequent coordinated internal and external forces through the core structure and the peripheral limbs. (Not to confuse the issue, but note that although the musculature is labeled a stabilizer, it still has mobilizing properties, just as mobilizing musculature has stabilizing properties. More on this later.) Both the core structure and the peripheral limbs play important roles in the body, providing dynamic stabilization and efficient force allocation, leading to optimal production of movement.

Transversus Abdominis (TVA)

The transversus abdominis, or TVA, lies deep in the abdominal section of the core and directly under the internal oblique (figure 2.2). The TVA originates from the front of the hip, specifically the iliac crest and inguinal ligament, as well as ribs 7 to 12. When trained appropriately the TVA can generate a large surface, which is the underpinning for enhanced stabilization. Its insertion (or end) points are in the linea alba and contralateral rectus sheaths—the midline of the body. What truly enables the TVA to act as a stabilizer are its attachment points in the back, specifically to the thoracolumbar fascia (this is also true for the internal oblique). This creates a hoop-like

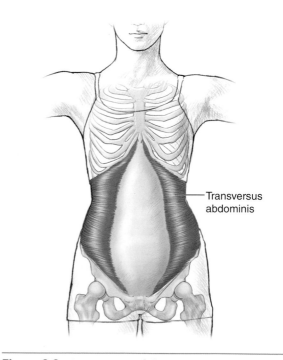

Transversus abdominis

Figure 2.2 Transversus abdominis.

tension, which causes a complete brace throughout the core. (Remember our cylinder?)

As a deep stabilizer, one of the main functions of the TVA is to play a role in the "bracing" function of the core. Bracing occurs when all the muscles of the core work together to create stiffness and stability of the LPHC and thoracic regions. In the case of the TVA, this comes from compressing the ribs and visceral bodies by working in direct conjunction with the internal oblique, multifidus, and deep erector spinae.

Internal Oblique

The internal oblique lies directly between the TVA and the external oblique (figure 2.3). Its origins and insertion points are almost identical to that of the TVA; the major difference is that while the TVA *originates* on ribs 7 to 12, the internal oblique *inserts* on ribs 9 to 12. This is an important distinction because when a muscle contracts, its insertion is pulled toward its origin, causing slightly differing lines of pull from both muscles.

As an individual muscle, the internal oblique's primary task is to create spinal flexion in multiple directions as well as rotational movements. However, within the framework of the core unit, the internal oblique works synergistically with the TVA to enable overall stability to the lumbar spine.

Multifidus

The multifidus is comprised of a series of small muscles that run the entire length of the spine from the sacrum to the axis (figure 2.4). They are divided into two additional groups: the superficial and deep multifidi, each crossing three joint segments. They originate from the spinous processes (the backward-pointing protrusions of the spine that create its ridge-like appearance) of the various different regions that forge the S-shaped curvature of the spine (lumbar, thoracic, and cervical). Individually, their insertion points are one to four vertebral segments above the point of origin.

Acting very much like tent guide wires, the multifidi aid in taking strain off the vertebral discs so that body weight can be distributed proportionately along the spine. The superficial multifidi aid in keeping our vertebrae aligned, and the deeper multifidi contribute to the stability of the spine.

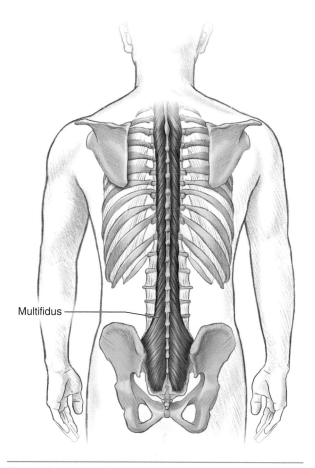

Figure 2.4 Multifidus.

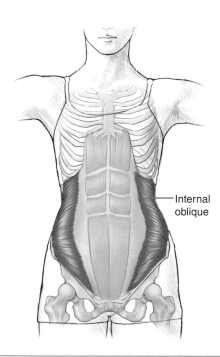

Figure 2.3 Internal oblique.

Quadratus Lumborum

The quadratus lumborum, or QL, lies bilaterally on each side of the lower back, initially arising from the iliac crest and the iliolumbar ligament (set deep in between the ilium and the sacrum; see figure 2.5). Ultimately, the QL inserts into the 12th rib and lumbar vertebrae 2 to 5.

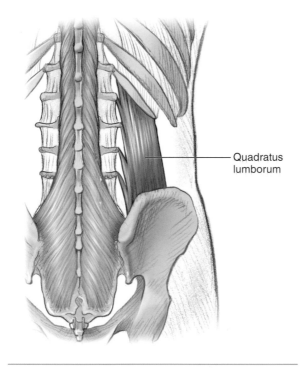

Quadratus
lumborum

Figure 2.5 Quadratus lumborum.

Working in isolation, the QL serves to flex the spine laterally in the case of a one-sided hip hike. More important, it works together with the gluteus medius, tensor fascia latae, and adductor complex to serve as a major LPHC stabilization mechanism.

Thoracoabdominal Diaphragm

Commonly called the *diaphragm*, this parachute-shaped, musculotendinous mass separates the thoracic cavity from the abdominal cavity (figure 2.6). It has origins and insertions throughout that region, from the xiphoid process in the lower aspect of the sternum to points on the lumbar vertebrae.

Often referenced in activities such as singing, the diaphragm's primary function is to aid in respiration. During inhalation the diaphragm contracts, enlarging the thoracic cavity and drawing air inward. The diaphragm can also assist in anterior spinal stability and posture via its control of intra-abdominal pressure.

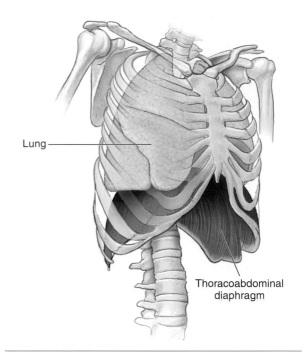

Lung

Thoracoabdominal
diaphragm

Figure 2.6 Thoracoabdominal diaphragm.

Pelvic Diaphragm

The pelvic diaphragm lies at the opposing end of the torso to the thoracoabdominal diaphragm, and thus is often called the *pelvic floor*. It is also a muscular partition, in this case between the pelvic cavity and perineal region. It is comprised of fibers from the levator ani, the coccygeus, and ancillary connective tissue, which cover the area underneath the pelvis (figure 2.7).

Usually referenced in discussions about pregnancy because of its critical importance in the overall support of the pelvic viscera, the pelvic diaphragm affects spinal stability and postural control in a similar way to the thoracoabdominal diaphragm.

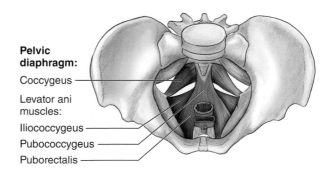

**Pelvic
diaphragm:**

Coccygeus

Levator ani
muscles:

Iliococcygeus

Pubococcygeus

Puborectalis

Figure 2.7 Pelvic diaphragm.

Gluteus Medius

As opposed to the gluteus maximus, which is clearly situated on the back of the hip and will be discussed later in the chapter, the gluteus medius is located on the outer surface of the pelvis (figure 2.8). It originates under the gluteus maximus out of the gluteal surface of the ilium. It inserts into the femur or thigh bone by way of the greater trochanter, which is a raised section of bone at the top of the femur that serves as an attachment site.

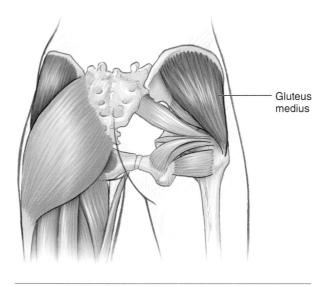

Figure 2.8   Gluteus medius.

During locomotion, the gluteus medius helps to control much of the action of the thigh bone. When the leg is straight or in a neutral position, the gluteus medius and the gluteus minimus function together to pull the thigh in an outward, or abducted, motion. When walking or running, these same two muscles work principally to support the body on one leg to prevent the pelvis from sinking to the opposite side. Again, when isometrically contracted, the gluteus medius helps stabilize this region.

Outer Mobilizers

The outer mobilizers are characterized for creating movement and should engage secondarily to the deep stabilizers (stability before strength). They are generally more superficial and thus are easily seen through the skin in well-conditioned individuals. Because they are readily visible, the outer mobilizers are typically more aesthetically prized than their stabilizing brethren, and thus are commonly trained more diligently and with higher frequency. As we will explain later, this is not only a poor training strategy but one fraught with injury risk and decreased performance.

Rhomboid

Another muscle categorized in two parts, the rhomboid includes the rhomboid major and minor. The rhomboid major and minor connect the scapula to the spinal column and lie beneath the trapezius (figure 2.9).

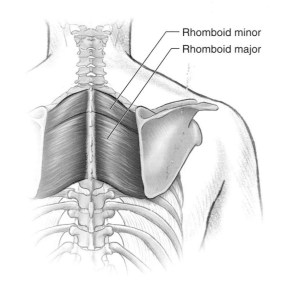

Rhomboid minor
Rhomboid major

Figure 2.9   Rhomboid.

The rhomboid minor is located under the levator scapulae (which assists in scapular elevation) and directly above (superior to) the rhomboid major originates from the nuchal ligament as well as the seventh cervical and first thoracic vertebrae. Covering only a minor area, the rhomboid minor inserts into a small point at the top of the medial border of the scapula.

The rhomboid major is set a little lower than (inferior to) the rhomboid minor and arises from the spinous process of the early section of the thoracic spine (T2 to T5) as well as the supraspinous ligament. It inserts along the inner portion of the scapula, extending down the medial side to the inferior angle.

Working synergistically, the rhomboids maintain appropriate scapular retraction, pulling them inward toward the vertebral column as well as ensuring that the scapula lay flat against the thoracic wall and do not wing outward. Because of their influence over the scapula, the rhomboids also play an important role in rotator cuff stabilization.

Middle and Lower Trapezius

The trapezius is a large superficial upper-back muscle made up of three distinct sections, all with differing roles. Our interest here, and of primary focus in the text, is the middle and lower trapezius (figure 2.10).

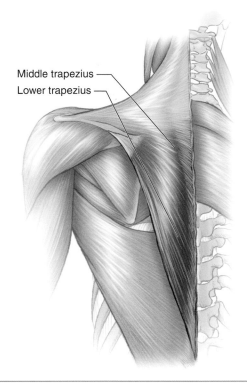

Figure 2.10   Middle and lower trapezius.

The middle trapezius is sometimes called the intermediate region. It originates from the processes of thoracic vertebrates 1 through 5, inserting into the acromion process of the shoulder blade as well as the spine of the scapula. The middle trapezius's primary functions are to retract the shoulder blades and to stabilize the area when other back and shoulder muscles are acting on the scapula.

The lower trapezius originates from the last six thoracic vertebrae (T6 to T12) and also inserts into the spine of the scapula. It is responsible for depressing or pulling down the scapula as well as working along with the upper trapezius and serratus anterior to abduct the scapula when elevation occurs. As with many of these muscles, the lower trapezius also functions as a stabilizer for the scapulae.

Serratus Anterior

The serratus anterior is a set of muscles that lie on top of the rib cage under the chest, vaguely resembling fingers (figure 2.11). Depending on the individual, they originate from either the first to eighth or first to ninth ribs and insert all along the inside or medial border of the scapula.

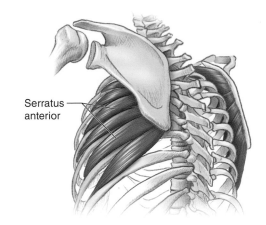

Figure 2.11   Serratus anterior.

The serratus anterior is primarily responsible for the protraction of the scapula, which moves the blades forward and around the rib cage. As previously mentioned, serratus anterior also works together with the upper and lower trapezius to provide scapular mobility and stability during shoulder elevation. Isometrically, it stabilizes the scapulothoracic joint.

Latissimus Dorsi

The latissimus dorsi is the largest muscle in the upper body; the Latin translation literally means broadest muscle of the back. The latissimus dorsi muscles sit on the back like folded bird wings, lying behind the arm and partially covered at one point by the trapezius (figure 2.12).

Because of its large size, the muscle has a broad surface area of origins: T7 to T12, iliac crest, thoracolumbar fascia, and ribs 9 to 12. It inserts into the lower, or inferior, angle of the scapula as well as into the humerus under the armpit. This means that when activated, it has the ability to affect the arm and the movement of the scapula, as well as the lower back area.

Often called the handcuff muscle, the latissimus dorsi's primary responsibilities are adduction, extension, and internal rotation of the arm (essentially putting your arms behind your back, as if you have been cuffed).

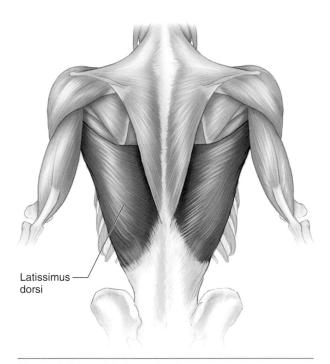

Figure 2.12   Latissimus dorsi.

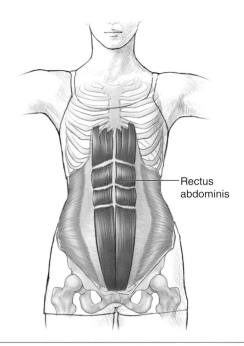

Figure 2.13   Rectus abdominis.

However, because of its attachment points on the scapula and lower back, the latissimus dorsi is also involved in the movement of the shoulder blades as well as lateral flexion and extension of the lumbar spine. When trained appropriately, the latissimus dorsi, along with the thoracolumbar fascia, notably stabilizes the LPHC.

Rectus Abdominis

The rectus abdominis is one of the more attractive muscles of the core section because of its aesthetic appearance. It originates from the pubic symphysis, a small joint that joins the two ears, or ilium, of the hips at their base. This muscle runs the full length of the abdomen and inserts into the fifth, sixth, and seventh ribs as well as the xiphoid process of the sternum. The rectus abdominis is a two-part muscle, running vertically and separated by the connective tissue of the linea alba (figure 2.13). It is commonly crossed by three fibrous bands, creating the highly prized six-pack appearance.

Functionally, the isolated role of the rectus abdominis is to bring the hips toward the rib cage via spinal flexion. It also aids in lateral flexion and rotation. During abdominal bracing, mentioned earlier, the rectus abdominis aids in overall stability of the LPHC via increased intra-abdominal pressure.

External Oblique

The external oblique is the most superficial of all the lateral abdominal muscles, and also the largest of the three. It originates from ribs 4 through 12 and inserts into the anterior iliac crest, linea alba, and inguinal ligament (figure 2.14).

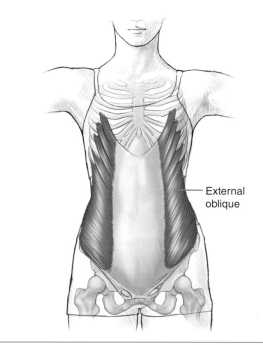

Figure 2.14   External oblique.

The external oblique's central function is to increase intra-abdominal pressure by drawing the chest downward and compressing the abdominal cavity. It also has a lesser role in both flexion and rotation of the spine. When contracting individually, the oblique can create lateral flexion.

Erector Spinae

The erector spinae is similar in some respects to the multifidus, as it runs the length of the torso and is situated close to the vertebral column. In actuality, the erector spinae is not a singular muscle but a grouping of muscles and tendonous structures extending through the lumbar, thoracic, and cervical regions (figure 2.15). The thickness of the tissues differ throughout depending on location and is generally thicker in the lumbar section and thinner as the tissues move upward. Some of the erector spinae's distal fibers are seamless with the fibers from the origin of the gluteus maximus, once again showing how the unified core is truly interlinked.

The erector spinae originates on the iliac crest as well as the sacrum and spinous processes of

T11 through Tl5. However, in the upper lumbar region, the erector spinae splits into three columns—the iliocostalis, longissimus, and spinalis—thus creating many effectual insertion points:

Iliocostalis—inserts into ribs 1 to 12, as well as into cervical vertebrae 4 to 6

Longissimus—inserts into T1 to T12, ribs 2 to 12, cervical vertebrae 2 to 6, and the mastoid process at the very base of the skull

Spinalis—inserts into the spinous process of C2 to C3 and T4 to T7, as well as into the occipital bone at the back of the skull

Because of its vast array of attachment points, the erector spinae's functions relate to the extension, rotation, and lateral flexion of the spine. However, working in conjunction with the rectus abdominis as a brace, it helps create full spine stabilization when required.

Gluteus Maximus

The gluteus maximus is the largest and most external of the three gluteal muscles (which also include the medius and minimus). Because of its large size, it has multiple points of origin, including the outer ilium, posterior gluteal line, aponeurosis (broad, flat connecting tendons) of the erector spinae and gluteus medius muscles, sacrum, coccyx, and sacrotuberous and sacroiliac ligaments.

The gluteus maximus is heavily involved in hip extension and external rotation of the hip. It is considered one of the primary force producers in the body and as such should be

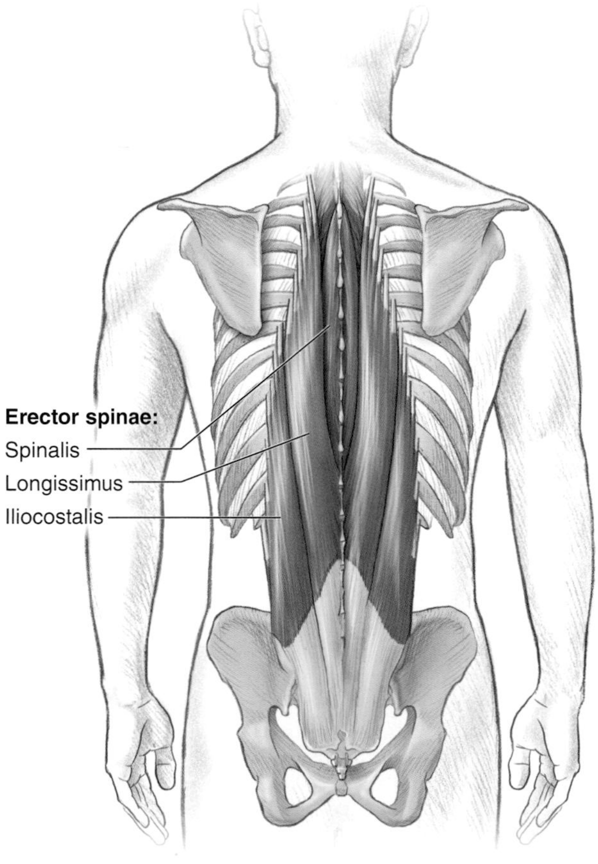

Erector spinae:
Spinalis
Longissimus
Iliocostalis

Figure 2.15 Erector spinae.

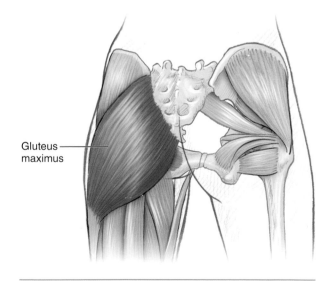

Gluteus maximus

Figure 2.16 Gluteus maximus.

respected, fully developed, and functionally utilized. Additionally, through its many attachment points, it works synergistically with a variety of additional hip musculature to aid in the overall LPHC stabilization.

Iliopsoas

The iliopsoas refers to three individual muscles: the psoas major, psoas minor, and iliacus (figure 2.17). Curiously, the psoas minor is present in only about 40 percent of the population. Both the psoas major and minor originate through L1 to L5 as well as the associated invertebral discs; differing only slightly, the psoas major also has origins on T12. The iliacus arises from the iliac fossa on the interior of the hip bone as well as the anterior-inferior iliac spine. The psoas major unites with the iliacus at the level of the inguinal ligament and crosses the hip joint to insert on the lesser trochanter of the femur (the lesser trochanter is at the lower end of the same bony outcrop as the greater trochanter). The psoas minor inserts at the iliopectineal arch, which is a thick band of the iliac fascia.

The iliopsoas group is primarily involved in hip flexion, often in a powerful manner, making it an essential piece in the training of sprinters. It also aids in the control of external rotation and overall LPHC stabilization. It is important to understand that although the iliopsoas inserts into and affects movement in front of the body, it actually begins in the back of the body. In particular, it connects into the lower back; an overactive or chronically tight hip flexor can thus lead to a myriad of uncomfortable back problems.

Thoracolumbar Fascia

Of the many muscles involved in core activity, one of the major players is a large and complex, nonmuscular fascial structure. The thoracolumbar fascia is a paper-thin membrane that covers the deep muscles of the lower back (figure 2.18). It extends from the back of the pelvis to the rib cage, serving as a bridge between upper and lower torso. The internal oblique, TVA, and latissimus dorsi all originate from this fascia, and as these muscles contract, the fascia tightens to create a very important brace for the lower back. When the deep stabilizers and outer mobilizers perform together with help from the thoracolumbar fascia, we are left with our woven basket, where each piece of the cylinder works together to create a strong, stable structure.

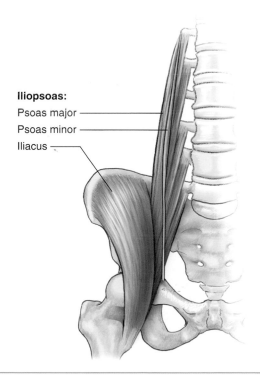

Figure 2.17   Iliopsoas.

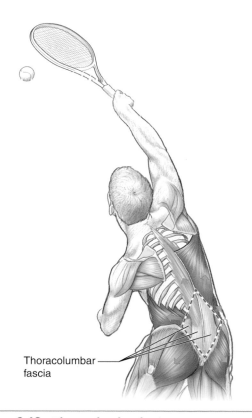

Figure 2.18   Thoracolumbar fascia.

You must understand that the human body incorporates *all* of these core muscles in one role or another at *all* times during *all* activities. With this in mind, we can ascertain that the aforementioned core musculature is involved heavily in producing efficient, crisp, and powerful global movement patterns. These patterns are intertwined in all of us and are structured almost identically in each human, yet the infinite combination of muscle functionality enables us to create uniqueness in our movements, be it the unorthodox throwing motion of South African bowler Paul Adams or the fluid pitching motion of San Francisco Giants pitcher Tim Lincecum. Our core allows us to create athletic movements that, while visually similar, are contextually different. As such, isolated muscle training does little toward the enhancement of complex, global movement patterns throughout the body's purposeful kinetic chain.

The core is so integrated in everything we do on a daily basis that a significant injury can have devastating effects and even end an athletic career in an instant. Athletes and nonathletes alike are told constantly to strengthen their core, no matter what their deficiencies are (and whether the deficiencies are mechanical or on the field of play). No other area of the body has received the same level of interest as the core, and research is consequently unlocking more and more of its secrets. The serious-minded athlete must stay on top of this constantly evolving information.

Your core—the complex link between your upper and lower limbs—must have the ability to be rigid when called on, pliable if needed, and efficient at all times. Nothing in your core musculature is a creation of chance; everything has its place, working in perfect synergy to ultimately allow you to live. Your core plays a personal orchestral performance every day of your life.

Injury Reduction

In recent years, phrases such as "prehab" and "injury prevention" have become ubiquitous in listings of exercise programming benefits. In reality, the only way to prevent sport injuries from occurring is to prevent athletes from training, practicing, and playing. Far too many risks are involved in athletics to guarantee that someone will be injury free. It is much more realistic to focus on reducing injury incidence and severity. Even this can be frustratingly difficult to achieve.

Though not all injuries can be avoided, injury reduction is a very important reason for training the core. A strong core allows athletes to gain and maintain body control, be it controlling the movement of the hips and vertebrae or controlling the forces that pass through the region.

Let's examine how a properly conditioned core increases the body's resilience to injury. We can perform this examination in three ways. In the first—postural modification—we look at how imbalances in the body can lead to aggravation and injury. In the second—a stronger, more stable core—we explain the functional timing and patterning of muscle activation and enhance load transfer efficiently with discriminating purpose. Finally, in the third—effective distribution of forces—we examine how superfluous external forces can lead to a variety of biomechanical and orthopedic issues.

POSTURAL MODIFICATION

A hugely recognizable force in today's NBA scene is Dwight Howard. Following in the footsteps of Wilt Chamberlain, Kareem Abdul-Jabbar, Patrick Ewing, Shaquille O'Neal, and other trend-setting basketball centers before him, Howard is once again revolutionizing the position. With his chiseled frame and remarkable explosiveness, he is a circadian highlight reel of dunks and blocked shots. However, if you could rewind back to the year 2000, you would see Dwight Howard, high school freshman: tall, skinny, and unpolished, yet radiating potential. You would also see a classic ectomorph, the hunched posture of a teenager who had yet to step onto an NBA floor. This position, known as upper-crossed syndrome, is common in tall athletes. These individuals exist as giants in a little person's world, constantly fighting the forces of gravity through their long spines, which causes them to protract their shoulders and slouch over in a bent, or kyphotic, posture. This posture is not a strong position to be in either structurally (in relation to the joints) or functionally (in relation to performance). To be able to fend off all-star centers and post up against the best, Howard had to overcome this syndrome and transform a solid, resilient structure to build strength on. Today we see the results: an erect, stable framework with powerful muscles layered over it.

All postural distortion patterns affect the integrity of the kinetic chain; this in turn leads to the development of muscle imbalances and dysfunction of the joints. Upper- and lower-crossed syndrome are the two biggest culprits, with upper crossed, as just mentioned, characterized by protracted shoulders and a slouched posture (figure 3.1). This syndrome can cause deterioration of the shoulder caused by the position of the humeral head in the glenoid process or can even lead to breathing dysfunction. Lower-crossed syndrome is characterized by a rotation of the pelvis either posteriorly (in a butt tucked under position) or, much more frequently, anteriorly, causing an increased arch in the lumbar spine (figure 3.2).

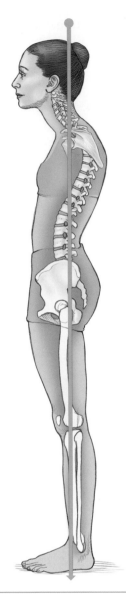

Figure 3.1   Upper-crossed syndrome.

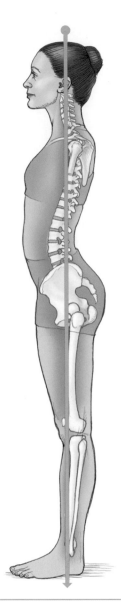

Figure 3.2   Lower-crossed syndrome.

At a cellular level, these syndromes cause altered length-tension relationships within the individual muscle fiber or bundles of muscle fiber. Simply stated, an optimal length-tension relationship refers to the length at which a muscle can produce its greatest amount of force. If this relationship is altered, less force is produced, creating imbalances that can lead to asynchronous and inefficient movement patterns—thus, a weak link in the kinetic chain. Deep within each fiber are sarcomeres that contain myofilaments (actin and myosin) that slide on top of one another (figure 3.3). A perfect relationship is when the myofilaments are stacked neatly. If these fibers are pulled apart or squeezed further together, the muscle is placed in a weakened

state. A simple analogy is Velcro laces—if the tips are barely touching and you pull, the Velcro tears easily away from itself. But if the laces meet neatly where they should and cover both surfaces, pulling the Velcro apart is more difficult because the bond is stronger. Core integrity can rectify sarcomere problems by helping to realign these areas and increase structural efficiency and neuromuscular control.

Ignoring these syndromes and allowing for bad posture to perpetuate leads not only to poor athletic output but also causes a cycle of soft-tissue trauma throughout the kinetic chain. This sequence is referred to as the cumulative injury cycle and is something all athletes deal with on a frequent basis if not effectively treated and

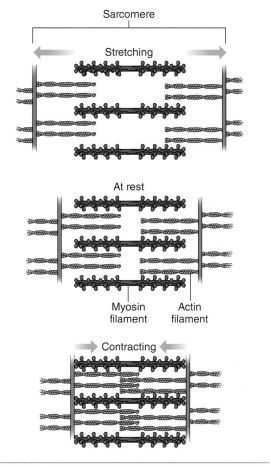

Figure 3.3 Sarcomeres at various lengths.

reeducated through sound exercise programming. For example, a softball pitcher with poor shoulder-joint position will eventually cause damage to the soft tissues surrounding the shoulder joint. The immediate biological response is inflammation, which we feel through the skin as heat (in some cases, we see it as swelling). This triggers the body's protective mechanisms, and the surrounding muscles increase their tension (often in the form of a spasm), and the whole area stiffens. This tension causes inelastic adhesions (or knots) to form in the soft tissue, which in turn alters the length-tension relationships we have just discussed. Once this happens, the correct sequence the muscles are supposed to work in is thrown off, leading to altered body mechanics and more injury. The cycle thus continues (figure 3.4).

With a well thought-out core training plan, many of the everyday aches and pains can be avoided. For muscles in a shortened, or hypertonic, state, a sound flexibility program is first imperative to reset the length; once established, a legitimate core-strengthening program will maintain this optimal fiber layout. The same is true for the need to strengthen an elongated muscle to reestablish the appropriate length-tension relationship. This will also realign the filaments, or sliding surfaces, of the muscle (actin and myosin, our Velcro laces), allowing the user to realize the full benefits of such training.

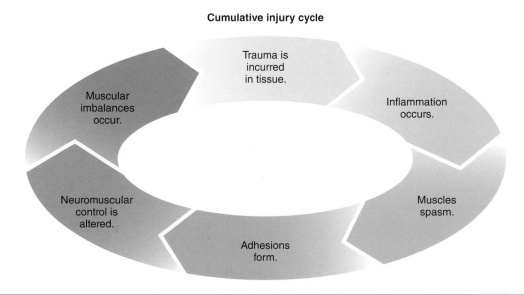

Figure 3.4 Cumulative injury cycle.

Shortened muscles can be addressed by implementing a sound joint range of motion or flexibility program along with integrated core development. Elongated muscles are ultimately corrected by an unrelenting focus on proper foundational posture and correct joint alignment throughout each training session. The integral strength created by training in the fashion we are describing will reset the necessary length-tension relationship and also heighten both functional static and functional dynamic motor control that is essential to all sport performance.

A STRONGER, MORE STABLE CORE

Many options are available for motivated athletes to facilitate preparation for their chosen activities. However, modalities such as conventional strength training, cardio, power yoga, and boot camp classes only scratch the surface of the potential opportunities toward enhanced physical development. From a purely physiological standpoint, the anchor to all fitness and sports performance activities is adequate core strength, dynamic balance, and functional control.

Contests missed because of injury can dramatically affect an otherwise successful season, regardless of the level of participation. Injuries are frustrating for athletes and teammates and can cost teams millions of dollars. Injury is, however, an unfortunate reality of sports and should be confronted head-on with a sound plan of anticipatory action. Although the core cannot be directly linked to every injury, many common injuries can be eliminated or their severity greatly reduced simply by intelligently training this critically important region of the body.

Over 80 percent of adults have suffered low back pain at one time or another. Research shows that individuals with chronic low back pain have decreased activation of the deep core stabilizers, particularly the transversus abdominis, internal oblique, pelvic floor muscles, multifidus, diaphragm, and deep erector spinae. Despite what we know, these muscle groups are the least likely to have been trained. It is clear, then, that if this musculature is significantly weak, overall core programming should begin with training to improve the deep stabilizers before systematically moving to the outer mobilizers using a stability-to-strength-to-power format. This is precisely the approach we will guide you through in this book.

Among the athletic community, knee pain is one of the more frequent complaints. Typically, this pain manifests in the front portion of the knee. Anterior knee pain is often referred to as patella-femoral pain syndrome, patellar tracking disorder, or iliotibial band (ITB) tendonitis. Regardless of the moniker, treatment protocols have traditionally focused solely on and around the knee itself; ultimately, this has been proven unsuccessful. It has recently been discovered that the position of the hip joint as it relates to the femur carries much of the blame (ankle alignment issues can be just as devastating to the knee, but they are out of the scope of this book). This links directly back to the core because the muscles that attach to and control the femur are all located there.

All three gluteal muscles (maximus, medius, and minimus) provide internal and external rotation of the femur as well as the ability to abduct. This is important to understand because often the glutes are duly affected by prior injury, incorrect training, and in some cases physiological adaptations, and can become ineffectual in their primary function. This leads to an inhibition of sorts, making other muscles that are ill-equipped for the task work harder to accomplish the physical pursuit we are requesting—often called compensation.

For example, in football, linemen spend a great deal of time bent at the waist in a hip-flexed position. Over the years, their hip flexors become chronically tight because they have adapted to being in that position. Physiologically, this leads to compensation, in which the central nervous system constantly sends signals to the flexors to remain short. At the same time, the glutes lengthen, putting them in a weak or ineffective position. The glutes' primary function is hip extension, and whenever linemen must extend quickly at the hips, their glutes often don't assist in the manner they were designed to. In this case, the athlete is still requiring the hip to extend, so the body calls on the hamstrings to become primary movers when they are better equipped to simply aid in the movement. All of this leads to the overload of a muscle unprepared for the task and, more often than not, a hamstring pull.

Another example of compensation is when the tensor fascia latae (TFL) becomes dominant over the glutes. In this scenario, the ITB connects directly into the TFL and is pulled taut, which causes friction at the knee joint and often leads to ITB syndrome. Such a circumstance leads to many types of knee pain, so it is essential that professionals in this field understand the relationships among the knees, hips, and core.

The core is clearly not the root of all injuries, but a weak or functionally inept core may well lead to injury intensification. For example, a growing area of concern is the sports hernia. Much like anterior knee pain, sports hernias fall into different categories—namely, athletic pubalgia, athletic hernia, Ashby's inguinal ligament enthesopathy, incipient hernia, and osteitis pubis. All of these conditions are characterized by chronic pain in the lower abdominal and high inner thigh area. This pain is aggravated by rapid rotational or kicking movements and quick direction changes. The actual injury is thought to come from a variety of sources, with the most common being a weakening of the posterior inguinal wall that lies in the area commonly called the groin. The injury mechanism itself is not fully understood, but most experts agree that the hip flexors and adductors are at the root of involvement. This involvement can range from compensation issues that result from muscular strength imbalances to asynchronous muscle firing patterns. This directly leads to excessive anterior rotation of the pelvis and internal rotation of the hip, both of which are likely to be the biggest factor for injury. These two areas of the body attach directly into the hip complex, thus physical therapists strongly suggest that sufferers focus on core stabilization training to balance out the deficits between the hip flexors and extensors and the internal and external rotators, many of which lie within the gluteal complex and are stabilized by the anterior core musculature.

Many other areas of the body can also be aided by quality core training. Ankle sprains, for example, have been linked to gluteal dysfunction, and low-back spasms are very likely caused by a chronically tight piriformis, which lies neatly under the gluteus maximus. So, as we have seen, the kinetic chain can work in two ways: from a positive functional and performance-enhancement standpoint and, conversely, from a referred injury perspective.

As we mentioned in chapter 2, traditional core training seeks to isolate a single area, the result of which is a program designed to strengthen in a solitary fashion. This leads to strength gains in that particular area alone, which is a fundamental flaw. Instead of creating a high-functioning and efficient unit that is strong at the core, the athlete's body will have weak links throughout, leading to unproductive movement and possible injuries.

Many athletes have overtrained their rectus abdominis, external oblique, and erector spinae but neglected their deep stabilizing musculature, resulting in the superfluous movement of the vertebral segments. More often than not, this unwanted surplus of motion plays out in pain or injury.

Stuart McGill, a Canadian researcher and leading voice in lower back health, has furthered the concept of the body damaging itself through poor programming. He has determined that repeated spinal flexion is a key contributor to disc herniations. In *Ultimate Back Fitness and Performance*, he writes, "The traditional sit-up imposes approximately 3300 N or about 730 pounds of compression on the spine," and that "the National Institute of Occupational Safety and Health has set the action limit for low back compression at 3300 N. Repetitive loading about this level is linked with higher injury rates in workers, yet this is imposed on the spine with each repetition of the sit-up." Research from other independent studies has supported McGill's findings.

Science is critical in guiding the decisions we make when training our athletes. However, although our understanding of the human body has increased dramatically, a significant shift in consciousness is needed to retire concepts of the past and openly embrace what is new and backed by fresher research. This shift is a major challenge for coaches and athletes alike. That said, many of the traditional core exercises still hold prominence in today's contemporary core programming. Recognizing which exercises achieve the results we strive for is the challenge. This book is an attempt to cut through the confusion.

EFFECTIVE DISTRIBUTION OF FORCE

Most injuries in sport occur during deceleration or rotational movements. Surprisingly high numbers of these are noncontact injuries. For instance, a rugby player might sprain an ankle by simply planting his foot and cutting sharply in another direction. A well-conditioned core might have allowed for a more appropriate distribution of force and reduced the extent of the injury, if not possibly prevented the injury in the first place.

When discussing force distribution, we might best make our point by considering knee injuries, particularly injuries to the anterior cruciate ligament (ACL). Obviously, the knee is a vital link between the hip and the ground. The ability to decelerate explosive movements is critical not only to provide a platform for the next movement, but also to avoid injury. Between 80,000 and 100,000 ACL injuries occur annually, and about 70 percent of them are noncontact in nature. Understanding the mechanisms of these injuries reinforces the importance of the core's ability to dynamically stabilize the body.

As ACL injury rates have risen sharply, especially among female athletes, a great deal of research has dealt with these injuries over the last few years. Much has been brought to light, but there is still much to learn. The classic "danger" position for the ACL is landing or changing direction with the femur adducted and internally rotated and the tibia abducted and externally rotated. Essentially, this is a knock-kneed position, clinically called genu valgum (figure 3.5).

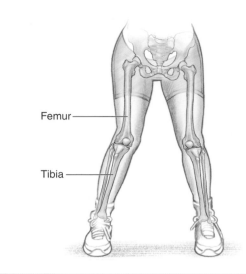

Figure 3.5 ACL danger position: genu valgum.

Women and ACL Tears

Women appear to be at higher risk of ACL injury for several reasons:

- The knock-kneed position is an indication of poor stability within the core musculature. A valgus knee is a combination of core instability and Q-angle. The angle created by the difference between the descending line of the femur as it drops from the hip to knee as compared to a vertical line (perpendicular to the ground) is called the Q-angle. The consequent biomechanic of the lower leg (tibia and fibula) is to flare out. This angle at the knee is called genu valgum, and if it is noticeably pronounced the individual is often labeled as knock-kneed. Because women tend to have a proportionally wider hip, this angle at the knee can at times be quite severe. This does not suggest automatic instability. However, this greater descending angle can be a precursor for valgus knee issues.

- Ligament dominance occurs in women more than men. In this instance, females stress their ligaments prior to muscular activation to absorb ground reaction forces. The lack of core muscular control at the hip joint leads to increased valgus motion, greater force, and higher torque that can stress the passive structures of the knee joint.

- Women tend to be more quadriceps-dominant than men. This gender difference occurs because females activate their knee extensors preferentially over their knee flexors during dynamic activities to aid in stabilizing the knee joint. ACL injuries most often occur when the knee is close to full extension, so quadriceps-dominance might put the ligament at increased risk.

- Females have a smaller intercondylar notch at the end of the femur where the ACL attaches. This would suggest a thinner ACL with less area for freedom of movement, which could lead to a higher chance of damage.

- Preliminary research has indicated that the ACL itself may have hormone receptor sites attached to it, which could mean that women are more likely to suffer this type of injury during and around menstruation.

What does all this have to do with core strength? One indicator of poor levels of stability is genu valgum, the knock-kneed position. The body must be trained in a way so that, during landing and cutting, the knee line does not shift inward; it must be stabilized in an almost straight line from hip to ankle. This leads to fewer injuries and allows for more highly proficient direction changes.

A poorly functioning gluteal complex produces a dominance of the hip flexors and shifts the pelvis into an anterior tilt, which can cause a whole host of problems, most notably lower back pain. Plus, as the pelvis rolls forward, the dominant flexors (some of which help to adduct and internally rotate) pull and twist the femur inward, creating the beginning point of our ACL danger position. Developing enhanced neuromuscular efficiency to the gluteal area allows the body to preserve a brace throughout movement; the body will then "call on" the brace automatically whenever the spine needs additional stability. We will return to this discussion in part II.

The ability to overcome external forces and muscular imbalance is important to a long and successful athletic career. If you develop, streamline, and control your body's ability to generate and withstand dynamic forces with a strong and stable core, you will find yourself far less often on the injured list.

Essential Strength and Power Source

If you are not happy with the current fitness fad, then just wait a minute, because some trends are just that . . . fads. However, some methods of training are quite effective and are in fact scientifically verified. Often, advances in science allow us the opportunity to justify traditional conditioning systems that have been hypothesized for many years. Since physiology hasn't changed much over the past 40,000 years, it is relatively predictable that when a stress is imposed to the biological system, a calculable adaptation to that stress can be expected. Training modalities that were once thought to be speculative and possibly detrimental, yet appeared to realize positive outcomes, are now becoming a standard of industry practice. Over the past decade one such training theory has been extensively researched, and overwhelmingly the data supports the importance of core stabilization and its relationship to all facets of movement and performance.

Thus far we have built a case supporting the importance of core development from a functionality standpoint. Let's now turn our focus to the core's role in enhanced sport performance. More specifically, we will look at the core's influence on the origin and transfer of strength and power, two prerequisites for superior performance that all serious athletes covet. You need only glance at a daily sports page or listen to Mike Breen announce a game to understand the importance of strength and power in sport (e.g., "That was a strong move to the basket" . . . "His hits are the most powerful in the league"). In this chapter, we look beyond the hyperbole and determine what strength and power mean as they relate to athletics and why the core is an essential source for both.

TRAINING FOR STABILIZATION

The muscular structures of the abdominal and back regions play a dominant role in postural control, lumbar stabilization, and proprioception (what we call total body balance). As we have said, a well-functioning core can help reduce the risk and severity of injury and promote greater efficiency. Precise movements such as lifting a baby from a crib or throwing a dart would not be possible without effective involvement of the core musculature. Tasks that demand synchronous strength, such as standing in strict military posture for an extended time or maintaining balance while exiting a ski lift, similarly require core involvement. In addition, power-based tasks such as sprinting, swinging a golf club, or dunking a basketball would be impossible without a stable core.

You might ask how the core is involved in throwing a dart. The answer is that we must use the deep stabilizers to isometrically and dynamically sustain the kinetic chain during energetic movements within all three planes of motion. More simply stated, stabilization provides a strong foundation through which an action (such as throwing a dart) can occur most efficiently, powerfully, and accurately. Action is never plane-specific. That is, even though your movement is taking place in one plane, the other two planes must be stabilized for the action to be successful. How accurate can a dart-throw be from a core foundation as wobbly as a cube of Jell-O? Force reduction, stabilization, and force production within all planes of movement is the template for training the entire kinetic chain. In training, as we have stated before, stability is trained before strength, and strength is trained before power.

A stable core is no doubt important to everyday activities, but for optimal athletic performance stabilizing the core is imperative. Eastern philosophers have been preaching core stability for thousands of years. Trunk and torso stabilization techniques are as much a daily ritual for them as are eating and sleeping. The view is that you enhance your quality of life through maximizing efficiency of physical function. Eastern martial artists routinely focus the greatest percentage of their training time on the development of the "Hara" (the core), the physical center of being.

Relaxation of the muscles promoted by a strong core allows for greater freedom of movement, better control of power within a movement, less extraneous movement, and most important, the conservation of energy through efficient movement. Controlled body movement is also a prerequisite for accuracy of skill. The power developed in the core must eventually travel through the musculoskeletal system to the more precision-oriented distal musculature of the extremities. Only after achieving this ability to channel energy can you begin to realize your tremendous physical potential—and it all starts with the core.

Characteristics of Good Balance

Balance is the result of correct body alignment and fully functioning sensory mechanisms. The proper synergism between the core and the legs, arms, feet, hands, and head is essential to achieving correct body alignment.

From an athletic perspective, someone who is standing and is balanced (in an athletic stance) typically demonstrates the following:

1. The knees are flexed rather than straight, creating a slightly lower center of mass.
2. The base of support is comfortably wide, with feet parallel.
3. Body weight is slightly forward of the midpoint of the foot.

4. The center of mass is dynamic; that is, the athlete continually uses rapid yet controlled motion to respond to sudden changes of direction.

The ability to accurately adjust to changes in your position or to an unstable equilibrium and to sense your limitations in the constant battle against gravity indicates accomplished balance. Most great athletes possess such balance without even realizing it.

Dynamic Balance

Maintaining balance and stability is a dynamic process. With no conscious effort, your body's muscular system is continually contracting and relaxing in order to sustain sitting, standing, walking, running, or any other posture. Your body is continually trying to achieve a state of equilibrium. Several mechanisms within the body continually process information in an effort to attain this state. Two of the more athletically relevant sources of feedback include the vestibular apparatus within the inner ear and proprioceptors within the muscles and joints.

- The *vestibular apparatus* relays information to the central nervous system concerning the body's spatial awareness, including any deviations from the vertical position.
- *Proprioceptors,* such as the muscle spindle and Golgi tendon organ, sense the magnitude and speed of a stretched muscle and changes in joint angles.

These sensors provide input necessary to make immediate and essential adjustments in balance. A good example of your receptors at work is that disturbing feeling of just beginning to nod off, only to be abruptly jerked back to reality. For example, while sitting in the film room listening to an unbearably boring lecture on postural assessments and realizing that you can never possibly get back these wasted four hours of your life, you begin to doze off and your head starts to drop forward. The muscle spindles in the back of your neck sense the stretch placed on the neck musculature and quickly make a correction by firing those same muscles and returning your head to upright position. From a stabilization, balance, and postural standpoint, refining your proprioceptor sensors enhances athletic performance and reduces injury risk.

The Importance of Good Posture

Poor posture affects not only balance but all other athletic performance variables. Keep in mind that force is more effectively transferred through a straight line. Obviously, there are natural curvatures throughout the body, but generally speaking, you should strive for proper body alignment between segments—particularly during the push or explosive phase of a movement. A person with poor posture lacks that straight line.

The preferred path of force transfer is through the skeletal system. Poor posture, however, causes detours in the force transfer because the smaller and weaker muscles outside the core must act as the force conduit. Much wasted energy results, and subsequent and usually more severe breakdowns are inevitable. Poor posture leads to countless mechanical and structural problems, some of which we touched on in chapter 3.

TRAINING FOR STRENGTH

We can break strength down into two categories: muscular strength and muscular endurance. In its strictest sense, muscular strength is the maximum amount of force that a muscle can generate against resistance in a single effort. In contrast, muscular endurance is the ability of a muscle or group of muscles to exert force for a sustained time, such as when running, raking leaves, or hitting hundreds of forehands over the course of a tennis match. From an athletic perspective, both muscular strength and muscular endurance are critical for

- performance enhancement,
- functional stabilization and dynamic postural control of the spine, and
- efficient biomechanical movement throughout the kinetic chain.

Most people think of strength in terms of *how much can I lift?* In fact, strength—and specifically core strength—is an integral protective mechanism that helps eliminate postural distortions that can lead to ineffective neuromuscular proficiency. Low strength levels at any point within the kinetic chain place the athlete at risk for compensation issues that can elicit extra stresses

placed on the contractile and noncontractile tissues, which will adversely affect functional movement patterns and place the athlete at greater risk of injury. Conversely, strong muscles provide efficient dynamic stabilization, decrease the risk of serial distortion patterns, and transmit forces to the bones, acting as levers and resulting in precise and effectual movement.

Unfortunately, most coaches and athletes view strength in its absolute sense—the greater weight that can be lifted translates to heightened performance on the court or field. Strength is but one component within a complex system of a multisensory sport performance. Without stabilization, strength cannot be fully developed. Without strength, stabilization—or the lack thereof—will decrease performance and expose the weak link in the kinetic chain. Without both stability and strength and the refined neuromuscular efficiency associated with the systematic functioning of their relationship, athletes cannot hope to fully develop their power potential.

If you are new to strength training, we encourage you to take the same approach to training for strength as for the global development of all physiological processes. As we have mentioned, enhanced motor skill development evolved following a proximal-to-distal progression. Your strength training should follow a similar course, with emphasis on developing core strength before implementing extremity exercises. Once you have established a foundation of strength, you can then focus on the quality of technique and execution over quantity (with regard to load and repetitions). Quality is nearly impossible without the proper foundation from which to execute the activity. In addition, once foundational core development has been established, you can begin to focus on sport specific–related movements without risking deleterious technical inaccuracies.

TRAINING FOR POWER

Assimilating stability and strength is an important part of developing your center of power. Sport movements, however, typically require explosive, ballistic, and well-coordinated muscular actions. The ability to take strength gained from the weight room and apply it effectively on the playing field is the goal of any performance-enhancement program. Power and strength are not synonymous. As such, the strongest athlete is not necessarily the most powerful athlete.

Power conditionally relies on the correlation between strength and speed—thus the clever phrase "speed strength." For athletes to maximize their power gains, they must include a *speed* component in their training. Simply put, power is a relationship between strength and speed. To this point we have discussed strength, but what exactly is speed? How important is speed? How is speed developed?

Speed can be broadly defined as the elapsed time it takes to move from point A to point B. The distance between point A and point B could be the 26.2 miles of a marathon, the 10 feet from the floor to the basketball rim, or, when at bat, from the "cocked" position to the contact point with the ball. Once you combine speed with strength, the long hours of strength training in the weight room start to pay off, and sport-specific, or *functional,* strength starts to translate to power. Thus power is the product of force (the weight room) and velocity (the functional application). It should come as no surprise that all of this begins at the core.

Developing Speed

Developing the speed component of power differs dramatically from standard programs designed to enhance strength. Typically, you increase your muscular strength through consistent and progressive overload training (increasing load). Training for enhanced speed can certainly be influenced by regular trips to the weight room; however, the level of change is more often a predisposition of unseen factors. These considerations, along with diligent workouts, determine the ultimate level of speed development. These factors are

- individual genetic characteristics and
- the physiology of the muscular system.

Individual Genetic Characteristics and Their Relation to Speed

An athlete's proportional configuration of muscle fiber type (i.e., muscle cell types) has a profound influence on his or her potential for speed. For our purposes here, we will simplify the physiology and discuss two types of muscle fiber: fast-twitch and slow-twitch.

Fast-twitch muscle fibers exert great power but fatigue quickly. The body generates the energy required to contract a fast-twitch fiber anaerobically, or without oxygen. These fibers are best suited for short, explosive actions, such as sprints, Olympic lifting, or volleyball spikes. In contrast, slow-twitch muscle fibers require oxygen for sustained contraction and are thus ideal for endurance activities, such as cross-country skiing, marathon running, or road cycling.

Athletes who participate in endurance sports typically have a higher percentage of slow-twitch fibers. Conversely, the muscles of athletes whose sports require explosive actions tend to contain a higher percentage of fast-twitch fibers. Most elite-level athletes gravitate toward sports that are compatible with their genetic makeup (remember that we are simplifying the physiology).

All of us were born with a certain ratio of fast-twitch to slow-twitch fibers. Even if your muscles are predominantly slow-twitch, however, does not mean you are destined to remain slow. Clearly, you will never become as fast as a cheetah, but you can always become faster than you are right now. You simply learn to maximize what you have inherited.

Muscle Physiology and Its Impact on Speed

Power performance is a consequence of the relationship between muscles and the nervous system. The muscles provide the gas to generate the force, and the nervous system monitors how much gas is needed to execute the task. One way to tap into your vast reservoir of power is to further develop your naturally occurring physiological processes—to "step on the gas." Training the core's neural response mechanisms helps to facilitate this speed component. (Keep in mind that we are not talking about winning a race, necessarily, but, rather, drawing on your vast potential of untapped athleticism.)

The neural adaptation to strength training takes the shape of increased activation of the primary movers, or the agonist muscles. The neural response also includes a heightened involvement of the synergist muscles—the muscles that support the prime movers. Common sense suggests that the opposing torque developed by the coactivation of the antagonist muscles would decrease the net torque intended by the agonists, but on the contrary, it is the antagonist that provides the stability—primarily within the acting joint or joints—necessary to elicit maximum force and, from a power perspective, the rate of that force. Thus for performance to have a chance of success, the agonists (prime movers), synergists (coordinators), and antagonists (stabilizers) must work in concert, and when they do, great things can happen. All of this must occur against a backdrop of sensory feedback in the form of perception and reflexes.

The Stretch Reflex

The speed component of power is directly influenced by a highly trainable attribute called the *stretch reflex*. Within a bundle of muscle are tiny sensory mechanisms called muscle spindles. These spindles are about the size of a muscle fiber (or cell) and are located in, among, and parallel to the muscle fibers (figure 4.1). A spindle's primary duty is to prevent injury to its associated muscle fibers in situations in which the fibers might be placed on an excessively rapid or overly forceful stretch—well beyond the muscle's tolerance. An extreme stretch such as this can certainly occur as a result of the ballistic nature of many athletic movements.

However, muscle spindles can also be used to the athlete's advantage to generate a more powerful muscle contraction. For example, during the drop or descent of a jump (the countermovement phase), those muscles that span the shoulder, hip, knee, and ankle joints are placed on a *rapid stretch*, primarily as a result of gravity and body weight. Because the muscle spindles lie parallel to the muscle fibers, they too experience a rapid stretch. The spindles consequently "sense" the stretch and send a message to the central nervous system (brain or spinal cord). In turn, the central nervous system instructs the stretched muscles to contract forcefully, relative to the speed and magnitude of the prestretch. If this sensory mechanism did not exist or for some reason was not functioning, the rapid stretch could possibly exceed the extensibility of the fiber and would most certainly result in an injury to the muscle. The muscle spindle response, subsequently combined with an intended voluntary contraction, can maximize peak force with athletic movements.

Stored Elastic Energy

Another important physiological phenomenon of muscle is the process of *stored elastic energy*. Think of stretching a rubber band. Imagine that the elasticity of the rubber is similar to the elastic properties of muscle (the fibers and its tendon). As you stretch the rubber band, energy is stored in the elastic properties of the rubber. When you release one end, you release that energy stored. However, there is an essential difference between a rubber band and muscle fiber. With the rubber band, the longer the stretch, the more energy is stored and then released. But with muscle fiber, it is not the magnitude but rather the speed of the eccentric stretch that determines how much energy can be used during the immediate ensuing concentric contraction.

Athletes can take advantage of this inherent elastic quality of the muscle tendon unit. The baseball batter cocking the body with the bat held high just before swinging or the discus thrower

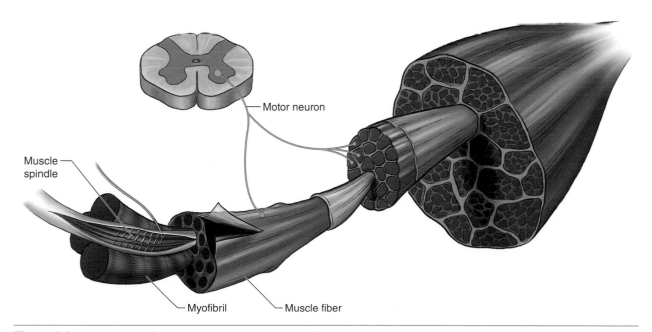

Figure 4.1 Muscle spindles located within the muscle fibers.

Labels: Motor neuron, Muscle spindle, Myofibril, Muscle fiber snapping (rotating the hips) just prior to release are prime examples of this *stretch-shortening cycle*. The elastic energy is stored in the active muscles as a result of a rapid prestretch. This physiological process is trainable, and most progressive regimens employ drills and activities designed to enhance it.

Additionally, the stretch-shortening cycle (muscle spindle response) can help facilitate the recruitment of a greater percentage of muscle to perform a given task. With greater motor unit involvement, the potential for intensified power output is thus more thoroughly exploited. Superior power in the core region directly enhances all athletic movements. Remember that no matter what your current ability, you can improve. Training the speed component is one more weapon in the training arsenal.

Transfer of Power

Without the efficient transfer of your newfound power potential, your core training might as well be focused on beach abs. Thus the number one training objective for every athlete should be to develop an efficient coupling system in which the tremendous power potential of the core can be expressed distally to the extremities, the goal being to functionally transfer this core power through progressively smaller and weaker musculature without a contemporaneous loss of energy. For example, if you were to lock your elbow and wrist and extend your index finger, and then attempt to push your friend, the force generated from the pelvic muscles will efficiently transfer from your core through your straight arm to your fingertip with little energy loss. The resulting push would cause at least minor discomfort, if not knock your friend off balance. If, however, you were to bend one of the joints along the chain, such as your elbow, the force generated by the core would dissipate through the bend in the elbow. The strong muscles of the core would become less effective, and the resulting push might feel like an aggressive tickle.

Today's flaccid approach to athletic development, which is often prescribed by physiotherapists and trainers, alienates us from our individual health and fitness goals, and of more critical concern, our athletic potential. We have become a collective ethos in which coddling and the sedentary methodology concerning athletic development has led to a generation of athletes whose performance is declining. Many athletes will experience some degree of intensified physical and structural breakdown on a regular basis during their career. In contrast, intelligently organized and purposefully executed training regimens that are progressively challenging will help maintain proper, efficient, and synchronous functioning of all body systems. Freedom of movement in harmony with the body's design, without the constraints of poor posture and unresponsive modalities, will help eliminate inferior function, thereby enhancing performance.

You must regain control of your fitness and performance potential. Proactivity, as opposed to passivity, will lead to a greater influence over your stability, strength, and power. Motion will become robustly efficient with a minimum of wasted energy, leading to enhanced control and spectacular performance. This controlled energy enables you to deal better with the physical and emotional stress of competition and to perform at a higher intensity for a longer duration with less fatigue—in other words, more productive time competing and less pampering time in the training room.

Exercise Selection and Training Considerations

As an athletic-minded person, you should be progressive when selecting exercises and developing a training program. As we have said before, nothing in your training routine should be selected arbitrarily. Everything must have reasoning behind it. You should select exercises based on your level of conditioning and then intelligently progress over the course of the training cycle. This book will guide you through the development process, relying on a variety of progression methodologies. Changing body position, incorporating instability features, working against external resistance, adding or decreasing a speed element, or any combination of the aforementioned will contribute toward progression.

As you will see throughout this book, no matter where you start, your training program will be recurring. That is, at various points you will train recurrently in each phase (stability, strength, and power) throughout given cycles. To this end, we provide logical progressions and regressions to each of the highlighted exercises so that as you move through the phases you will constantly be challenged. As you complete the strength and then the power phase, you will be required to cycle back to stability; however, your exercise selection will be more demanding than the original. The same will be true of each level as you rotate back through strength and then power. One of our goals is for you to become your own coach as you progress in your training. In other words, you will eventually be able to identify exercises not included in this book and determine whether they are valid, safe, and effective and where they would fit in a comprehensive training program.

EXERCISE CATEGORIES

Parts II through IV contain an assortment of exercises for the various levels of core training. All exercises in this book fall into one of five categories:

1. Anti-extension
2. Anti-rotation
3. Scapulothoracic
4. Lumbo-pelvic hip complex
5. Total core (strength phase only)

At this point, it is important to discuss the nature and reasoning behind training to resist extension and rotation. As we explained in chapter 2, of all the defined core musculature (and those of the periphery), only the rectus abdominis and spinalis muscles have fibers lined vertically. The many remaining muscles have fibers that align in an oblique direction. This shows that on a purely anatomical level, the core is designed mainly to reduce rotational movement. To be specific, we are attempting to restrict this movement in the lumbar spine but promote it in the thoracic spine.

Overall, your lumbar vertebrae have roughly only 13 degrees of rotation. Individually, T10 to L5 has 2 degrees. The greatest rotational range is between L5 and S1, which is only 5 degrees. This is obviously an incredibly small amount, so between the muscle structure described in chapter 2 and the actual segmental range, forcing explosive rotation in an area not equipped for it is a prescription for trouble. Conversely, thoracic rotation can be as much as 70 degrees, and rotation in the midthoracic region (T3 to T9) can be as much as 10 degrees. We will respect these structural limitations, yet our training must reflect the range. Thus, anti-rotation movements such as those presented should involve a high level of thoracic rotation but as little lumbar movement as possible.

The same is true for the anti-extension exercises. If you look at the natural S-shaped curve of the spine, the lumbar spine is gently arched in a natural curve (lordotic curve), and the thoracic spine is rounded forward (kyphotic curve). Intervertebral discs lie between adjacent vertebrae in the spine and provide an articulating surface that allows for slight movement of the spine. In addition to helping maintain structural integrity of the vertebral column, the discs provide a cushion, which is extremely important to athletes from an impact and axial load perspective. Excessive extension in the lumbar spine (an anterior pelvic tilt), intentional or not, serves only to put added compressive pressure on the posterior vertebral discs. These compressive forces to the gel-like discs can make them bulge outward, causing all manner of issues. At the other end of the spine, gentle and controlled extension of the thoracic vertebrae is appropriate; there is a naturally occurring space for the discs to move in without any major compression on either side of the disc.

We can see a pattern for an equal, if not greater, need to train the core to *resist* movement in addition to creating movement. With this in mind, understand that most exercises in the book will be *anti* in nature—anti-extension based and anti-rotation based. These will be combined with exercises to strengthen the scapulothoracic musculature, along with lumbopelvic hip exercises to ensure high levels of neural drive and overall quality of movement in that area.

SPECIFIC BENEFITS OF THE EXERCISES

As a conscientious trainee, you need a good working knowledge of why you are selecting certain exercises and not others. The testing we outline in chapter 18 will create the parameters of your training program and help you to know when to progress if you are unsure. But what of the exercises themselves? Why are some more beneficial than others? And why do some seem impossible at times and others too easy?

Having a basic working knowledge of the specific benefits of each of the exercises we have presented will allow you to see behind the curtain and get a better feel for what your body is going through and what it needs next in the training paradigm. We set out to make this book different from other training texts that have charted similar waters, and this section is no different. The benefits we have chosen to highlight (in truth there are multiple benefits for each exercise, from physiological to neural) do not concern isolated muscle actions or basic fitness concepts. Instead, they follow our consistent message about the global approach to training and therefore more comprehensively cover what is beneficial about each exercise and in most cases what to expect from each.

Each exercise in chapters 6 through 17 lists one or more of the following specific benefits by number. Once you are familiar with the exercises (and your body), you will not only be able to assess your needs based on core assessment testing but also based on the training benefits you are seeking.

Specific Benefits

 1 | **Unstable surface** | *Unstable surfaces create a task complexity situation whereby a relatively simple activity becomes more difficult.*
Using unstable devices of any variety immediately places an additional proprioceptive and dynamic stabilization demand on the physiological and musculoskeletal systems. The ultimate benefit is the challenge to the body's stabilizing mechanisms; these systems will work harder in an unstable environment as opposed to a fully stable environment where the stimulation to the stabilizers is lessened. Additionally, due to the changeable height of various stability balls, while the firing sequence, synergism, and specific muscle involvement remain the same as a floor exercise, the difference in the line of pull as a result of the alteration in contact points creates an alternatively unique challenge.

2	**Upper-body incline**	*Unless specifically noted for a particular exercise, in most instances, the greater the height of the upper-body incline, the easier the challenge.* Progressively inclining the upper body changes the line of gravitational pull, thereby decreasing the challenge to the body. Specifically, an upper incline is somewhat less challenging and allows the bigger musculature of the chest and shoulder complex to stabilize the body.
3	**Lower-body incline**	*In most instances, from a prone and supine perspective, the greater the height of the lower-body incline, the harder the challenge.* Progressively inclining the lower body creates a more challenging scenario and places more adaptive stress (load) away from the bigger musculature of the chest and higher onto the shoulder girdle.
4	**Single-leg hip extension**	*The strength requirements of the gluteal structure will be enhanced regardless of the criteria imposed.* A single-leg hip extension creates an asymmetrical base of support. This disproportionate body position will enhance the rotational demand to the core musculature whereby the body now has to control this added stress.
5	**Abduction and adduction**	*The strength requirements of the gluteal structure and shoulder complex, as well as the various abducting and adducting musculature involved in those regions, will be enhanced regardless of the criteria imposed.* A single-leg limb abduction movement dramatically shifts the center of gravity laterally, away from the midline of the body (in the frontal plane). To counter this shift, engage the deep stabilizers necessary for maintaining straight spinal alignment and avoid deleterious postural distortions. Additionally, the opposing adducting musculature (whether it be attached at the hip or shoulder) must isometrically work to maintain overall pelvic or shoulder girdle stability.
6	**Suspension**	*Suspension training will challenge stability, strength, kinesthesis, and proprioception.* Similar to the adaptive qualities of benefit 1, using a suspension apparatus eliminates any advantage of control one might receive from the unstable device being in contact with the floor or other solid surface. There are many ways to make suspension training more or less challenging. For example, with the handle grips elevated and the feet closer to the hanging gravitational straight line, the easier the activity (push-up, I-pattern, single-leg hip extension). Conversely, if the handles are low (close to the floor) and the feet are elevated and farther away from the gravitational line, the exercise would be extremely demanding, especially so the higher the feet are elevated.
7	**Upper-body walking and total-body displacement**	*This disproportionate body position will enhance the rotational demand to the core musculature whereby the deep stabilizers will work together with the outer mobilizers to develop control.* Arm walking that incorporates the feet from both a stationary and mobile device (including displacement) will continually challenge the region between the two contact points (typically the forearms or hands and the feet). A larger area between the two contact points will create a longer lever arm, while a shorter distance between these two points will lessen the lever arm. You will feel the various difficulty levels immediately after experimenting with ipsilateral, bilateral, and contralateral transfer of fluctuating degrees of difficulty and within varying planes of movement. Moreover, moving the limbs forward and backward in an alternating process will generate an additional rotational emphasis to the body.

(continued)

⑧	Lower-body movement	*Walking and marching will globally challenge the entire kinetic chain and specifically targets the deep stabilizers of the core.* Anti-extension, anti-rotation, and shoulder stabilization are just a few of the physiological adaptive benefits of marching. The body is accustomed to having a symbiotic relationship between its upper and lower half with locomotion occurring in synchronous fashion with the lower limbs as drivers. By selecting exercises that primarily require lower-body movement as part of a rudimentary core program, you are beginning to refine that symbiotic process from the ground up.
⑨	Unilateral action	*Unilateral training will expose any asymmetries in the body, thereby leaving the weaker extremity no choice but to perform the same ratio as the stronger extremity. This generates better total balance in the body.* Force production, force reduction, and certainly stabilization can be further challenged through the implementation of a fluctuating single-extremity posture or movement patterns. Sporadic disparate body positions will enhance the rotational demand to the core musculature whereby the body now has to control this added stress in an effort to maintain dynamic balance while still performing the prescribed action. When employing unilateral (single-limb) postures or movements, a bilateral deficit occurs: One limb has more coordinated control than that of its counter. Also, athletes typically have a dominant and nondominant extremity. That is, one extremity is stronger or more coordinated than the other. Adhering to our philosophy of specificity of training, rarely in sport (if ever) is an athlete positioned in a symmetrically bilateral stance with an equally balanced extremity effort. An infinite number of movement patterns are available. As such, there must be safe disproportionate variety in training.
⑩	Ipsilateral action	*Raising both limbs on the same side of the body raises the difficulty level of a prone exercise to its maximum.* This creates a situation whereby the center of mass is outside and lateral to the base of support. To counter this, shift your weight toward the midline of the base of support while concurrently engaging the anti-rotators of the core. Opposing-limb activities, such as contralateral exercises, typically help to provide the counterbalance necessary to stabilize the spine and maintain dynamic balance with multilimb extension exercises or situations involving a two-point base of support.
⑪	Contralateral action	*Movement patterns involving cross-body extremities illicit an anti-rotational response in the body in an attempt to maintain structural homeostasis, balance, and kinesthetic awareness.* The act of raising opposing limbs changes the types of stress on the body and compels the body in the redistribution of forces in an unfamiliar way, forcing the body to adapt. Resisting this force creates the need for a more complex physiological strategy and therefore raises the difficulty level of the exercise.
⑫	Axis and lever modification	*The farther away from the axis the load is placed on the lever arm, the more challenging an exercise can be and the more the stabilizers around the axis point must be engaged.* Bones, ligaments, and muscles form the three lever classes found in the human body. Together they create movement around a fulcrum, or axis point. From a biomechanical perspective, the fulcrum is the center of rotation of a joint. Basic examples of this premise would be simply extending your arms from a plank to a straight-arm plank position. This can be even more profound in the case of the Pallof Press series of movements in chapter 10, where initially the load is held isometrically at arm's length. In subsequent progressions the arms extend and retract throughout the movement, smoothly changing the length of the lever arm and increasing the involvement of the stabilizers around the axis point (in this case the shoulder joint) to deal with the constantly changing stresses.

⑬	**Lateral and side-lying action**	*Lateral and side-lying postures and actions shift the training focus and incorporate often-overlooked areas of the upper back and shoulder.* With so much emphasis deliberately and inadvertently placed on the development of the upper trapezius, lateral and side-lying postures and actions shift the training focus to the middle and lower portion of the trapezius and incorporate the critical serratus musculature. Working alone, the serratus pulls the scapula forward; however, when working synergistically with the rhomboids, this musculature keeps the scapula pressed against the thorax. Inhibition of the lower trapezius and serratus musculature can lead to problems such as upper-cross syndrome. Likewise, athletes with a high degree of imbalance between the upper and lower trapezius often have subacromial impingement, not to mention poor shoulder functionality.
⑭	**Reaction and response**	*Athletes who exhibit refined reaction and response often have a high degree of agility.* Common qualities of superior athleticism are reaction and response. Often thought of as one and the same, reaction is the recognition of a stimulus, and response is characterized as the necessary, and hopefully effective, consequential action. Drills that are based on temporal stress (reduced decision-making time) have a high carryover to sport where everything happens in an instant. Tying that to core training can have positive effects where the body sees, thinks, and reacts as one whole unit much more quickly, thereby improving the overall output.
⑮	**Contrast sensitivity function (CSF)**	*The ability to process spatial and temporal objects, their movements, the surrounding background, and peripheral data indicates a high-functioning contrast sensitivity function (CSF) and is a precursor to movement discrimination and functional performance.* Contrast sensitivity refers to the ability to quickly and clearly identify objects in varying lighting conditions and against backgrounds of varying color. The ability to observe fast movements is an asset. Through vision, information is sent to the brain where an integrated three-dimensional process takes place and often-subconscious interpretation and action ensue.
⑯	**Hanging with secure upper body**	*Benefits of hanging exercises include increased latissimus dorsi and scapular stabilization, grip and forearm strength, and pelvic control.* Pelvic discipline is required during all sport performance. As such, the kinesthetic awareness associated with controlling the anterior and posterior tilt of the pelvis is important to the mechanical success of all hanging exercises with lower-body action. With the hands in a locked position above the head, the shoulders are forced to become major stabilizers as the body's weight pulls on the shoulder capsule. To maintain a strong and consistent position the scapula have to remain retracted and depressed throughout, forcing stability throughout the kinetic chain. At the same time, the latissimus muscles, one of the major crossbridges between the upper and lower body that connect under the armpit and into the lower back, also engage in a high-stability strategy to compliment the scapulae in creating full torso stability, allowing the action to occur appropriately and with less risk. Improving grip strength has many positive outcomes. The lowered need for high-threshold neural drive to the hand and forearm muscles creates room for bigger lifts, better tackles, and a higher transfer of force to and through your racket or bat. Additionally, improvements in grip strength have shown to have serious ramifications for elbow and rotator cuff strength due to the muscular attachments at the elbow and timing of muscular contractions between the hand and shoulder.
⑰	**External resistance**	*Adding external resistance to any exercise will make it more difficult because more force is required to move it, control it, or slow the resistance down.* Adaptation takes the form of strength, power, or proprioceptive development and is specific to the load imposed. Rubber bands around the knees, dumbbells in the hands, a stretching strap around the ankles, and suspended body weight are a few examples of integrated external resistance that require you to perform a prescribed movement pattern against a resistance while maintaining structural dynamic stabilization.

(continued)

18	Total-body complex	*The advantage of incorporating a total-body compound movement into a training regimen is that the entire spectrum of stabilization and mobilization is encompassed.* During these complexes the agonists, antagonists, and synergists work congruently to maintain dynamic postural control in conjunction with the accurate sequential firing and neural drive processes necessary for the efficient application of the prime movers. It is preferential to have command of the correct muscular sequencing and spinal stabilization to minimize detrimental spine forces before developing the mobilizers.
19	Slideboard	*The use of a slideboard will further challenge stabilization, strength, power, and proprioception.* When used properly and with attentiveness, a slideboard can produce spectacular results. Precision in the performance of a drill when using a slideboard will greatly enhance the functionally adaptive qualities of the movement. Throughout the book we demonstrate many drills and movement patterns that employ this piece of equipment. We encourage you to examine a particular drill of your liking and determine whether a slideboard will make that drill more challenging and thereby make the adaptive qualities more functionally worthwhile.
20	Implement acceleration	*Including acceleration in your power training allows for the addition of speed. Speed is a premium in all sports and should be trained accordingly.* Genetics and body type often are the final determiners of top-end speed; however, everyone can improve the ability to accelerate. If you can improve the early phases of the speed continuum, you will hold your own with the best of them. It is typically associated with phase 3, or the concentric phase, of a plyometric exercise. Acceleration is the rate of force development and the maintenance of that maximal force throughout the intended range of motion.
21	Implement deceleration	*Speed may be at a premium, but uncontrolled speed can lead to disastrous outcomes. Improving your brakes will allow for maximum output in the long run.* An often-overlooked yet critical athletic trait is the capacity to rapidly decrease velocity. The ability to precipitously alter speeds on command is a characteristic of exceptional agility. Should it become necessary to make a rapid change of direction or even to simply stop, you may never reach maximum speed primarily because of a perceived inability to control that speed. Many injuries, specifically ACL injuries, are the result of this inability to decelerate and safely. Deceleration is not limited to total-body displacement; it can also involve activities focusing on muscle-specific activities and actions that involve manipulation. Deceleration is also considered to be the eccentric phase, or phase 1, of the three phases of a plyometric exercise.
22	Stretch–shortening cycle and stored elastic energy	*Every attempt to minimize the time between your muscles' initial stretch and subsequent contraction affects explosiveness and agility.* The stretch–shortening cycle is simply the time between the eccentric (or decelerative) and concentric (accelerative) phases of a movement, technically referred to as the amortization phase. During the eccentric phase, energy is stored in the elastic properties of the muscle–tendon unit. During the concentric phase, this energy is released in an equal and opposite action. The process of elastic energy storage and the neural receptors' response is the stretch–shortening cycle. The ability to decrease the time during the amortization phase allows you to produce more power quickly and therefore create more explosive movements.
23	Gravity load	*The height of the drop (extent of gravity's influence) is an external force that challenges your adaptive and developmental qualities.* Gravity is resistance. As such, simply dropping off of an elevated platform generates velocity at 32.2 feet (9.8 m) per second. This, combined with absorbing your body weight, creates a force equaling 6 to 10 times your body weight. All of this energy must be efficiently transferred through the core. The ability to decelerate gravity's force and counter with a subsequent movement indicates efficient energy transfer such as that required to rapidly change direction.

| 24 | Multiplanar movement | *Multiplanar movements tend to be more complex and correlate well to circumstances frequently occurring in sport or daily activity. Drills that are multiplanar are considered more functional in nature than drills that are uniplanar.*

Dynamic planes of motion in the human body can be broken down into three flat-surface imaginary lines that divide the body in half:
1. Sagittal plane, also called the lateral plane, divides the body into halves from side to side. Movement specific to this plane typically involves flexion and extension.
2. Coronal plane, also called the frontal plane, divides the body into halves from front to back. Movement of any part of the body in this plane usually involves abduction and adduction of the extremities and side bends.
3. Transverse plane divides the body into top and bottom halves (superior and inferior).

You would be hard pressed to find a sport where movement occurs strictly in one plane. The obvious assertion is track running or sprinting (known as athletics in Europe). However, even though movement takes place in one plane, the other two planes are in a constant state of dynamic stabilization. Gone are the days of muscle isolation and uniplanar movements. Functional movements are always multijoint (involving more than one muscle group) and are, at the very least, biplanar if not triplanar actions. |

TRAINING GUIDELINES

Once you ascertain your starting level (see chapter 18 for core assessment tools), you must incorporate an appropriate training progression, maintain correct technique, and establish a frequent routine to gain the most benefits from the time and effort invested. To get the most benefit from the exercises in this book and to understand how to comfortably and safely progress them (after testing), follow these basic procedures:

1. Master the specific mechanics of each exercise before attempting heavier resistance or increasing the volume. *Never* sacrifice technique for added resistance or repetitions! If you deviate from precise technique, you will rehearse incorrect movement patterns, develop muscle imbalances (asymmetrical development of strength), or incur an injury. The only way to maximize your workout is to adhere to the drill descriptions.

2. Begin with light resistance and low-repetition training. Gradually build up to greater resistance or higher-repetition protocols. This book demonstrates a variety of exercises with progressively more difficult variations; ultimately it will be up to *you* to determine whether your technique allows for advancement.

3. Chapter 18 outlines how to determine where you are in a training continuum. It is also important in between retests to know how to advance yourselves with each exercise. In chapters 6-17, we instruct you to repeat each exercise for a predetermined number of repetitions or time interval. How do you know how to determine the appropriate number of repetitions or adequate time interval without the trained eye of a coach working with you? To simplify, you need a brief understanding of technical failure. When you are performing an exercise (for time or repetitions) and the form we've outlined for each of the exercises breaks down or changes and you are not performing the exercise with technical proficiency, you've reached technical failure. On the other side of the coin, if you have chosen a certain time frame or repetition number and you reach that limit without feeling slightly challenged to maintain that technical proficiency, then it is time to increase the number of repetitions, weight, or the amount of time.

4. Exercise often enough to create a significant effect. Initially, we recommend that you exercise four or five days per week for several months. Once you have achieved your goal—such as dynamic postural stabilization, improved athletic control, greater strength and power, elimination of low back pain—you can decrease the duration (number of repetitions per set) and the frequency of your training to as few as two sessions per week and still maintain your accomplishments. However, intensity of the training sessions should never wane. *Frequency* refers to how often you train the center of power, while *duration* refers to the length of a workout (measured by the number of sets and repetitions per session).

Intensity is the level of difficulty, which is determined by adding or subtracting resistance or varying the speed of the exercise. As you move closer to realizing individual goals, the training can shift to fewer workouts per week but intensity must never waver. If you decrease intensity, you will most certainly have a detraining effect. Dramatic accomplishments through months of hard work can be quickly lost with training cessation or simply decreased intensity. Sporadic exercise will never fully develop the core, nor will it enhance performance or decrease the incidence or severity of low back pain. Only if you make the commitment to a lifestyle of regular training will you reap its benefits. If the neuromuscular system is not fully functioning and continually challenged at a high intensity, you will be unable to respond to the extreme demands placed on it during high-level functional performance.

EQUIPMENT OPTIONS

Many of the drills we include in parts II through IV incorporate a slideboard or suspension or hanging apparatus. Here are some additional options to consider as you look to incorporate these apparatus into your training program.

Slideboard

Wear gloves and socks for all slideboard activities to minimize friction and assist with ease of sliding. Specially designed slideboard booties are an even better option; these are available from the UltraSlide Company at ultraslide.com. It is very important to only allow your body to slide into ranges of motion you can control. The nature of this piece of equipment is to dramatically lower the coefficient of friction, thereby increasing the body's ability to slide beyond normal ranges. This is clearly beneficial but must be done so with intelligence and control; if the ranges of motion are not controlled you can put your body in compromising positions that lead to injury.

Suspension Apparatus

As noted in specific benefit 6, suspension training will challenge your stability, strength, kinesthesis, and proprioception. For most of the suspension drills in this book, we use a suspension apparatus commonly known as a TRX, but there are other options available, including Blast Straps, Jungle Gym, gymnastics rings, or something similar.

The height of the handles and hand and foot placement determine load demand and exercise difficulty.

- As a general rule, for supine exercises in which pulling is involved, the higher the feet and the lower the shoulders, the more challenging the exercise. Therefore, with the feet on the floor, the joints aligned, and the body near perpendicular (to the floor), the exercise is relatively easy.

- With the feet elevated (on a box, bench, or platform) and the shoulders low to the floor, the exercise becomes quite difficult.

- Select a handle height and foot position that challenges your strength without compromising exercise mechanics.

- When performing exercises in either the prone or supine positions it is important to make sure your shoulders remain in a strong, neutral position throughout. No matter where the action or movement is, do not allow the shoulders to sublux. Instead, strive to maintain depression and retraction of the scapulae throughout each exercise.

- A great deal of your focus will be on your hands and shoulders during exercises with this piece of equipment, which is appropriate. However do not lose track of your hips and lower back. Compensating at the LPHC can be a problem when performing prone exercises where the hips sag to the floor or the lower back slips into extension. The same can be said for performing exercises where the feet are suspended and the focus shifts to controlling through the hips and creates poor awareness of shoulder positioning. Always be aware of your alignment checkpoints (ears, shoulders, hips, and ankles all in alignment) and do not sacrifice quality in one area due to hyperfocus on another.

Hanging Apparatus

We demonstrate many of the hanging exercises in the book with a chin-up bar or arm slings/straps, but as long as the apparatus is secure and meets the manufacturer's standards, then Jungle Gym handles with chains, gymnastics rings, a rope, or other similar hanging apparatus can also work. Sufficient strength, a spotter, and a padded floor are strongly recommended.

The following dynamics should be contemplated prior to integrating these exercises into a training regimen:

- **Underhand or overhand grip.** There is an ongoing debate as to whether an overhand or underhand grip is better. While specific musculature might be emphasized a bit more when using one method rather than another, they both have their advantages. Our advice is to incorporate both within a total training philosophy. Never in sport are there two identical situations. Defenders, temperature, fans, strategies, wind, and injuries are just a few situations that are continuously fluctuating. Therefore the athlete must likewise continuously adapt to this ever-changing assortment of uncontrollable scenarios. As such, why train within the realm of one specific circumstance when in actuality the athlete will face an infinite combination of circumstances?

- **Narrow or wide grip.** The grip width will vary among individuals, and both the narrow and wide grip have their advantages. However, one important consideration is shoulder and scapular stabilization. Avoid subluxation of the shoulder (extreme protraction). Do not let the body weight pull on the joint. Maintain a retracted scapulae as much as possible. Discontinue the drill if the athlete is unable to maintain this retracted position.

- **Straight arms or bent arms.** As with grip type and width, there are advantages and disadvantages to having straight or bent arms during a hanging drill. With the arms straight, the focus of spinal dynamic stabilization shifts noticeably; however, maintaining scapulae retraction and avoiding subluxation (especially when fatigued) can be difficult. A bent-arm hang (usually with an underhand grip) makes it easier to retract the shoulder blades; however, this positioning typically is less challenging from a stabilization perspective.

While equipment choices can greatly vary and limb placement, grip choice, and body positioning will change, one constant is stabilizing the scapula through retraction and depression as well as neutralizing the pelvis. It is important to avoid an extreme kyphotic lumbar curve as well as protracting or elevating the shoulder blades and putting them in a vulnerable position.

SAFETY CONSIDERATIONS

The exercises in this book range from passive to active to explosive. We identify the exercises that may be perilous if you're a novice fitness enthusiast. However, we cannot account for all body types, specific diseases, injuries, and mechanical deviations. Therefore, if you have concerns with this or any other new program, consult your physician, coach, trainer, or a qualified fitness instructor to determine if any of the drills you choose pose a risk to your specific situation and at which level you should begin your training. The assessments in the book will certainly help you determine the latter issue. If apprehension prevails, then undergo a comprehensive postural evaluation to determine if you have an underlying biomechanical issue in the kinetic chain or additional compensatory issue that might require attention before program implementation.

Many exercise enthusiasts seek that burning sensation when working the core. To achieve that effect, they do excessive repetitions. However, you should be left with only a tightening feeling after a core training session. Any discomfort beyond that indicates overtraining. The results you seek might be small and incremental, but they accumulate over time and should leave you with no true discomfort or delayed-onset muscle soreness.

Training can both build up and break down systems in the body; you must understand both processes to create the most effective program for you. A strongly recommended exercise might be appropriate for a high-level athlete, but the same exercise will be ill advised for novices. Therefore, before you get started on developing your center of power, note a few precautions.

- Receive clearance from your doctor before initiating any new program.
- Make sure equipment is regularly cleaned and disinfected, undamaged, and maintained to meet the manufacturer's standards.
  - Cables, bands, plates, medicine balls, and balance apparatus should be free of wear and pose no danger with repeated high-intensity use.
  - Before incorporating a stability ball, ensure that the ball is free of nicks, gouges, holes, rips, or anything that might further expand it and cause it to

burst. Likewise, keep the training area free of obstructions or debris that might cause the ball to rupture.

- Never use iron plates, dumbbells, kettlebells, and the like while on a stability ball. Additionally, never extend these unforgiving external loads overhead or over the face.

- Ensure the environment has adequate space and is free of potential hazards.

- Warm up before implementing any exercise program no matter how advanced you are.

- Always use a spotter during some of the more complex exercises and those that involve external resistance.

- Have a coach or trainer monitor mechanics and assess the performance of the tests.

- During all exercises, keep your breathing rhythmic and natural. Never hold your breath. Typically, you should exhale during the contraction, or lifting, phase and inhale during the relaxation, or lowering, phase. If possible, perform the exercises in front of a mirror. This provides immediate visual feedback, helping you to more quickly develop proper technique.

- Drills performed on a hard surface such as the floor or a plyometric box pose a slight, but nevertheless possible, risk to the joints, specifically the knees and elbows. A folded towel, exercise mat, or similar item will provide comfort and protection to the bony joints during the exercise.

- Use only solid walls when executing any of the medicine ball throwing exercises.

- The location of the load (resistance), whether it be your arms and hands, a medicine ball, or a kettlebell, will make a significant difference on the adaptive stress placed on the working musculature of the core and, ultimately, in the effectiveness of the exercise. The farther the resistance is located from the point of axis, the greater the demand on the abdominals. The point of axis varies, depending on the exercise, but it is generally located between the hip and the waist. If you are new to core training, you should start all your exercises with either no additional resistance or the added resistance as close to the axis point as possible. As your strength develops, progressively move the arms to more demanding positions. Never, however, compromise technique when determining the correct position for your arms or added load. This is especially important as fatigue sets in. It is usually at this point, when trying to squeeze out a few additional reps, that mechanical breakdown occurs. Pulling on the head and neck, hyperextending the low back, and throwing the legs into the lift will do little to train the intended musculature and will in fact interfere with correct technique leading to a potential injury. Do power exercises at the beginning of practice so that fatigue doesn't influence the neural response.

- Never train through an injury. Know the differences between discomfort, pain, and injury.

- If you are a novice, a less physically developed athlete, or an athlete coming off a back injury or if you have a history of back injury, avoid bilateral (double) straight-leg lifts, straight-leg sit-ups, Roman chair exercises, or any exercise that disproportionately arches the low back. The psoas muscles run from the upper legs through the pelvis and attach to the low back. When the legs are in a straight position, the psoas muscles are placed in high tension and pull on the low back. If you are free from back pain, try an experiment. Lie on the floor on your back with your legs extended. Slowly raise your legs off the floor a couple of inches and try to slide your hand under your low back. If there is a space between the floor and your low back, then your spine is in hyperextension and therefore subjected to potentially dangerous posterior intradisc compressive stress. Some might argue about the importance of training in dangerous positions that might be encountered during athletic performance. First, you cannot account for all scenarios that might place you at risk of injury. Second, there are hundreds of drills in this book and probably a thousand more that can safely and effectively provide a stimulus for development, so why pick one or two drills that might place your structural integrity at risk? Avoid compromising exercises altogether. There are plenty of ways to accomplish your goals safely.

CORE STABILIZATION TRAINING

Whether they are as impressive as the Empire State Building or as simple as a bungalow, all structures must begin with a solid foundation. The same is true of the human body. No matter what level of sport you are striving for, a conscious commitment toward developing your personal groundwork is critical. The architects of New York City knew better than to build their skyscrapers on soft, spongy ground. Likewise, you must not seek to build your athletic framework on an unstable foundation.

A SOLID CORE FOUNDATION

In referring to a solid core foundation, we are *not* simply talking about a great six-pack. In fact, we have both worked with countless athletes who have the outward appearance of a great set of abs. But when it comes to functionality, their core foundation is astonishingly unstable. The majority of the general population and, surprisingly, many elite-level athletes lack the necessary core integral stability to adequately perform daily tasks, let alone to take their athleticism to the next level without an increased risk of injury. As such, performance mediocrity becomes the accepted norm, and further development wanes. Core enhancement should be first and foremost when initiating the beginning phase of any training program.

Regrettably, when we think about stability and its relation to balance and performance, most of us immediately think *static* rather than dynamic. This could not be further from the functional truth. Yes, static balance is important, but very little strength is required to maintain the isometric contractions involved in low-level force application. In fact, the deep stabilizers rarely produce movement. However, from a performance-functionality perspective, balance is dynamic and requires a persistent, coordinated interaction of all core musculature, deep stabilizers, and outer mobilizers correspondingly.

As we have mentioned, adaptation to stress is specific to the stress imposed. In other words, to improve free-throw shooting, you shoot free throws. To improve vertical jumping, you do jumping drills. To improve your golf putt, you do not rake leaves. The central nervous system plays a critical role in establishing and maintaining dynamic postural control (stability). The development of greater levels of neuromuscular control provides the stability necessary to efficiently perform force reduction, force production, stabilization, and manipulative skills through the kinetic chain. Athletes who excel in these performance variables consistently maintain a reinforced concentration of dynamic postural stabilization.

BRACING THE CORE

Learning to brace your core is an important part of gaining stability. We stress this repeatedly in our descriptions of exercises and tests. The act of bracing is simply a conscious activation of the core musculature as described in chapter 2. To achieve this brace, set your abdominal area as if expecting to receive a blow to the midsection. At the same time, maintain effective posture and tighten your glutes, no matter what position your body is presently in. A strong brace is the first step on the road to high-level core functioning. As you gain proficiency, the conscious effort to brace becomes automatic as you instinctively maintain dynamic control of your core (figure 1).

Before you begin, you need to establish your neutral position through the application of the isolated and co-contraction exercises of the core muscles in chapter 5. Stand tall with your hands on your hips and contract the low-back musculature while simultaneously bracing the abdominals. Develop a feel for the muscles involved. There should be no noticeable movement of the pelvis either forward (anteriorly) or backward (posteriorly). If you look at yourself in a mirror, you should see the natural curves of the spine; but if you were to draw a straight line, the line should intersect your ear, shoulder, hip, knee, and ankle. This straight line should be natural, not forced.

Next, relax the abdominals just enough to allow tension from the low-back muscles to anteriorly tilt the pelvis (figure 2a). Feel how well you can control this action. Return to neutral with the aforementioned co-contraction. Now relax the low-back muscles, allowing the abdominals to pull at their inferior (low) attachment site, which will slowly tilt the pelvis posteriorly (figure 2b).

Understanding the function of the muscles involved is important from the standpoint of total trunk stabilization. You will initially have to make an effort to apply this newfound control to the exercises presented. As you become proficient, conscious effort will not be needed to maintain the neutral position.

GOALS OF STABILIZATION TRAINING

The benefits of the exercises described in parts III and IV of this book relate to the enhanced relevance of force and power production. The exercises presented in this part, however, were designed to promote basic trunk and torso stabilization. Stabilization exercises are intended to challenge your senses. You will begin to discriminate among subtle changes in your body's equilibrium, automatically adjusting to those changes in a conservative, yet effective, effort. Certainly, the goal of stability exercises is not to structurally develop the abdominals to generate greater force and power or to augment your emerging washboard abs. These exercises are a safe, effective way of reinforcing the elements of good posture through a wide range of movement.

In some exercises we make a relatively simple action more complex by incorporating a challenging modality, such as requiring the task be performed on a large stability ball. Here, rudimentary actions become dynamically multifaceted. This triggers your postural-maintenance musculature to continually work to maintain balance and provide a foundation of stability. Eventually, you will make these adjustments automatically, as your sensory mechanisms (proprioceptors) learn to maintain your equilibrium.

Generally speaking, all of the exercises that fall into the core stability phase will have controlled movement and no external resistance. The aim is to teach the body to support itself, eliminate extraneous movement, and improve force transfer.

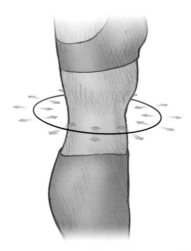

Figure 1 Bracing is a critical technique that needs to be mastered.

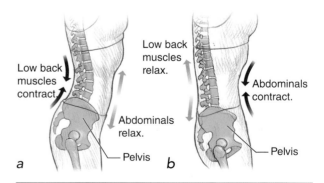

Figure 2 (a) Anterior pelvic tilt; (b) Posterior pelvic tilt.

Anti-Extension Exercises

A frequent mistake people make about stabilization is that effective athletic performance and, for the purposes of this book, successful performance of the core stability exercises, is predicated on absolutely no movement. A principal function of the central nervous system is not the selection of individual muscles but rather to optimize the use of integrated muscle interaction. It is this efficient integration that stabilization facilitates. No single muscle works in isolation to perform tasks such as osteoarticular maintenance and functional dynamic stabilization. Similarly, although the core is the focus of this book, elements of stabilization are realized throughout the entirety of the kinetic chain, from proximal to distal, deep stabilizers to outer mobilizers. Efficient functional movement,

high-intensity sport performance, compensation suppression, and many other benefits are derived from a stable spine. In this chapter we focus on stabilization from simple uniplanar bracing activities to increasing range of motion via multidirectional patterns and, finally, to progressively manipulating instability, load, frequency, duration, and intensity. A strong and stable core will improve neuromuscular efficiency throughout the kinetic chain and lay the groundwork for intensified sport performance and reduced injury risk.

The following exercise finder lists the benefits, difficulty level, and equipment needed for every exercise that appears in this chapter. Primary exercises are highlighted in beige with their progressions in blue. The primary exercises are also noted in the text with a blue title bar.

Anti-Extension Stability Exercise Finder

Exercise Name	Specific Benefits (see chapter 5)	Easy	Medium	Hard	Equipment
Elbow Plank	⑫	X	.		
Straight-Arm Plank	⑫	X			
Elbow Plank, Unstable Upper	❶ ⑫		X		Unstable apparatus*
Straight-Arm Plank, Unstable Upper	❶ ⑫		X		Unstable apparatus
Elbow Plank, Unstable Upper, Arms Elevated	❶ ❷ ⑫		X		Stability ball
Straight-Arm Plank, Unstable Upper, Arms Elevated	❶ ❷ ⑫		X		Stability ball
Elbow Plank, Feet Elevated	❸		X		Raised platform**
Straight-Arm Plank, Feet Elevated	❸ ⑫		X		Raised platform
Elbow Plank, Unstable Lower, Feet Elevated	❶ ❸		X		Stability ball or unstable apparatus on raised platform

* Many options are available for the unstable apparatus, including a thick foam pad, wobble board, balance disc, pillows, or stability ball.
** Many options are available for the raised platform, including a box, bench, stair, or step.

(continued)

Exercise Name	Specific Benefits (see chapter 5)	Difficulty Level Easy	Difficulty Level Medium	Difficulty Level Hard	Equipment
Straight-Arm Plank, Unstable Lower, Feet Elevated	❶ ❸ ⑫		X		Stability ball or unstable apparatus on raised platform
Elbow Plank, Unstable Upper and Lower	❶			X	Two unstable apparatus
Straight-Arm Plank, Unstable Upper and Lower	❶ ⑫			X	Two unstable apparatus
Elbow Plank, Single-Leg Hip Extension	❹	X			
Straight-Arm Plank, Single-Leg Hip Extension	❹ ⑫	X			
Elbow Plank, Single-Leg Hip Extension, Feet Elevated	❸ ❹		X		Raised platform
Straight-Arm Plank, Single-Leg Hip Extension, Feet Elevated	❸ ❹ ⑫		X		Raised platform
Elbow Plank, Unstable Upper, Single-Leg Hip Extension	❶ ❹		X		Unstable apparatus
Straight-Arm Plank, Unstable Upper, Single-Leg Hip Extension	❶ ❹ ⑫		X		Unstable apparatus
Elbow Plank, Unstable Upper, Single-Leg Hip Extension, Feet Elevated	❶ ❸ ❹		X		Unstable apparatus, raised platform
Straight-Arm Plank, Unstable Upper, Single-Leg Hip Extension, Feet Elevated	❶ ❸ ❹ ⑫		X		Unstable apparatus, raised platform
Elbow Plank, Unstable Upper, Single-Leg Hip Extension, Arms Elevated	❶ ❷ ❹		X		Stability ball
Straight-Arm Plank, Unstable Upper, Single-Leg Hip Extension, Arms Elevated	❶ ❷ ❹ ⑫		X		Stability ball
Elbow Plank, Single-Leg Hip Abduction	❺	X			
Straight-Arm Plank, Single-Leg Hip Abduction	❺ ⑫	X			
Elbow Plank, Single-Leg Hip Abduction, Feet Elevated	❸ ❺		X		Raised platform
Straight-Arm Plank, Single-Leg Hip Abduction, Feet Elevated	❸ ❺ ⑫		X		Raised platform
Elbow Plank, Unstable Upper, Single-Leg Hip Abduction	❶ ❺		X		Unstable apparatus
Straight-Arm Plank, Unstable Upper, Single-Leg Hip Abduction	❶ ❺ ⑫		X		Unstable apparatus
Elbow Plank, Unstable Upper, Single-Leg Hip Abduction, Feet Elevated	❶ ❸ ❺		X		Unstable apparatus, raised platform
Straight-Arm Plank, Unstable Upper, Single-Leg Hip Abduction, Feet Elevated	❶ ❸ ❺ ⑫		X		Unstable apparatus, raised platform
Elbow Plank, Unstable Upper, Single-Leg Hip Abduction, Arms Elevated	❶ ❷ ❺		X		Stability ball
Straight-Arm Plank, Unstable Upper, Single-Leg Hip Abduction, Arms Elevated	❶ ❷ ❺ ⑫		X		Stability ball
Straight-Arm Plank, Suspended Upper	❻ ⑫		X		Suspension trainer
Straight-Arm Plank, Suspended Upper, Feet Elevated	❸ ❻ ⑫			X	Suspension trainer, raised platform

Exercise Name	Specific Benefits (see chapter 5)	Difficulty Level			Equipment
		Easy	Medium	Hard	
Straight-Arm Plank, Suspended Upper, Single-Leg Hip Extension	4 6 12			X	Suspension trainer
Straight-Arm Plank, Suspended Upper, Single-Leg Hip Extension, Feet Elevated	3 4 6 12			X	Suspension trainer, raised platform
Straight- Arm Plank, Suspended Upper, Single-Leg Hip Abduction	5 6 12			X	Suspension trainer
Straight-Arm Plank, Suspended Upper, Single-Leg Hip Abduction, Feet Elevated	3 5 6 12			X	Suspension trainer, raised platform
Elbow Plank, Leg Abduction and Adduction	5		X		
Straight-Arm Plank, Leg Abduction and Adduction	5 12		X		
Elbow Plank, Stationary Walk Out and Back	7		X		
Straight-Arm Plank, Stationary Walk Out and Back	7 12		X		
Elbow to Straight-Arm Plank, Box Walk Up	2 7		X		Raised platform
Straight-Arm Plank, Box Walk Up	2 7 12		X		Raised platform
Straight-Arm Plank, Ball Walk Up	1 2 7 12		X		Medicine ball
Elbow Plank, Unstable Lower, Walk Out and Back	1 7			X	Unstable apparatus
Straight-Arm Plank, Unstable Lower, Walk Out and Back	1 7 12			X	Unstable apparatus
Straight-Arm Plank, Suspended Lower, Walk Out and Back	3 6 7 12			X	Suspension trainer
Elbow Plank, Full-Body Walk	7		X		
Straight-Arm Plank, Full-Body Walk	7 12		X		
Elbow Plank, Stability Ball Circle Walk	1 2 5 7		X		Stability ball
Straight-Arm Plank, Stability Ball Circle Walk	1 2 5 7 12		X		Stability ball
Mountain Climber	8 12	X			
Mountain Climber, Incline	2 8 12	X			Raised platform
Mountain Climber, Unstable Upper	1 8 12		X		Unstable apparatus
Mountain Climber, Suspended Upper	2 6 8 12			X	Suspension trainer
Mountain Climber, Suspended Lower	3 6 8 12			X	Suspension trainer
Mountain Climber, Unstable Lower, Feet Elevated, Double Knee Tuck	1 3 8 12		X		Stability ball
Mountain Climber, Unstable Lower, Feet Elevated, Single Knee Tuck	1 3 8 9 12			X	Stability ball
Mountain Climber, Suspended Lower, Abduction and Adduction, Double Knee Tuck	3 5 6 12			X	Suspension trainer
Mountain Climber, Suspended Upper, Unstable Lower, Double Knee Tuck	1 3 6 12			X	Suspension trainer, stability ball

51

ELBOW PLANK

MOVEMENTS

1. Lie face down on the floor in a prone position with the feet together.
2. Place upper-body weight on the forearms; dorsiflex the feet and toes toward the shins.
3. Lock the knees, tighten the glutes, and brace the core.
4. Lift the body so the only contact points are the balls of the feet, toes, elbows, and forearms on the floor.
5. Maintain a completely straight line in the body with the ears, shoulders, hips, knees, and ankles in alignment. Hold this position of a predetermined amount of time.

CONSIDERATIONS

1. Do not sag the hips (pelvis should not drop toward the floor).
2. Do not pike the hips (pelvis and butt should not arch toward the ceiling).
3. Keep the chin pushed back (think double chin) and avoid dropping the head (cervical vertebrae are straight, with the head tilted neither forward or back).

SPECIFIC BENEFITS

12

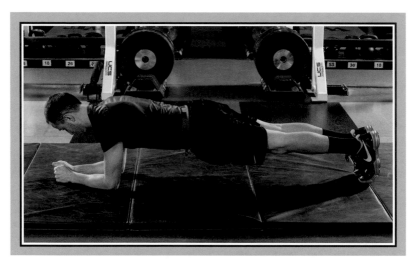

■ STRAIGHT-ARM PLANK ■

Modifications

1. Position the hands on the floor directly under the shoulders with the arms perpendicular to the floor.

2. Lift the body so the only contact points are the balls of the feet, toes, and hands on the floor.

Specific Benefits **12**

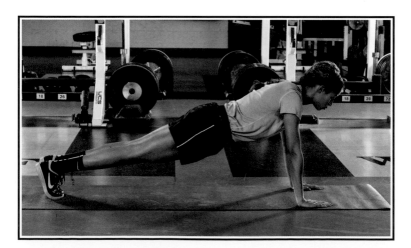

■ ELBOW PLANK ■
UNSTABLE UPPER

Modifications

1. Place the elbows and forearms on a moderately unstable apparatus (thick foam pad, wobble board, balance disc, pillows, etc.).
2. Lift the body so the only contact points are the balls of the feet and toes on the floor and the elbows and forearms on the unstable apparatus.

Specific Benefits

■ STRAIGHT-ARM PLANK ■
UNSTABLE UPPER

Modifications

1. Straighten the arms with the hands on a moderately unstable apparatus (thick foam pad, wobble board, balance disc, pillows, etc.). Position the hands directly under the shoulders with the arms perpendicular to the floor.
2. Lift the body so the only contact points are the balls of the feet and toes on the floor and the hands on the unstable apparatus.

Specific Benefits

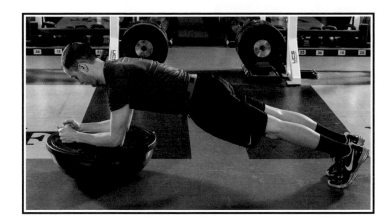

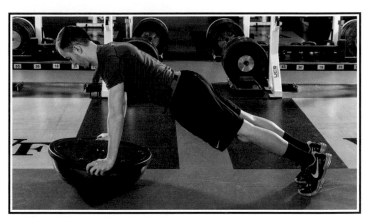

■ ELBOW PLANK ■
UNSTABLE UPPER, ARMS ELEVATED

Modifications

1. Position the elbows and forearms on a stability ball.

2. Lift the body so the only contact points are the balls of the feet and toes on the floor and the elbows and forearms on the stability ball.

Specific Benefits

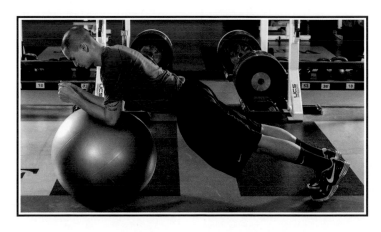

■ STRAIGHT-ARM PLANK ■
UNSTABLE UPPER, ARMS ELEVATED

Modifications

1. Straighten the arms with the hands on a stability ball. Position the hands under the shoulders with the arms perpendicular to the floor (the size of the ball dictates the degree of perpendicularity).
2. Lift the body so the only contact points are the balls of the feet and toes on the floor and the hands on the stability ball.

Specific Benefits

Note Try different hand positions for additional control or difficulty. For example, point the fingers forward for greater difficulty, or point the fingers lateral toward the floor for greater control. Always be mindful of joint stability and control; never place a joint or body part in a compromised position (which is unique to the individual) that might lead to injury.

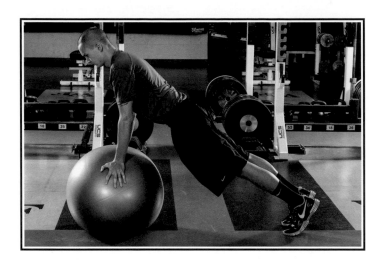

■ ELBOW PLANK ■
FEET ELEVATED

Modifications

1. Place the feet on a raised platform (box, bench, or stair).
2. Lift the body so the only contact points are the elbows and forearms on the floor and the balls of the feet and toes on the platform.

Specific Benefits ❸

■ STRAIGHT-ARM PLANK ■
FEET ELEVATED

Modifications

1. Place the feet on a raised platform (box, bench, or stair).
2. Straighten the arms with the hands on the floor. Position the hands directly the under shoulders with the arms perpendicular to the floor.
3. Lift the body so the only contact points are the hands on the floor and the balls of the feet and toes on the platform.

Specific Benefits ❸ ⑫

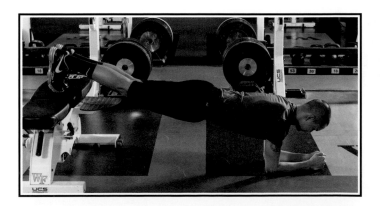

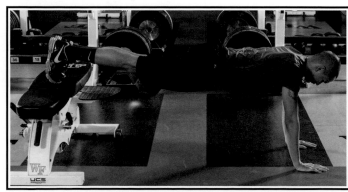

▪ ELBOW PLANK ▪
UNSTABLE LOWER, FEET ELEVATED

Modifications

1. Place the feet on a stability ball or a moderately unstable apparatus positioned on a raised platform. Note: Make sure that the unstable apparatus is relatively secure on the raised platform.
2. With the elbows and forearms on the floor, lift the body so some part of the lower body is in contact with the unstable apparatus.

Specific Benefits

Note There are many kinds of unstable apparatus. As an example, if using a stability ball, the difficulty progression might look something like this:

1. Knees on ball
2. Ankles on ball
3. Balls of feet and toes on ball

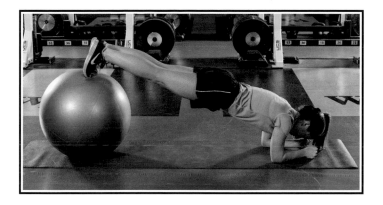

▪ STRAIGHT-ARM PLANK ▪
UNSTABLE LOWER, FEET ELEVATED

Modifications

1. Place the feet on a stability ball or moderately unstable apparatus positioned on a raised platform. Note: Make sure that the unstable apparatus is relatively secure on the raised platform.
2. Straighten the arms with the hands on the floor. Position the hands directly under the shoulders with the arms perpendicular to the floor.
3. With the hands on the floor, lift the body so some part of the lower body is in contact with the unstable apparatus.

Specific Benefits

Note See a sample difficulty progression in the previous exercise.

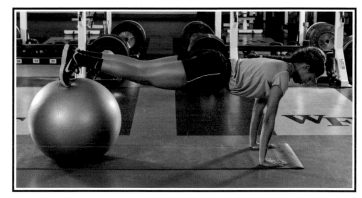

▪ ELBOW PLANK ▪
UNSTABLE UPPER AND LOWER

Modifications

1. Carefully place the forearms on a moderately unstable apparatus.
2. Place the feet on another moderately unstable apparatus (it does not have to be the same type of moderately unstable apparatus used for the upper body).

3. Lift the body so all contact points (balls of the feet, toes, elbows, forearms) are on the unstable apparatus.

Specific Benefits

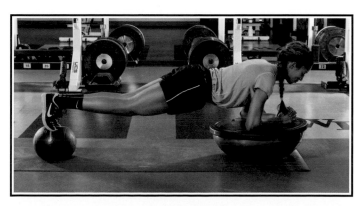

■ STRAIGHT-ARM PLANK ■
UNSTABLE UPPER AND LOWER

Modifications

1. Carefully place the hands on a moderately unstable apparatus.
2. Place the feet on another moderately unstable apparatus (it does not have to be the same type of moderately unstable apparatus used for the upper body).
3. Lift the body so all contact points (balls of the feet, toes, hands) are on the unstable apparatus.

Specific Benefits

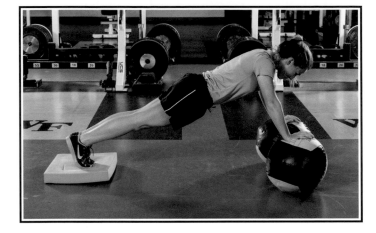

■ ELBOW PLANK ■
SINGLE-LEG HIP EXTENSION

Modifications

1. With the elbows and forearms on the floor, lift the body so only the ball of one foot and that foot's toes contact the floor.
2. Engage the glutes and extend the hip to raise the opposite straight leg off the floor.
3. Avoid extension of the lumbar spine.

Specific Benefits

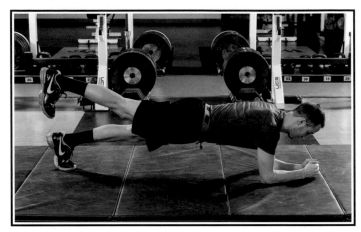

■ STRAIGHT-ARM PLANK ■
SINGLE-LEG HIP EXTENSION

Modifications

1. Position the hands on the floor directly under the shoulders with the arms straight and perpendicular to the floor.
2. With the hands on the floor, lift the body so only the ball of one foot and that foot's toes contact the floor.

3. Engage the glutes and extend the hip to raise the opposite straight leg off the floor.
4. Avoid extension of the lumbar spine.

Specific Benefits

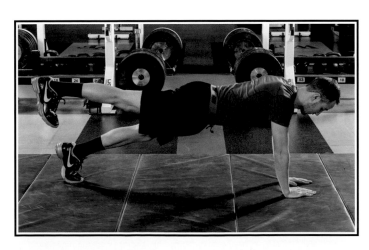

■ ELBOW PLANK ■
SINGLE-LEG HIP EXTENSION, FEET ELEVATED

Modifications

1. Place one foot on a raised platform.
2. Lift the body so the only contact points are the elbows and forearms on the floor and the ball of one foot and that foot's toes on the raised platform.
3. Engage the glutes and extend the hip to raise the opposite straight leg off the floor.
4. Avoid extension of the lumbar spine.

Specific Benefits

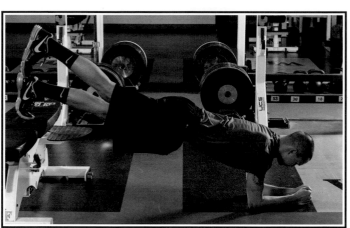

■ STRAIGHT-ARM PLANK ■
SINGLE-LEG HIP EXTENSION, FEET ELEVATED

Modifications

1. Place one foot on a raised platform. Arms are straight and perpendicular to the floor.
2. Lift the body so the only contact points are the hands on the floor and the ball of one foot and that foot's toes on the raised platform.
3. Engage the glutes and extend the hip to raise the opposite straight leg off the floor.
4. Avoid extension of the lumbar spine.

Specific Benefits

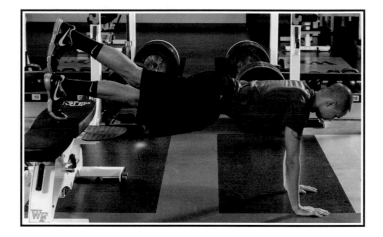

■ ELBOW PLANK ■
UNSTABLE UPPER, SINGLE-LEG HIP EXTENSION

Modifications

1. With the elbows and forearms on a moderately unstable apparatus, lift the body so only the ball of one foot and that foot's toes contact the floor.

2. Engage the glutes and extend the hip to raise the opposite straight leg off the floor.
3. Avoid extension of the lumbar spine.

Specific Benefits

■ STRAIGHT-ARM PLANK ■
UNSTABLE UPPER, SINGLE-LEG HIP EXTENSION

Modifications

1. Position the hands on a moderately unstable apparatus. The hands are directly under the shoulders with the arms perpendicular to the floor.
2. Lift the body so the only contact points are the hands on the moderately unstable apparatus and the ball of one foot and that foot's toes on the floor.
3. Engage the glutes and extend the hip to raise the opposite straight leg off the floor.
4. Avoid extension of the lumbar spine.

Specific Benefits

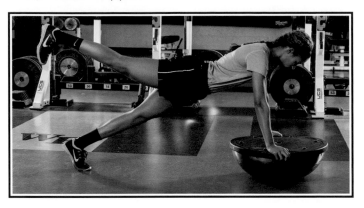

■ ELBOW PLANK ■
UNSTABLE UPPER, SINGLE-LEG HIP EXTENSION, FEET ELEVATED

Modifications

1. Place the elbows and forearms on a moderately unstable apparatus. Place one foot on a raised platform.
2. Lift the body so the only contact points are the forearms and elbows on the moderately unstable apparatus and the ball of one foot and that foot's toes on the raised platform.
3. Engage the glutes and extend the hip to raise the opposite straight leg off the floor.
4. Avoid extension of the lumbar spine.

Specific Benefits

■ STRAIGHT-ARM PLANK ■
UNSTABLE UPPER, SINGLE-LEG HIP EXTENSION, FEET ELEVATED

Modifications

1. Position the hands on a moderately unstable apparatus. The hands are positioned directly under the shoulders with the arms perpendicular to the floor. Place one foot on a raised platform.
2. Lift the body so the only contact points are the hands on the moderately unstable apparatus and the ball of one foot and that foot's toes on the raised platform.
3. Engage the glutes and extend the hip to raise the opposite straight leg off the floor.
4. Avoid extension of the lumbar spine.

Specific Benefits

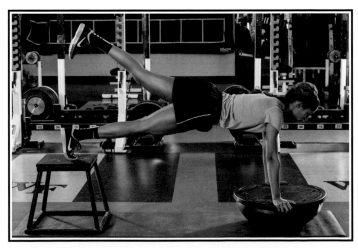

■ ELBOW PLANK ■
UNSTABLE UPPER, SINGLE-LEG HIP EHTENSION, ARMS ELEUATED

Modifications

1. Position the elbows and forearms on a stability ball.
2. Lift the body so the only contact points are the elbows and forearms on the stability ball and the ball of one foot and that foot's toes on the floor.

3. Engage the glutes and extend the hip to raise the opposite straight leg off the floor.
4. Avoid extension of the lumbar spine.

Specific Benefits   ❹

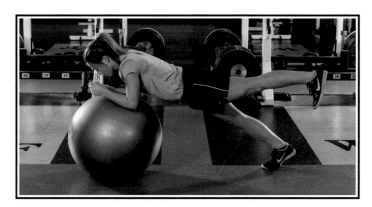

■ STRAIGHT-ARM PLANK ■
UNSTABLE UPPER, SINGLE-LEG HIP EHTENSION, ARMS ELEUATED

Modifications

1. Straighten the arms with the hands on a stability ball. Position the hands under the shoulders with the arms perpendicular to the floor (the size of the ball dictates the degree of perpendicularity).
2. Lift the body so the only contact points are the hands on the stability ball and the ball of one foot and that foot's toes on the floor.
3. Engage the glutes and extend the hip to raise the opposite straight leg off the floor.
4. Avoid extension of the lumbar spine.

Specific Benefits   ⑫

Note Try different hand positions for additional control or difficulty. For example, point the fingers forward for greater difficulty, or point the fingers lateral toward the floor for greater control. Always be mindful of joint stability and control; never place a joint or body part in a compromised position (which is unique to the individual) that might lead to injury.

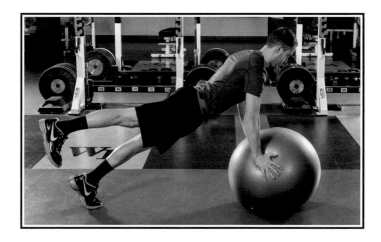

▪ ELBOW PLANK ▪
SINGLE-LEG HIP ABDUCTION

Modifications

1. With the elbows and forearms on the floor, lift the body so only the ball of one foot and that foot's toes contact the floor.

2. Engage the hip abductors of the opposite leg and move the straight leg laterally (within the frontal plane).

3. Avoid the tendency to rotate in opposition of the abducted leg. Maintain level hips and a straight line in the body.

Specific Benefits **5**

▪ STRAIGHT-ARM PLANK ▪
SINGLE-LEG HIP ABDUCTION

Modifications

1. Position the hands on the floor directly under shoulders with the arms straight and perpendicular to the floor.

2. With the hands on the floor, lift the body so only the ball of one foot and that foot's toes contact the floor.

3. Engage the hip abductors of the opposite leg and move the straight leg laterally (within the frontal plane).

4. Avoid the tendency to rotate in opposition of the abducted leg. Maintain level hips and a straight line in the body.

Specific Benefits **5** **12**

▪ ELBOW PLANK ▪
SINGLE-LEG HIP ABDUCTION, FEET ELEVATED

Modifications

1. Place one foot on a raised platform.

2. With the elbows and forearms on the floor, lift the body so only the ball of one foot and that foot's toes contact the raised platform.

3. Engage the hip abductors of the opposite leg and move the straight leg laterally (within the frontal plane).

4. Avoid the tendency to rotate in opposition of the abducted leg. Maintain level hips and a straight line in the body.

Specific Benefits **3** **5**

▪ STRAIGHT-ARM PLANK ▪
SINGLE-LEG HIP ABDUCTION, FEET ELEVATED

Modifications

1. Place one foot on a raised platform. Arms are straight and perpendicular to the floor.

2. Lift the body so the only contact points are the hands on the floor and the ball of one foot and that foot's toes on the raised platform.

3. Engage the hip abductors of the opposite leg and move the straight leg laterally (within the frontal plane).

4. Avoid the tendency to rotate in opposition of the abducted leg. Maintain level hips and a straight line in the body.

Specific Benefits **3** **5** **12**

▪ ELBOW PLANK ▪
UNSTABLE UPPER, SINGLE-LEG HIP ABDUCTION

Modifications

1. Place the elbows and forearms on a moderately unstable apparatus.
2. Lift the body so only the ball of one foot and that foot's toes contact the floor.
3. Engage the hip abductors of the opposite leg and move the straight leg laterally (within the frontal plane).
4. Avoid the tendency to rotate in opposition of the abducted leg. Maintain level hips and a straight line in the body.

Specific Benefits ❶ ❺

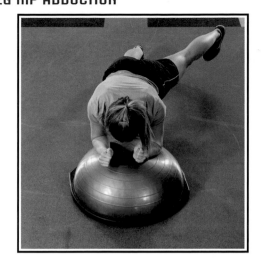

▪ STRAIGHT-ARM PLANK ▪
UNSTABLE UPPER, SINGLE-LEG HIP ABDUCTION

Modifications

1. Straighten the arms with the hands on a moderately unstable apparatus. Position the hands directly under the shoulders with the arms perpendicular to the floor.
2. Lift the body so only the ball of one foot and that foot's toes contact the floor.
3. Engage the hip abductors of the opposite leg and move the straight leg laterally (within the frontal plane).
4. Avoid the tendency to rotate in opposition of the abducted leg. Maintain level hips and a straight line in the body.

Specific Benefits ❶ ❺ ⓬

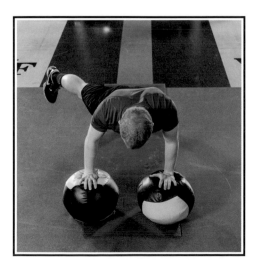

▪ ELBOW PLANK ▪
UNSTABLE UPPER, SINGLE-LEG HIP ABDUCTION, FEET ELEVATED

Modifications

1. Place one foot on a raised platform.
2. Place the elbows and forearms on a moderately unstable apparatus.
3. Lift the body so only the ball of one foot and that foot's toes contact the raised platform.
4. Engage the hip abductors of the opposite leg and move the straight leg laterally (within the frontal plane).
5. Avoid the tendency to rotate in opposition of the abducted leg. Maintain level hips and a straight line in the body.

Specific Benefits ❶ ❸ ❺

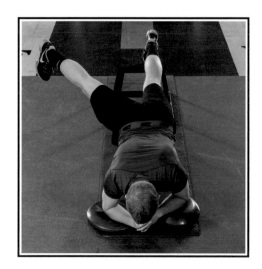

■ STRAIGHT-ARM PLANK ■
UNSTABLE UPPER, SINGLE-LEG HIP ABDUCTION, FEET ELEVATED

Modifications

1. Place one foot on a raised platform.
2. Straighten the arms with the hands on a moderately unstable apparatus.
3. Lift the body so only the ball of one foot and that foot's toes contact the raised platform.
4. Engage the hip abductors of the opposite leg and move the straight leg laterally (within the frontal plane).
5. Avoid the tendency to rotate in opposition of the abducted leg. Maintain level hips and a straight line in the body.

Specific Benefits ❶ ❸ ❺ ⓬

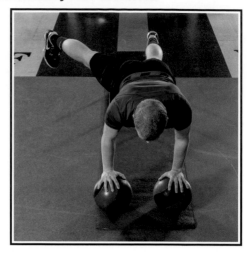

■ ELBOW PLANK ■
UNSTABLE UPPER, SINGLE-LEG HIP ABDUCTION, ARMS ELEVATED

Modifications

1. Position the elbows and forearms on a stability ball.
2. Lift the body so the only contact points are the elbows and forearms on the stability ball and the ball of one foot and that foot's toes on the floor.
3. Engage the hip abductors of the opposite leg and move the straight leg laterally (within the frontal plane).
4. Avoid the tendency to rotate in opposition of the abducted leg. Maintain level hips and a straight line in the body.

Specific Benefits ❶ ❷ ❺

■ STRAIGHT-ARM PLANK ■
UNSTABLE UPPER, SINGLE-LEG HIP ABDUCTION, ARMS ELEVATED

Modifications

1. Straighten the arms with the hands on a stability ball. Position the hands under the shoulders with the arms perpendicular to the floor (the size of the ball dictates the degree of perpendicularity).
2. Lift the body so the only contact points are the hands on the stability ball and the ball of one foot and that foot's toes on the floor.
3. Engage the hip abductors of the opposite leg and move the straight leg laterally (within the frontal plane).
4. Avoid the tendency to rotate in opposition of the abducted leg. Maintain level hips and a straight line in the body.

Specific Benefits ❶ ❷ ❺ ⓬

Note Try different hand positions for additional control or difficulty. For example, point the fingers forward for greater difficulty, or point the fingers lateral toward the floor for greater control. Always be mindful of joint stability and control; never place a joint or body part in a compromised position (which is unique to the individual) that might lead to injury.

The suspension exercises on the following pages will employ an apparatus commercially known as a TRX, Blast Straps, or something similar. As long as the apparatus is secure and meets the manufacturer's standards, then Jungle Gym handles with chains, gymnastics rings, or some other similar suspension apparatus can also work. Sufficient strength, a spotter, and a padded floor are always strongly recommended. For all of the following suspended drills, the height of the handles and the degree of foot elevation determine load demand and, ultimately, exercise difficulty.

■ STRAIGHT-ARM PLANK ■
SUSPENDED UPPER

Modifications

1. Place the hands in the grips (or straps). Arms are straight with fairly rigid elbows.
2. Assume a straight body alignment (ears, shoulders, hips, knees, and ankles are in a straight line, with no arching or sagging of the midsection). Only the balls of the feet and toes contact the floor.

Specific Benefits ⑫

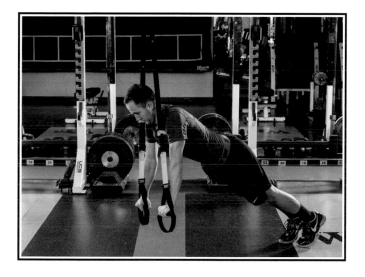

■ STRAIGHT-ARM PLANK ■
SUSPENDED UPPER, FEET ELEVATED

Modifications

1. Place the hands in the grips (or straps). Arms are straight with fairly rigid elbows.
2. Once the hands are in the grips, carefully position one foot on a raised platform, followed by the opposite foot.
3. Assume a straight body alignment (ears, shoulders, hips, knees, and ankles are in a straight line, with no arching or sagging of the midsection). Only the balls of the feet and toes contact the raised platform.

Specific Benefits ③ ⑥ ⑫

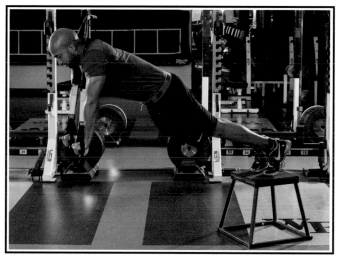

■ STRAIGHT-ARM PLANK ■
SUSPENDED UPPER, SINGLE-LEG HIP EXTENSION

Modifications

1. Place the hands in the grips (or straps). Arms are straight with fairly rigid elbows.

2. Assume a straight body alignment (ears, shoulders, hips, knees, and ankles are in a straight line, with no arching or sagging of the midsection). Only the ball of one foot and that foot's toes contact the floor.

3. Engage the glutes and extend the hip. Raise the opposite straight leg off the floor.

4. Avoid extension of the lumbar spine.

Specific Benefits

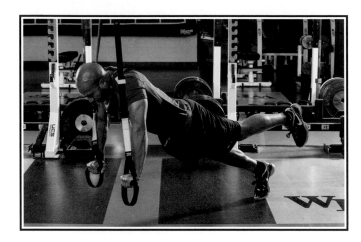

■ STRAIGHT-ARM PLANK ■
SUSPENDED UPPER, SINGLE-LEG HIP EXTENSION, FEET ELEVATED

Modifications

1. Place the hands in the grips (or straps). Arms are straight with fairly rigid elbows.

2. Once the hands are in the grips, carefully position one foot on a raised platform, followed by the opposite foot.

3. Assume a straight body alignment (ears, shoulders, hips, knees, and ankles are in a straight line, with no arching or sagging of the midsection). Only the balls of the feet and toes contact the raised platform.

4. Engage the glutes and extend the hip. Raise the opposite straight leg off the floor. Only the ball of one foot and that foot's toes remain in contact with the raised platform.

5. Avoid extension of the lumbar spine.

Specific Benefits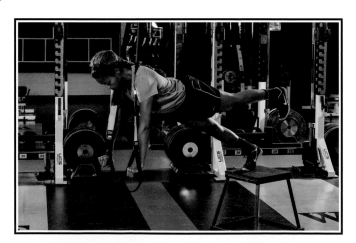

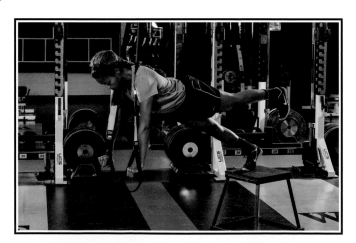

■ STRAIGHT-ARM PLANK ■
SUSPENDED UPPER, SINGLE-LEG HIP ABDUCTION

Modifications

1. Place the hands in the grips (or straps). Arms are straight with fairly rigid elbows.
2. Assume a straight body alignment (ears, shoulders, hips, knees, and ankles are in a straight line, with no arching or sagging of the midsection). Only the ball of one foot and that foot's toes contact the floor.
3. Engage the hip abductors of the opposite leg and move the straight leg laterally (within the frontal plane).
4. Avoid the tendency to rotate in opposition of the abducted leg. Maintain level hips and a straight line in the body.

Specific Benefits **5** **6** **12**

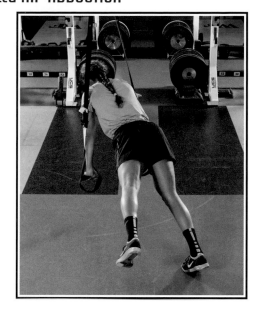

■ STRAIGHT-ARM PLANK ■
SUSPENDED UPPER, SINGLE-LEG HIP ABDUCTION, FEET ELEVATED

Modifications

1. Place the hands in the grips (or straps). Arms are straight with fairly rigid elbows.
2. Once the hands are in the grips, carefully position one foot on a raised platform, followed by the opposite foot.
3. Assume a straight body alignment (ears, shoulders, hips, knees, and ankles are in a straight line, with no arching or sagging of the midsection). Only the balls of the feet and toes contact the raised platform.
4. Engage the hip abductors of the opposite leg and move the straight leg laterally (within the frontal plane). Only the ball of one foot and that foot's toes remain in contact with the raised platform.
5. Avoid the tendency to rotate in opposition of the abducted leg. Maintain level hips and a straight line in the body.

Specific Benefits **3** **5** **6** **12**

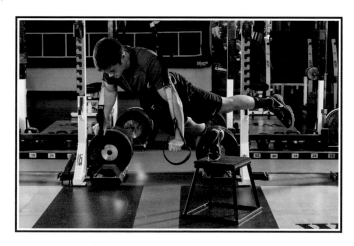

■ ELBOW PLANK ■
LEG ABDUCTION AND ADDUCTION

Modifications

1. Position the elbows and forearms on the floor.
2. Lift the body so only the balls of the feet, toes, elbows, and forearms are in contact with the floor.
3. Engage the hip abductors and move the straight left leg laterally (within the frontal plane). Avoid the tendency to rotate in opposition of the abducted left leg. Maintain level hips and a straight line in the body.

4. Return to neutral and place the left foot on the floor.
5. Immediately abduct the straight right leg and repeat steps 3 and 4.

Specific Benefits

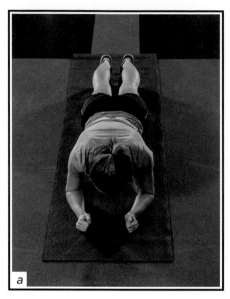 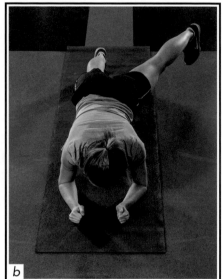

■ STRAIGHT-ARM PLANK ■
LEG ABDUCTION AND ADDUCTION

Modifications

1. Position the hands on the floor directly under the shoulders with the arms straight and perpendicular to the floor.
2. Lift the body so only the balls of the feet, toes, and hands are in contact with the floor.
3. Engage the hip abductors and move the straight left leg laterally (within the frontal plane). Avoid the tendency to rotate in opposition of the abducted left leg. Maintain level hips and a straight line in the body.

4. Return to neutral and place the left foot on the floor.
5. Immediately abduct the straight right leg and repeat steps 3 and 4.

Specific Benefits

STATIONARY WALK OUT AND BACK

MOVEMENTS

1. Lie face down in a prone position with the feet together.
2. Place upper-body weight on the forearms; dorsiflex the feet and toes toward the shins.
3. Lock the knees, tighten the glutes, and brace the core.
4. Lift the body so only the balls of the feet, toes, elbows, and forearms contact the floor.
5. Maintain a completely straight line in the body (ears, shoulders, hips, knees, and ankles are in alignment).
6. "Walk" forward and backward while maintaining the plank position. Move the right arm forward, left arm forward, right arm backward, and left arm backward.

CONSIDERATIONS

1. Do not sag the hips (pelvis should not drop toward the floor).
2. Do not pike the hips (pelvis and buttocks should not arch toward ceiling).
3. Keep the chin pushed back (think double chin) and avoid dropping the head (cervical vertebrae are straight, with the head tilted neither forward or back).

SPECIFIC BENEFITS

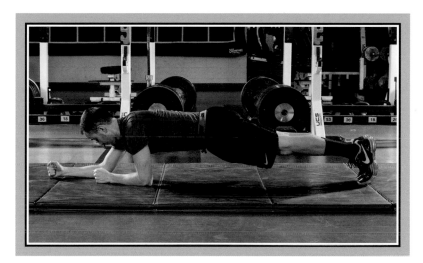

▪ STRAIGHT-ARM PLANK ▪
STATIONARY WALK OUT AND BACK

Modifications

1. Position the hands on the floor directly under the shoulders with the arms straight and perpendicular to the floor.
2. Lift the body so only the balls of the feet, toes, and hands are in contact with the floor.

3. "Walk" forward and backward while maintaining the plank position. Move the right hand forward, left hand forward, right hand backward, and left hand backward.

Specific Benefits

Modifications

1. The forearms are on the floor directly in front of a 6- to 18-inch (15-45 cm) box.

2. Extend the arms one at a time until in a straight-arm plank position.

3. Do not let the hips roll or sag during arm extension.

4. "Step" up onto the box (right arm up, then left arm up) to a straight-arm plank position with both hands on the box.

5. Return to the start position by reversing the action (right arm down, then left arm down).

6. Flex elbows one at a time to return to the elbow plank start position.

Specific Benefits ❷ ❼

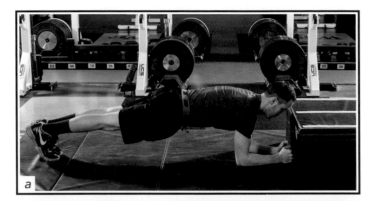

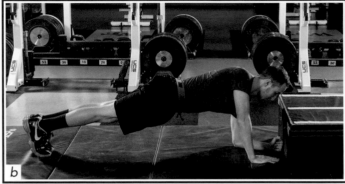

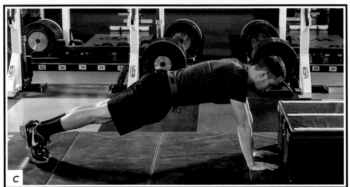

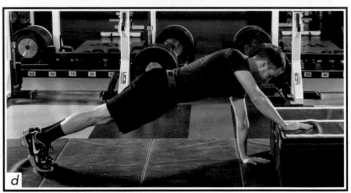

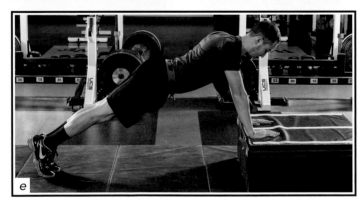

▪ STRAIGHT-ARM PLANK ▪
BOX WALK UP

Modifications

1. Position the hands on the floor directly under the shoulders and in front of a 6- to 18-inch (15-45 cm) box. Arms are perpendicular to the floor.
2. Lift the body so only the balls of the feet, toes, and hands are on the floor.
3. "Step" up onto a box (right arm up, then left arm up).
4. Return to the straight-arm plank start position by reversing the action (right arm down, then left arm down).

Specific Benefits

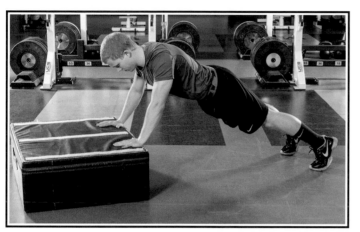

▪ STRAIGHT-ARM PLANK ▪
BALL WALK UP

Modifications

1. Position the hands on the floor directly under the shoulders and in front of a medicine ball, sand ball, basketball, volleyball, or other ball. Arms are perpendicular to the floor.
2. Lift the body so only the balls of the feet, toes, and hands contact the floor.
3. "Step" up onto the ball (right arm up, then left arm up).
4. Return to the straight-arm plank start position by reversing the action (right arm down, then left arm down).

Specific Benefits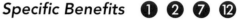

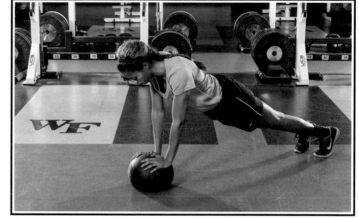

▪ ELBOW PLANK ▪
UNSTABLE LOWER, WALK OUT AND BACK

Modifications

1. Place the feet on a moderately unstable apparatus.
2. With elbows and forearms on the floor, lift the body so only the balls of the feet and toes contact the unstable apparatus. Maintain a completely straight line in the body (ears, shoulders, hips, knees, and ankles remain in alignment).

3. "Walk" forward and backward while maintaining the plank position:
   a. Move right hand forward, left hand forward, right hand backward, left hand backward.
   b. Alternate sets: Move left hand forward, right hand forward, left hand backward, right hand backward.

Specific Benefits

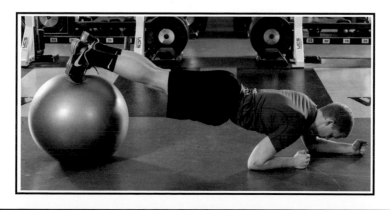

▪ STRAIGHT-ARM PLANK ▪
UNSTABLE LOWER, WALK OUT AND BACK

Modifications

1. Position the hands on the floor directly under the shoulders with the arms straight and perpendicular to the floor.
2. Place the feet on a moderately unstable apparatus.
3. With the hands on the floor, lift the body so only the balls of the feet and toes contact the unstable apparatus. Maintain a completely straight line in the body (ears, shoulders, hips, knees, and ankles remain in alignment).

4. "Walk" forward and backward while maintaining the plank position:
   a. Move right hand forward, left hand forward, right hand backward, left hand backward.
   b. Alternate sets: Move left hand forward, right hand forward, left hand backward, right hand backward.

Specific Benefits

▪ STRAIGHT-ARM PLANK ▪
SUSPENDED LOWER, WALK OUT AND BACK

Modifications

1. Position the hands on the floor directly under the shoulders with the arms straight and perpendicular to the floor.
2. Place the feet securely in the grips (or straps). This might initially require assistance from a training partner.
3. Assume a straight body alignment (ears, shoulders, hips, knees, and ankles are in a straight line, with no arching or sagging of the midsection). The only contact points are the feet in the grips and the hands on the floor.

4. "Walk" forward and backward while maintaining the plank position:
   a. Move right hand forward, left hand forward, right hand backward, left hand backward.
   b. Alternate sets: Move left hand forward, right hand forward, left hand backward, right hand backward.

Specific Benefits

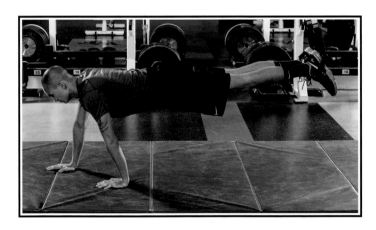

▪ ELBOW PLANK ▪
FULL-BODY WALK

Modifications

1. Lift the body so only the elbows, forearms, balls of the feet, and toes are in contact with the floor. Maintain a completely straight line in the body (ears, shoulders, hips, knees, and ankles are in alignment).
2. "Walk" forward with an alternating pattern: right arm simultaneous with left leg step; left arm simultaneous with right leg step.

Specific Benefits ❼

Note Adding moderate movement to a stability exercise creates an additional loading on the musculoskeletal system because of the compensatory control of the joint system in the presence of sagittal plane movement.

A difficulty progression might include the following:

1. Ipsilateral step: right arm simultaneous with right leg step; repeat opposite.
2. Upper/lower combo: right arm and left arm, right leg and left leg; repeat.
3. Lateral walk continuous: right arm and right leg simultaneous lateral step to the right; left arm and left leg simultaneous lateral step to the right; continue to the right.
4. Lateral walk back and forth: right arm and right leg simultaneous lateral step to the right; left arm and left leg simultaneous lateral step to the right; repeat to the opposite side.

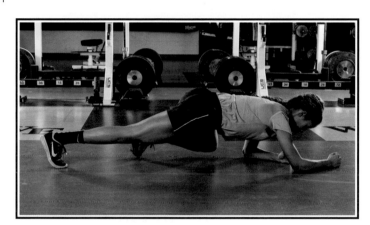

▪ STRAIGHT-ARM PLANK ▪
FULL-BODY WALK

Modifications

1. Position the hands on the floor directly under the shoulders with the arms straight and perpendicular to the floor.
2. Lift the body so only the balls of the feet, toes, and hands are on the floor. Maintain a completely straight line in the body (ears, shoulders, hips, knees, and ankles remain in alignment).

3. "Walk" forward with an alternating pattern: right arm simultaneous with left leg step; left arm simultaneous with right leg step.

Specific Benefits ❼ ⑫

Note The moderate movement variations listed in the Elbow Plank, Full-Body Walk apply.

▪ ELBOW PLANK ▪
STABILITY BALL CIRCLE WALK

Modifications

1. Position the elbows and forearms on a stability ball and lift the body so the balls of the feet and toes are on the floor. Maintain a completely straight line in the body (ears, shoulders, hips, knees, and ankles remain in alignment).

2. "Walk" laterally (circle) around the stability ball.

3. One complete orbit equals one repetition. Perform a predetermined number of repetitions in one direction, then repeat in the opposite direction.

Specific Benefits

Note Adding moderate movement to a stability exercise, such as walking around a stability ball, creates an additional loading on the musculoskeletal system because of the compensatory control of the joint system in the presence of frontal plane movement.

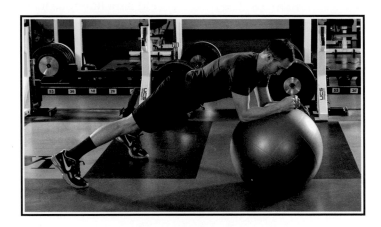

▪ STRAIGHT-ARM PLANK ▪
STABILITY BALL CIRCLE WALK

Modifications

1. Straighten the arms with the hands on a stability ball. Position the hands under the shoulders with the arms perpendicular to the floor (the size of the ball dictates the degree of perpendicularity).

2. Lift the body so the only contact points are the balls of feet and toes on the floor and the hands on the stability ball. Maintain a completely straight line in the body (ears, shoulders, hips, knees, and ankles remain in alignment).

3. "Walk" laterally (circle) around the stability ball.

4. One complete orbit equals one repetition. Perform a predetermined number of repetitions in one direction, then repeat in the opposite direction.

Specific Benefits

Note Adding moderate movement to a stability exercise, such as walking around a stability ball, creates an additional loading on the musculoskeletal system because of the compensatory control of the joint system in the presence of frontal plane movement.

Try different hand positions for additional control or difficulty. For example, point the fingers forward for greater difficulty, or point the fingers lateral toward the floor for greater control. Always be mindful of joint stability and control; never place a joint or body part in a compromised position (which is unique to the individual) that might lead to injury.

MOUNTAIN CLIMBER

MODIFICATIONS

1. Position the hands on the floor directly under the shoulders with the arms straight and perpendicular to the floor.
2. Lift the body so the only contact points are the balls of the feet, toes, and hands on the floor.
3. In rhythmic fashion, lift one knee up toward the chest, then return to the start position.
4. Repeat with the opposite leg.
5. Continue for a predetermined number of repetitions or time interval.

CONSIDERATIONS

1. Do not sag the hips (pelvis should not drop toward the floor).
2. Some compensatory lifting of the hips will occur to facilitate the knee drive, but avoid excessive arching of the pelvis and butt.
3. Keep the chin pushed back (think double chin) and avoid dropping the head (cervical vertebrae is straight with the head tilted neither forward or back).

SPECIFIC BENEFITS

8 **12**

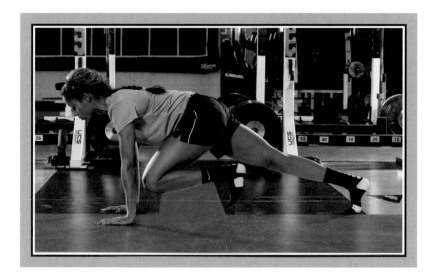

■ MOUNTAIN CLIMBER ■
INCLINE

Modifications

1. Place the hands on a raised platform or bench.

Specific Benefits **2** **8** **12**

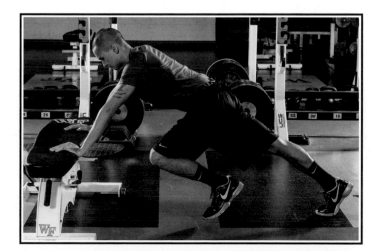

■ MOUNTAIN CLIMBER ■
UNSTABLE UPPER

Modifications

1. Straighten the arms with the hands on a moderately unstable apparatus.

Specific Benefits ❶ ❽ ⓬

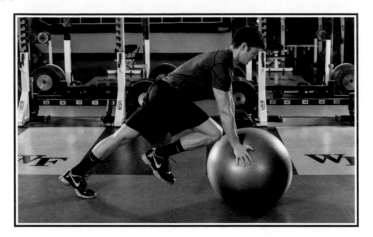

■ MOUNTAIN CLIMBER ■
SUSPENDED UPPER

Modifications

1. Place the hands in the grips (or straps). Keep the arms straight with fairly rigid elbows.

2. Assume a straight body alignment (ears, shoulders, hips, knees, and ankles are in a straight line, with no arching or sagging of the midsection). The only contact points are the balls of the feet and toes on the floor and hands on the straps.

3. Alternate driving the right knee to the chest, then the left knee to the chest. Avoid compensatory rotation as a result of lower-body movement. Controlled body alignment is the goal.

Specific Benefits ❷ ❻ ❽ ⓬

■ MOUNTAIN CLIMBER ■
SUSPENDED LOWER

Modifications

1. Position the hands on the floor directly under shoulders with the arms straight and perpendicular to the floor.

2. Place the feet securely in the grips (or straps). This might initially require help from a training partner.

3. Assume a straight body alignment (ears, shoulders, hips, knees, and ankles are in a straight line, with no arching or sagging of the midsection). The only contact points are the feet on the straps and the hands on the floor.

4. Alternate driving the right knee to the chest, then the left knee to the chest. Avoid compensatory rotation as a result of lower-body movement. Controlled body alignment is the goal.

Specific Benefits ❸ ❻ ❽ ⓬

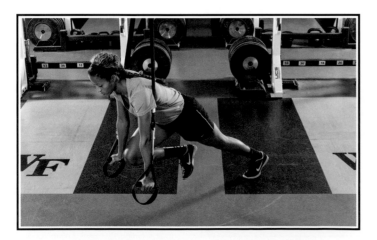

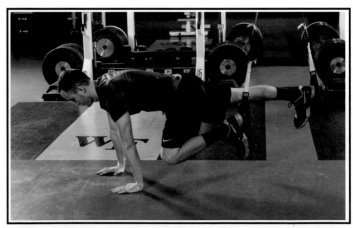

▪ MOUNTAIN CLIMBER ▪
UNSTABLE LOWER, FEET ELEVATED, DOUBLE KNEE TUCK

Modifications

1. Position part of the lower body on a stability ball.
2. Lift the body so the only contact points are the lower body on the stability ball and the hands on the floor.
3. Stabilize the upper body, specifically the shoulder complex.
4. Lift the hips toward the ceiling and draw (tuck) the knees toward the chest.
5. Extend the hips and knees and return to the start position. Maintain a tight core and proper mechanics throughout. Do not sag at the midsection.

Specific Benefits

Note The unstable apparatus must have a degree of mobility. There are many unstable apparatus options, including stability balls, for which a progression might look like this:

1. Knees on the ball
2. Ankles on the ball
3. Balls of the feet and toes on the ball

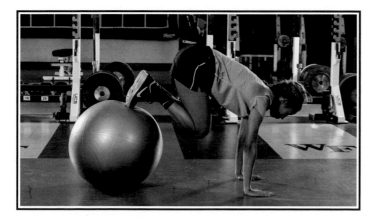

▪ MOUNTAIN CLIMBER ▪
UNSTABLE LOWER, FEET ELEVATED, SINGLE KNEE TUCK

Modifications

1. Position part of one leg on a stability ball. Flex the other leg at the hip.
2. Lift the body so the only contact points are the leg on the stability ball and the hands on the floor.
3. Stabilize the upper body, specifically the shoulder complex.
4. Lift the hips toward the ceiling and draw (tuck) the knee of the working leg toward the chest.
5. Extend the hip and knee of the working leg and return to the start position. Maintain a tight core and proper mechanics throughout. Do not sag at the midsection.

Specific Benefits

Note The unstable apparatus must have a degree of mobility. There are many unstable apparatus options, including stability balls, for which a progression might look like this:

1. Knee on the ball
2. Ankle on the ball
3. Ball of the foot and toes on the ball

Unilateral movements are harder to execute than their bilateral counterparts because of reduced balance from a point-specific or even an asymmetrical base of support. In this exercise, only one limb is used on the stability ball, creating an extreme balance situation that must be controlled by the core. Also, body weight is now moved to the working limb on one side of the body, rendering the other limb useless and causing the center of gravity to shift.

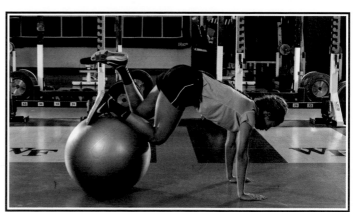

■ MOUNTAIN CLIMBER ■
SUSPENDED LOWER, ABDUCTION AND ADDUCTION, DOUBLE KNEE TUCK

Modifications

1. Position the hands on the floor directly under the shoulders with the arms straight and perpendicular to the floor.
2. Place the feet securely in the grips (or straps). This might initially require assistance from a training partner.
3. Assume a straight body alignment (ears, shoulders, hips, knees, and ankles in a straight line, with no arching or sagging of the midsection). The only contact points are the feet in the grips and the hands on the floor.

4. Simultaneously abduct both legs; then adduct both legs back to the start position.
5. Lift the hips toward the ceiling and draw (tuck) the knees toward the chest.
6. Extend the hips and knees back to the start position, maintaining a tight core and proper mechanics.

Specific Benefits ❸ ❺ ❻ ⓬

■ MOUNTAIN CLIMBER ■
SUSPENDED UPPER, UNSTABLE LOWER, DOUBLE KNEE TUCK

Modifications

1. Place the hands in the grips (or straps). Arms are straight with fairly rigid elbows.
2. Once the hands are in the grips, carefully place one foot and then the other on a stability ball. This might require assistance from a training partner.
3. Assume a straight body alignment (ears, shoulders, hips, knees, and ankles in a straight line, with no arching or sagging of the midsection). The only contact points are the feet on the stability ball and the hands in the grips.

4. Lift the hips toward the ceiling and draw (tuck) the knees toward the chest.
5. Extend the hip and knee back to the start position, maintaining a tight core and proper mechanics.

Specific Benefits ❶ ❸ ❻ ⓬

Anti-Rotation Exercises

When preparing for sport performance, a limited training methodology for many athletes is focused primarily on the development of absolute speed, absolute strength, and absolute power. Little if any attention is paid to the decelerative properties of athleticism. As we have mentioned in other chapters, from a neural perspective, having *confident* control of the rotational components does in fact facilitate the accelerators. In other words, if you know that you can stop a movement regardless of the velocity, then you can more confidently increase your velocity. Muscles are designed to produce force (acceleration), reduce force (deceleration), and stabilize articular structures. A critically important athletic trait is the forceful and accurate control of acceleration coupled with a precise command of deceleration. You see this trait in many athletes possessing superior agility skills.

Effective movement in one plane requires stabilization of the other two planes. For every subtle change in body position, translation, extremity movement pattern, or any combination of the infinite number of stabilization and movement scenarios, whether voluntary or reactive, the central nervous system is constantly monitoring homeostasis in an endeavor to provide the best possible strategy to achieve the intended outcome. Neuromuscular efficiency and its correlation to the proficient functioning of the deep stabilizers and outer mobilizers will improve kinetic chain performance. Accurate control of flexion, extension, and rotation when necessary will provide the foundation for acceleration, deceleration, and dynamic stabilization. The ultimate goal is of course improved performance.

Stabilizing and strengthening the broad spectrum of the osteoarticular spine from scapulothoracic to the lumbo-pelvic hip complex, from oblique emphasis on anti-rotation to mid- and low- trapezius and serratus scapular maintenance, we will provide a full range of functional anti-rotational examples necessary to start eliminating the weak links in the kinetic chain. Plank drills performed in a side-lying posture have many functional benefits that promote balanced muscular functioning through the entire kinetic chain. In this chapter we incorporate a variety of anti-rotation stabilization activities, which will further establish your athletic foundation—most of which are done in a side-lying position.

The following exercise finder lists the benefits, difficulty level, and equipment needed for every exercise that appears in this chapter. Primary exercises are highlighted in beige, with their progressions in blue. The primary exercises are also noted in the text with a blue title bar.

Anti-Rotation Stability Exercise Finder

Exercise Name	Specific Benefits (see chapter 5)	Difficulty Level			Equipment
		Easy	Medium	Hard	
Rolling Pattern 1: Soft Roll, Lower Body	10	X			
Rolling Pattern 1: Soft Roll, Upper Body	10	X			
Rolling Pattern 2: Hard Roll With Ball	11		X		Ball
Rolling Pattern 2: Hard Roll	11		X		
Lateral Elbow Plank	12 13	X			
Lateral Straight-Arm Plank	12 13	X			
Lateral Elbow Plank, Arm and Leg Abduction	5 12 13		X		
Lateral Straight-Arm Plank, Arm and Leg Abduction	5 12 13		X		
Lateral Elbow Plank, Unstable Upper	1 2 12 13		X		Unstable apparatus*
Lateral Straight-Arm Plank, Unstable Upper	1 12 13		X		Unstable apparatus
Lateral Elbow Plank, Unstable Upper, Arm and Leg Abduction	1 5 12 13			X	Unstable apparatus
Lateral Straight-Arm Plank, Unstable Upper, Arm and Leg Abduction	1 5 12 13			X	Unstable apparatus
Lateral Elbow Plank, Unstable Upper, Arm Elevated	1 2 12 13			X	Stability ball
Lateral Straight-Arm Plank, Unstable Upper, Arm Elevated	1 2 12 13			X	Stability ball
Lateral Elbow Plank, Unstable Upper, Arm and Leg Abduction, Arm Elevated	1 2 5 12 13			X	Stability ball
Lateral Straight-Arm Plank, Unstable Upper, Arm and Leg Abduction, Arm Elevated	1 2 5 12 13			X	Stability ball
Lateral Elbow Plank, Feet Elevated	3 12 13		X		Raised platform**
Lateral Straight-Arm Plank, Feet Elevated	3 12 13		X		Raised platform
Lateral Elbow Plank, Unstable Upper, Feet Elevated	1 3 12 13		X		Unstable apparatus, raised platform
Lateral Straight-Arm Plank, Unstable Upper, Feet Elevated	1 3 12 13			X	Unstable apparatus, raised platform
Lateral Elbow Plank, Unstable Upper, Arm and Feet Elevated	1 2 3 12 13		X		Stability ball, raised platform
Lateral Straight-Arm Plank, Unstable Upper, Arm and Feet Elevated	1 2 3 12 13			X	Stability ball, raised platform
Lateral Elbow Plank, Unstable Upper, Arm and Leg Abduction, Feet Elevated	1 3 5 12 13			X	Unstable apparatus, raised platform

* Many options are available for the unstable apparatus, including a thick foam pad, wobble board, balance disc, pillows, or stability ball.

** Many options are available for the raised platform, including a box, bench, stair, or step.

Exercise Name	Specific Benefits (see chapter 5)	Difficulty Level			Equipment
		Easy	Medium	Hard	
Lateral Straight-Arm Plank, Unstable Upper, Arm and Leg Abduction, Feet Elevated	(1)(3)(5)(12)(13)			X	Unstable apparatus, raised platform
Lateral Elbow Plank, Unstable Lower	(1)(12)(13)		X		Unstable apparatus
Lateral Straight-Arm Plank, Unstable Lower	(1)(12)(13)		X		Unstable apparatus
Lateral Elbow Plank, Unstable Lower, Arm and Leg Abduction	(1)(5)(12)(13)			X	Unstable apparatus
Lateral Straight-Arm Plank, Unstable Lower, Arm and Leg Abduction	(1)(5)(12)(13)			X	Unstable apparatus
Lateral Elbow Plank, Unstable Upper and Lower	(1)(12)(13)			X	Two unstable apparatus
Lateral Straight-Arm Plank, Unstable Upper and Lower	(1)(12)(13)			X	Two unstable apparatus
Lateral Elbow Plank, Arm Abduction, Foot Taps	(5)(12)(13)		X		
Lateral Straight-Arm Plank, Arm Abduction, Foot Taps	(5)(12)(13)		X		
Lateral Elbow Plank, Arm Abduction, Knee Drive to Chest	(5)(12)(13)		X		
Lateral Straight-Arm Plank, Arm Abduction, Knee Drive to Chest	(5)(12)(13)		X		
Lateral Elbow Plank, Ball Toss	(5)(12)(13)(14)(15)			X	Ball
Lateral Straight-Arm Plank, Ball Toss	(5)(12)(13)(14)(15)			X	Ball
Lateral Elbow Plank, Ball Toss, Feet Elevated	(3)(5)(12)(13)(14)(15)			X	Raised platform, ball
Lateral Straight-Arm Plank, Ball Toss, Feet Elevated	(3)(5)(12)(13)(14)(15)			X	Raised platform, ball
Lateral Elbow Plank, Ball Toss, Unstable Upper	(1)(5)(12)(13)(14)(15)			X	Unstable apparatus, ball
Lateral Straight-Arm Plank, Ball Toss, Unstable Upper	(1)(5)(12)(13)(14)(15)			X	Unstable apparatus, ball
Lateral Elbow Plank, Ball Toss, Unstable Lower, Arm Elevated	(1)(2)(5)(12)(13)(14)(15)			X	Raised platform, unstable apparatus, ball
Lateral Straight-Arm Plank, Ball Toss, Unstable Lower, Arm Elevated	(1)(2)(5)(12)(13)(14)(15)			X	Raised platform, unstable apparatus, ball
Lateral Elbow Plank, Top Leg Support, Bottom Leg Adduction	(5)(12)(13)			X	Raised platform
Lateral Straight-Arm Plank, Top Leg Support, Bottom Leg Adduction	(5)(12)(13)			X	Raised platform
Lateral Elbow Plank, Top Leg Support, Bottom Leg Adduction, Stability Ball	(1)(5)(12)(13)			X	Stability ball

(continued)

Exercise Name	Specific Benefits (see chapter 5)	Difficulty Level			Equipment
		Easy	Medium	Hard	
Lateral Straight-Arm Plank, Top Leg Support, Bottom Leg Adduction, Stability Ball	❶ ❺ ⑫ ⑬			X	Stability ball
Prone Rotary Stability Progression 1: Single-Leg Hip Extension	❹ ⑫	X			
Prone Rotary Stability Progression 2: Single-Leg Full Flexion	❾ ⑫		X		
Prone Rotary Stability Progression 3: Single-Leg Hip Internal Rotation and Tap	❾ ⑪ ⑫		X		
Prone Rotary Stability Progression 4: Single-Arm Full Flexion to Tap	❾ ⑫		X		
Prone Rotary Stability Progression 5: Single-Arm Overhead Shoulder Flexion	❾ ⑫		X		
Prone Rotary Stability Progression 6: Single-Arm Shoulder Extension to Hip Tap	❾ ⑫		X		
Prone Rotary Stability Progression 7: Contralateral Hip and Shoulder Extension	❹ ⑪ ⑫			X	
Prone Rotary Stability Progression 8: Contralateral Foot to Opposite Hand	❹ ❾ ⑪ ⑫			X	
Prone Rotary Stability Progression 9: Contralateral Knee to Opposite Elbow	❹ ❾ ⑪ ⑫			X	
Prone Rotary Stability Progression 10: Ipsilateral Elbow to Knee	❹ ❾ ⑩ ⑫			X	
Straight-Arm Plank Displacement Series Progression 1: Lower Body Abduction and Adduction Walk	❺ ❽ ❾ ⑫		X		
Straight-Arm Plank Displacement Series Progression 2: Upper Body Abduction and Adduction Walk	❺ ❼ ❽ ❾ ⑫		X		
Straight-Arm Plank Displacement Series Progression 3: Upper and Lower Body Abduction and Adduction Walk	❺ ❼ ❽ ❾ ⑪ ⑫		X		
Straight-Arm Plank Displacement Series Progression 4: Upper and Lower Body Abduction and Adduction Crab Walk	❺ ❼ ❽ ❾ ⑩ ⑫		X		
Straight-Arm Plank Displacement Series Progression 5: Upper and Lower Body Circle Pivot Walk	❺ ❼ ❽ ❾ ⑩ ⑫		X		
Low Prone Plank Spider-Man	❺ ❾ ⑫		X		
Low Prone Plank Spider-Man Push-Up	❺ ❾ ⑫			X	

ROLLING PATTERN 1

SOFT ROLL, LOWER BODY

MOVEMENTS

1. Lie on the floor in a supine position (face up) with the legs straight and arms extended overhead.
2. Brace the core and turn the head in the direction of the intended roll.
3. Remain completely relaxed in the upper body; try not to use the upper torso or arms to assist in the movement at any point.
4. Lift one leg up and across the body.
5. With the entire body, follow the momentum of the single leg and roll over to a prone position (face down).
6. Reverse the movement and roll back to the start position.
7. Repeat for a predetermined number of repetitions or time interval.
8. Repeat on the opposite side; note any asymmetry in stabilization, strength, or movement mechanics.

CONSIDERATIONS

1. Always roll in the direction of the head turn.
2. Maintain a braced core throughout.

SPECIFIC BENEFITS

NOTE

Variations might include the following:

- Roll over and back to one direction for the duration of the set. Repeat in the other direction.
- Roll continuously in one direction.
- Roll on command.

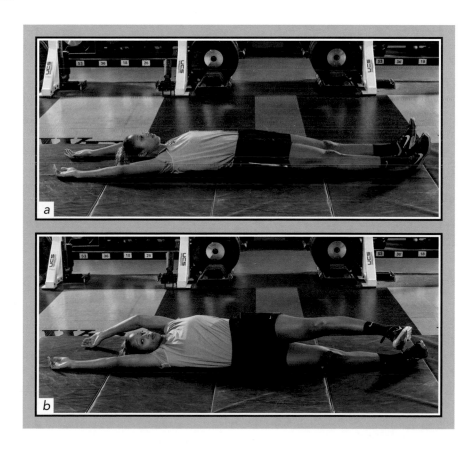

■ ROLLING PATTERN 1 ■
SOFT ROLL, UPPER BODY

Modifications

1. Lie supine on the floor with the legs straight and arms extended overhead.
2. Brace the core and turn the head in the direction of the intended roll.
3. Remain completely relaxed in the lower body; try not to use the legs to assist in the movement at any point.
4. Lift one arm up and across the body. The entire body follows the momentum of the arm and rolls over to a prone position.
5. Reverse the movement and roll back to the start position.

Specific Benefits   ⑩

Note

1. Always roll in the direction of the head turn.
2. Maintain a braced core throughout.
3. Using only the upper limbs as drivers avoids using the gross weight of the legs to simply flop the body over. Thus a greater emphasis on core muscular synergism is critical to the success of the movement.

■ ROLLING PATTERN 2 ■
HARD ROLL WITH BALL

Modifications

1. Lie supine on the floor with the arms extended overhead.
2. Bring one knee toward the chest; simultaneously move the opposite elbow toward that bent knee (contralateral).
3. Place a ball between the elbow and knee.
4. Brace the core; turn the head in the direction of the intended roll.
5. Maintaining a braced core, roll the body to the bent-leg side. Don't use the opposite straight arm and straight leg to assist the movement. Maintain tight contact with the ball throughout the movement.
6. Reverse the movement, always turning the head in the direction of the roll.

Specific Benefits ⑪

Note The contralateral action between the knee and elbow while holding the ball stimulates a deep stabilizer co-contraction simultaneous to the additional core action required to control the rolling motion. This exercise becomes a challenging and complex task that will further, and more completely, stress the physiological system.

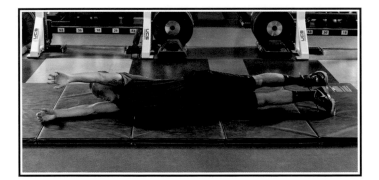

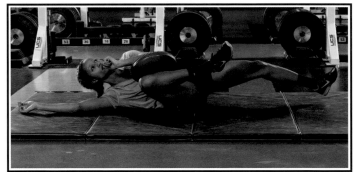

■ ROLLING PATTERN 2 ■
HARD ROLL

Modifications

1. This drill is identical to the previous exercise but without the ball.
2. Lift one knee up toward the chest; bring the opposite elbow toward the knee.
3. Maintain elbow and knee contact throughout the movement (contralateral).

Specific Benefits   ⑪

Note Performing this exercise without the ball places a greater demand on range of motion, which calls for a uniform co-contraction of the deep stabilizers. The result is challenging the core even further to maintain contact while controlling the rolling motion. This progressively increases overall task complexity and physiological demand on the involved systems.

LATERAL ELBOW PLANK

MOVEMENTS

1. Lie on one side with the legs straight and one leg and foot on top of the other leg and foot (stacked).
2. Place the bottom elbow and forearm on a soft surface, such as a gym mat or folded towel. The upper arm is perpendicular to the floor; the forearm of the bottom arm is perpendicular to the body. The bulk of the upper-body weight is supported by the bottom arm, so correct positioning is critical.
3. Place the opposite hand on the top hip (or the top arm can simply lie on top of the body).
4. Lock the knees, dorsiflex the feet and ankles, tighten the glutes, and brace the core.
5. While maintaining a lateral alignment, lift the body into a straight-line, neutral position (ear, shoulder, hip, knee, and ankle in a straight line). The contact points are the lateral side of the bottom foot and the bottom elbow and forearm on the floor.
6. Maintain a completely straight line in the body for a predetermined time interval.
7. Repeat on the opposite side.

CONSIDERATIONS

1. Athletes who feel stress in the ankle, knee, or hip joint should proceed with caution. Repositioning the body and feet can help reduce pain and injury risk. Try staggering the feet so that the top straight leg is a foot or two in front of the bottom leg (both feet on the floor). Or use the top hand and arm for additional support by placing it on the floor, thereby supporting some of the body weight and reducing the load on the bottom arm. Also, a spotter can help by placing an exercise strap around the athlete's waist and assist with lifting the body into a straight-line position. There are many ways to decrease load while maintaining acceptable posture and mechanics. The goal is to strive toward precision, maintaining a relatively straight-line mechanical form for this and all other plank drills, without the use of additional assistance.
2. Unless the drill calls for a hip-drop movement, avoid sagging the hips (the lower hip and buttock should not drop toward the floor).
3. Keep the chin pushed back (think double chin), and don't let the head drop laterally toward the floor. The cervical vertebrae should be straight, with the head tilted neither forward nor back. The tendency is to laterally tilt the head (frontal plane) when performing the side-lying plank. Avoid this by consciously aligning the body at the ear, shoulder, hip, knee, and ankle.

SPECIFIC BENEFITS

⑫ ⑬

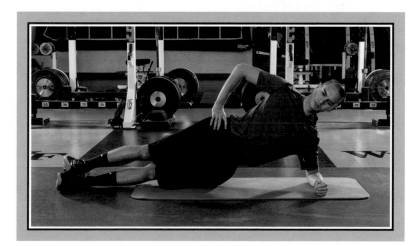

LATERAL STRAIGHT-ARM PLANK

Modifications

1. Lying on one side, position one hand on the floor directly under the shoulder with the arm perpendicular to the floor.
2. Lift the body so the only contact points are the lateral side of the bottom foot and the bottom hand on the floor.

Specific Benefits [12] [13]

Note If there is difficulty in maintaining a straight-line plank position, try placing the top hand on the floor, providing a three-point base of support (feet, bottom hand, top hand). This allows straight body alignment from ear to ankle, which is critically important in plank exercises.

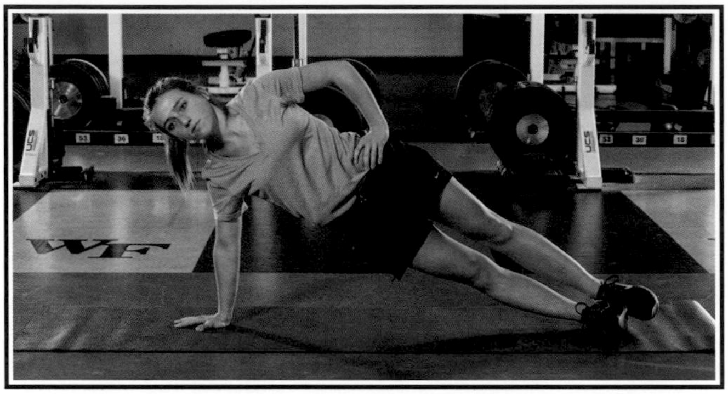

LATERAL ELBOW PLANK

ARM AND LEG ABDUCTION

Modifications

1. Assume the lateral elbow plank position.
2. Abduct the top arm straight toward the ceiling (frontal plane), perpendicular to the floor and aligned with the bottom arm.
3. Simultaneously lift the top leg up and away from the bottom leg. Keep the foot aligned and straight. A slight internal rotation of the top foot during abduction will more fully engage the gluteal complex (specifically the gluteus medius).

Specific Benefits [5] [12] [13]

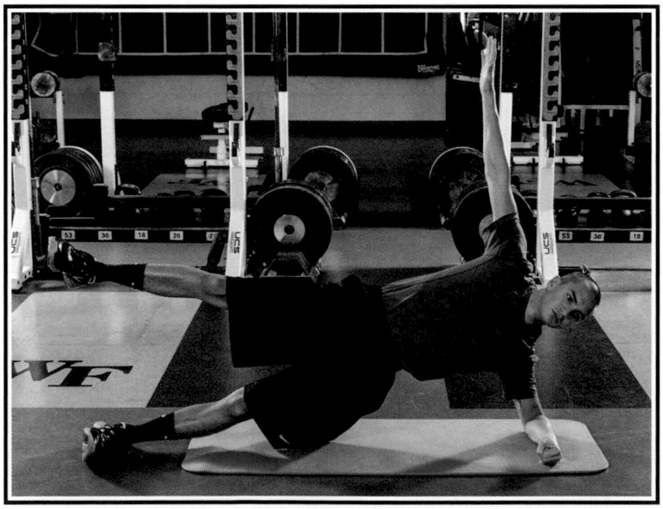

■ LATERAL STRAIGHT-ARM PLANK ■
ARM AND LEG ABDUCTION

Modifications

1. Lying on one side, position the bottom hand on the floor directly under the shoulder with the arm perpendicular to the floor.
2. Lift the body so the only contact points are the lateral side of the bottom foot and hand on the floor.

3. Abduct the top arm straight toward the ceiling (frontal plane) perpendicular to the floor and aligned with the bottom arm.
4. The action is the same as for the Lateral Elbow Plank, Arm and Leg Abduction.

Specific Benefits

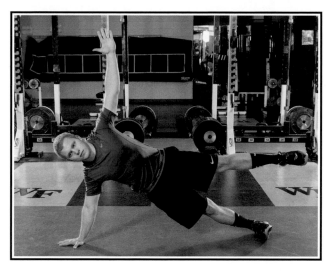

■ LATERAL ELBOW PLANK ■
UNSTABLE UPPER

Modifications

1. Assume the lateral elbow plank position with the bottom elbow and forearm on a moderately unstable apparatus (thick foam pad, wobble board, balance disc, pillows, etc.).
2. Lift the body so the only contact points are the elbow and forearm on the unstable apparatus and the lateral side of the bottom foot on the floor.

Specific Benefits

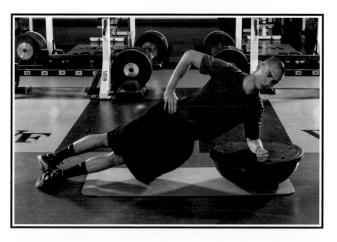

■ LATERAL STRAIGHT-ARM PLANK ■
UNSTABLE UPPER

Modifications

1. Lying on one side, position the bottom hand on a moderately unstable apparatus directly under the shoulder with the arm perpendicular to the floor. The legs are straight with one leg and foot on top of the other leg and foot (stacked).
2. Lift the body so the only contact points are the hand on the unstable apparatus and the lateral side of the bottom foot on the floor.

Specific Benefits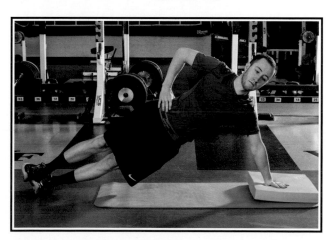

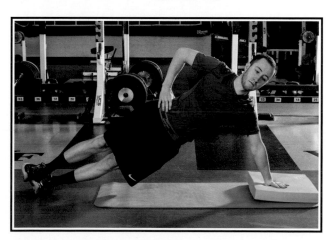

▪ LATERAL ELBOW PLANK ▪
UNSTABLE UPPER, ARM AND LEG ABDUCTION

Modifications

1. Assume the lateral elbow plank position with the bottom elbow and forearm on a moderately unstable apparatus. The upper arm is perpendicular to the floor; the forearm is perpendicular to the body.
2. Lift the body so the only contact points are the elbow and forearm on the unstable apparatus and the lateral side of the bottom foot on the floor.

3. Abduct the top arm straight toward the ceiling (frontal plane) perpendicular to the floor and aligned with the bottom arm (i.e., from top to bottom—wrist, elbow, shoulder, shoulder, elbow).
4. Simultaneously lift the top leg up and away from bottom leg. Keep the foot aligned and straight. A slight internal rotation of the top foot during abduction will more fully engage the gluteal complex (specifically the gluteus medius).

Specific Benefits   ❶ ❺ ⓬ ⓭

▪ LATERAL STRAIGHT-ARM PLANK ▪
UNSTABLE UPPER, ARM AND LEG ABDUCTION

Modifications

1. Lying on one side, position the bottom hand on a moderately unstable apparatus directly under the shoulder with the arm perpendicular to the floor. The legs are straight with one leg and foot on top of the other leg and foot (stacked).
2. Lift the body so the only contact points are the hand on the unstable apparatus and the lateral side of the bottom foot on the floor.
3. The action is the same as for the Lateral Elbow Plank, Unstable Upper, Arm and Leg Abduction.

Specific Benefits   ❶ ❺ ⓬ ⓭

▪ LATERAL ELBOW PLANK ▪
UNSTABLE UPPER, ARM ELEVATED

Modifications

1. In the lateral elbow plank position, place the bottom elbow and forearm on a stability ball.
2. Lift the body so the only contact points are the elbow and forearm on the stability ball and the lateral side of the bottom foot on the floor.

Specific Benefits   ❶ ❷ ⓬ ⓭

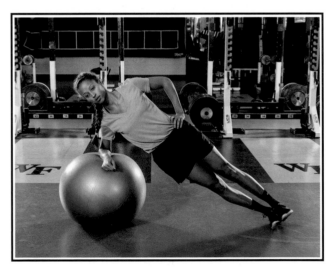

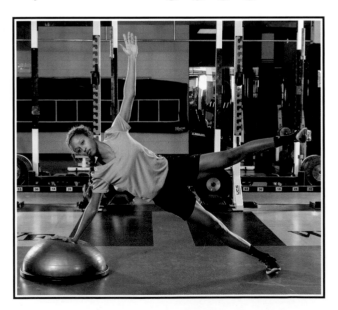

▪ LATERAL STRAIGHT-ARM PLANK ▪
UNSTABLE UPPER, ARM ELEVATED

Modifications

1. Lying on one side, straighten the bottom arm with the hand on a stability ball. Position the bottom hand directly under the shoulder with the arm relatively perpendicular to the floor (the size of the ball dictates the degree of perpendicularity).
2. Lift the body so the only contact points are the hand on the stability ball and the lateral side of the bottom foot on the floor.

Specific Benefits ❶ ❷ ⓬ ⓭

Note Try different hand positions for additional control or difficulty. For example, point the fingers forward for greater difficulty, or point the fingers lateral toward the floor for greater control. Always be mindful of joint stability and control; never place a joint or body part in a compromised position (which is unique to the individual) that might lead to injury.

▪ LATERAL ELBOW PLANK ▪
UNSTABLE UPPER, ARM AND LEG ABDUCTION, ARM ELEVATED

Modifications

1. In the lateral elbow plank position, place the bottom elbow and forearm on a stability ball.
2. Lift the body so the only contact points are the elbow and forearm on the stability ball and the lateral side of the bottom foot on the floor.
3. Abduct the top arm straight toward the ceiling (frontal plane) perpendicular to the floor and aligned with the bottom arm (i.e., from top to bottom—wrist, elbow, shoulder, shoulder, elbow).

4. Simultaneously lift the top leg up and away from the bottom leg. Keep the foot aligned and straight. A slight internal rotation of the top foot during abduction will more fully engage the gluteal complex (specifically the gluteus medius).

Specific Benefits ❶ ❷ ❺ ⓬ ⓭

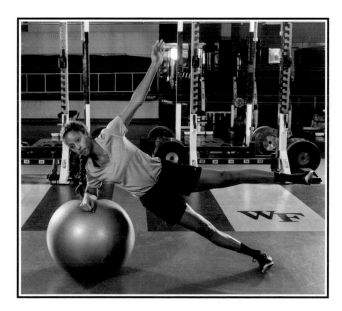

▪ LATERAL STRAIGHT-ARM PLANK ▪
UNSTABLE UPPER, ARM AND LEG ABDUCTION, ARM ELEVATED

Modifications

1. Lying on one side, straighten the bottom arm with the hand on a stability ball. Position the hand directly under the shoulder, relatively perpendicular to the floor (the size of the ball dictates the degree of perpendicularity).
2. Lift the body so the only contact points are the hand on the stability ball and the lateral side of the bottom foot on the floor.
3. The action is identical to the Lateral Elbow Plank, Unstable Upper, Arm and Leg Abduction, Arm Elevated

Specific Benefits   ⑬

Note Try different hand positions for additional control or difficulty. For example, point the fingers forward for greater difficulty, or point the fingers lateral toward the floor for greater control. Always be mindful of joint stability and control; never place a joint or body part in a compromised position (which is unique to the individual) that might lead to injury.

▪ LATERAL ELBOW PLANK ▪
FEET ELEVATED

Modifications

1. In the lateral elbow plank position, stack the feet on a raised platform (box, bench, stair step, etc.).
2. Lift the body so the only contact points are the bottom elbow and forearm on the floor and the lateral side of the bottom foot on the raised platform.

Specific Benefits ③ ⑫ ⑬

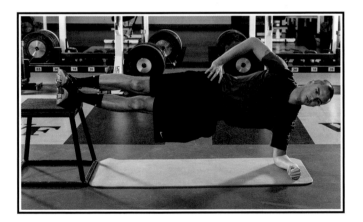

▪ LATERAL STRAIGHT-ARM PLANK ▪
FEET ELEVATED

Modifications

1. Lying on one side, position the bottom hand on the floor directly under the shoulder with the arm perpendicular to the floor.
2. Place the feet on a raised platform.
3. Lift the body so the only contact points are the bottom hand on the floor and the lateral side of the bottom foot on the raised platform.

Specific Benefits ③ ⑫ ⑬

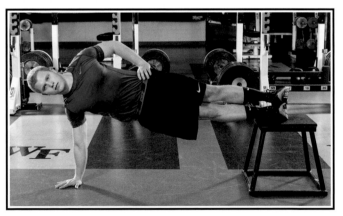

▪ LATERAL ELBOW PLANK ▪
UNSTABLE UPPER, FEET ELEVATED

Modifications

1. In the lateral elbow plank position, place the lower elbow and forearm on a moderately unstable apparatus.
2. Stack the feet on a raised platform.
3. Lift the body so the only contact points are the bottom elbow and forearm on the unstable apparatus and the lateral side of the bottom foot on the raised platform.

Specific Benefits

▪ LATERAL STRAIGHT-ARM PLANK ▪
UNSTABLE UPPER, FEET ELEVATED

Modifications

1. Lying on one side, straighten the bottom arm with the hand on a moderately unstable apparatus. Position the hand directly under the shoulder with the arm perpendicular to the floor.
2. Stack the feet on a raised platform.
3. Lift the body so the only contact points are the hand on the unstable apparatus and the lateral side of the bottom foot on the platform.

Specific Benefits

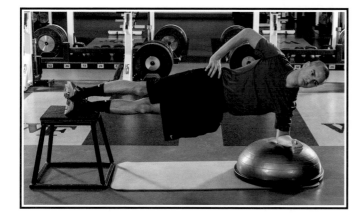

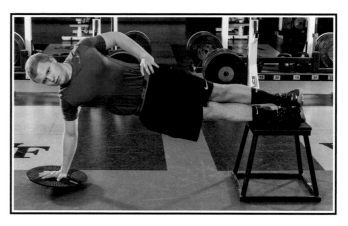

▪ LATERAL ELBOW PLANK ▪
UNSTABLE UPPER, ARM AND FEET ELEVATED

Modifications

1. In the lateral elbow plank position, place the bottom elbow and forearm on a stability ball and stack the feet on a raised platform.
2. Lift the body so the only contact points are the elbow and forearm on the stability ball and the lateral side of the bottom foot on the platform.

Specific Benefits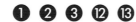

Note The benefit from this exercise is in the adaptive stress placed on the upper body, specifically the shoulder girdle. With the feet positioned on a raised platform and the arms elevated on a stability ball, the body is nearly parallel to the floor. This position makes the exercise much more challenging. In other words, keeping your body parallel on a stability ball is far more difficult than keeping your body inclined on a stability ball. In fact, if the feet were elevated higher than the stability ball, the body would be in a decline position, which creates an even more challenging movement pattern. Of course, along with the greater challenge comes greater risk potential.

■ LATERAL STRAIGHT-ARM PLANK ■
UNSTABLE UPPER, ARM AND FEET ELEVATED

Modifications

1. Lying on one side, straighten the bottom arm with the hand on a stability ball. Position the hand directly under the shoulder with the arm perpendicular to floor.
2. Stack the feet on a raised platform.
3. Lift the body so the only contact points are the hand on the stability ball and the lateral side of the bottom foot on the raised platform.

Specific Benefits   ⓫ ⓬ ⓭

Note Try different hand positions for additional control or difficulty. For example, point the fingers forward for greater difficulty, or point the fingers lateral toward the floor for greater control. Always be mindful of joint stability and control; never place a joint or body part in a compromised position (which is unique to the individual) that might lead to injury.

See also the note section for the previous exercise. This is a very challenging exercise, so take every precaution to prevent a mishap. A spotter is highly recommended.

■ LATERAL ELBOW PLANK ■
UNSTABLE UPPER, ARM AND LEG ABDUCTION, FEET ELEVATED

Modifications

1. In the lateral elbow plank position, place the lower elbow and forearm on a moderately unstable apparatus.
2. Stack the feet on a raised platform.
3. Lift the body so the only contact points are the elbow and forearm on the unstable apparatus and the lateral side of the bottom foot on the raised platform.
4. Abduct the top arm straight toward the ceiling (frontal plane) perpendicular to the floor and aligned with the bottom arm (i.e., from top to bottom—wrist, elbow, shoulder, shoulder, elbow).
5. Simultaneously lift the top leg up and away from the bottom leg. Keep the foot aligned and straight. A slight internal rotation of the top foot during abduction will more fully engage the gluteal complex (specifically the gluteus medius).

Specific Benefits ❶ ❸ ❺ ⓬ ⓭

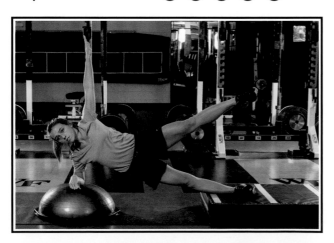

■ LATERAL STRAIGHT-ARM PLANK ■
UNSTABLE UPPER, ARM AND LEG ABDUCTION, FEET ELEVATED

Modifications

1. Lying on one side, position the bottom hand on a moderately unstable apparatus directly under the shoulder with the arm perpendicular to the floor.
2. Stack the feet on a raised platform.
3. Lift the body so the only contact points are the hand on the unstable apparatus and the lateral side of the bottom foot on the raised platform.
4. The action is the same as for the Lateral Elbow Plank, Unstable Upper, Arm and Leg Abduction, Feet Elevated.

Specific Benefits ❶ ❸ ❺ ⓬ ⓭

Note This is a very challenging drill, so take every precaution to avoid a mishap. A spotter is highly recommended.

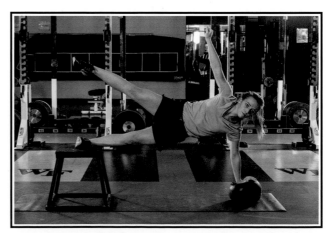

▪ LATERAL ELBOW PLANK ▪
UNSTABLE LOWER

Modifications

1. In the lateral elbow plank position, stack the feet on a moderately unstable apparatus.

2. Lift the body so the only contact points are the elbow and forearm on the floor and the lateral side of the bottom foot on the apparatus.

Specific Benefits

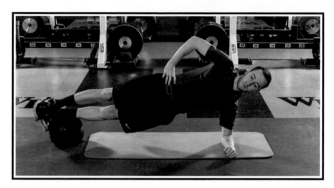

▪ LATERAL STRAIGHT-ARM PLANK ▪
UNSTABLE LOWER

Modifications

1. Lying on one side, position the bottom hand on the floor directly under the shoulder with the arm perpendicular to the floor.

2. Stack the feet on a moderately unstable apparatus.

3. Lift the body so the only contact points are the hand on the floor and the lateral side of the bottom foot on the apparatus.

Specific Benefits

▪ LATERAL ELBOW PLANK ▪
UNSTABLE LOWER, ARM AND LEG ABDUCTION

Modifications

1. In the lateral elbow plank position, stack the feet on a moderately unstable apparatus.

2. Lift the body so the only contact points are the elbow and forearm on the floor and the lateral side of the bottom foot on the apparatus.

3. Abduct the top arm straight toward the ceiling (frontal plane) perpendicular to the floor and aligned with the bottom arm (i.e., from top to bottom—wrist, elbow, shoulder, shoulder, elbow).

4. Simultaneously lift the top leg up and away from the bottom leg. Keep the foot aligned and straight. A slight internal rotation of the top foot during abduction will more fully engage the gluteal complex (specifically the gluteus medius).

Specific Benefits ❶ ❺ ⓬ ⓭

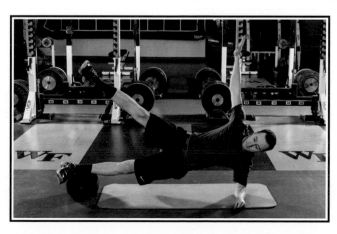

▪ LATERAL STRAIGHT-ARM PLANK ▪
UNSTABLE LOWER, ARM AND LEG ABDUCTION

Modifications

1. Lying on one side, position the bottom hand on the floor directly under the shoulder with the arm perpendicular to the floor.
2. Stack the feet on a moderately unstable apparatus.
3. Lift the body so the only contact points are the hand on the floor and the lateral side of the bottom foot on the apparatus.

4. The action is the same as for the Lateral Elbow Plank, Unstable Lower, Arm and Leg Abduction.

Specific Benefits ❶ ❺ ⓬ ⓭

▪ LATERAL ELBOW PLANK ▪
UNSTABLE UPPER AND LOWER

Modifications

1. In the lateral elbow plank position, stack the feet on a moderately unstable apparatus.
2. Carefully place the bottom elbow and forearm on a similarly moderately unstable apparatus.
3. Lift the body so all contact points (elbow, forearm, lateral side of the bottom foot) are on the apparatus.

Specific Benefits ❶ ⓬ ⓭

Note Using unstable devices of any kind places an additional proprioceptive demand on the physiological system and makes a simple task much more difficult. This is a very challenging drill, so take every precaution to avoid a mishap. A spotter is highly recommended.

A difficulty progression might include the following:

1. Knee and lower leg on the apparatus
2. Ankle on the apparatus
3. Lateral foot on the apparatus

▪ LATERAL STRAIGHT-ARM PLANK ▪
UNSTABLE UPPER AND LOWER

Modifications

1. Lying on one side, stack the feet on a moderately unstable apparatus.
2. Carefully place the bottom hand on another moderately unstable apparatus. The position of the bottom hand is directly under the shoulder with the arm relatively perpendicular to the floor.
3. Lift the body so the bottom hand and the lateral side of the bottom foot are on the apparatus.

Specific Benefits ❶ ⓬ ⓭

Note Using unstable devices of any kind places an additional proprioceptive demand on the physiological system and makes a simple task much more difficult. This is a very challenging drill, so take every precaution to avoid a mishap. A spotter is highly recommended.

A difficulty progression might include the following:

1. Knee and lower leg on the apparatus
2. Ankle on the apparatus
3. Lateral foot on the apparatus

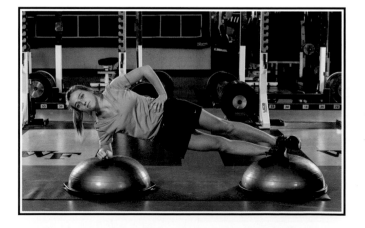

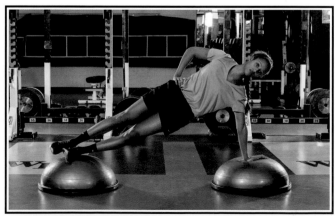

■ LATERAL ELBOW PLANK ■
ARM ABDUCTION, FOOT TAPS

Modifications

1. In the lateral elbow plank position, abduct the top arm toward the ceiling (frontal plane), perpendicular to the floor and aligned with the bottom arm (i.e., from top to bottom—wrist, elbow, shoulder, shoulder, elbow).
2. While bracing the core, lift the top leg up and forward and tap the floor with the foot a comfortable distance in front of the ground foot.
3. Repeat in reverse, tapping the floor behind the ground foot. Maintain a straight leg throughout.

4. Perform for a predetermined number of repetitions or time interval; repeat on opposite side.

Specific Benefits ⑫ ⑬

Note The range of motion of the top leg should be dictated by comfort and control. As strength and kinesthesis levels improve, try for greater lateral lift and more forward and backward leg reach.

■ LATERAL STRAIGHT-ARM PLANK ■
ARM ABDUCTION, FOOT TAPS

Modifications

1. Lying on one side, position the bottom hand on the floor directly under the shoulder with the arm perpendicular to the floor.
2. Lift the body so the only contact points are the hand and the lateral side of the bottom foot on the floor.
3. Abduct the top arm toward the ceiling (frontal plane) perpendicular to the floor and aligned with the bottom arm (i.e., from top to bottom—wrist, elbow, shoulder, shoulder, elbow).
4. While bracing the core, lift the top leg up and forward and tap the floor with the foot a comfortable distance in front of the ground foot.

5. Repeat in reverse, tapping the floor behind the ground foot. Maintain a straight leg throughout.
6. Perform for a predetermined number of repetitions or time interval; repeat on opposite side.

Specific Benefits ⑤ ⑫ ⑬

Note The range of motion of the top leg should be dictated by comfort and control. As strength and kinesthesis levels improve, try for greater lateral lift and more forward and backward leg reach.

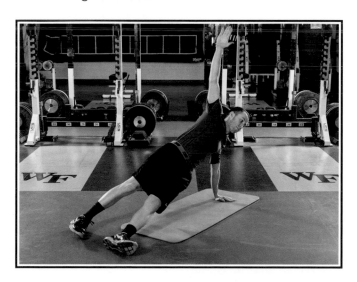

■ LATERAL ELBOW PLANK ■
ARM ABDUCTION, KNEE DRIVE TO CHEST

Modifications

1. In lateral elbow plank position, abduct the top arm toward the ceiling (frontal plane), perpendicular to the floor and aligned with the bottom arm (i.e., from top to bottom—wrist, elbow, shoulder, shoulder, elbow).
2. While bracing the core, lift the top leg slightly up and off the bottom leg while simultaneously flexing the top leg's hip and drawing the knee toward the chest. (Do *not* move the chest to the knee; maintain straight body alignment throughout the action.)
3. Return to the start position.

Specific Benefits **⑤** **⑫** **⑬**

■ LATERAL STRAIGHT-ARM PLANK ■
ARM ABDUCTION, KNEE DRIVE TO CHEST

Modifications

1. Lying on one side, position the bottom hand on floor directly under the shoulder with the arm perpendicular to the floor.
2. Lift the body so the only contact points are the lateral side of the bottom foot and the bottom hand on the floor.
3. Abduct the top arm straight toward the ceiling (frontal plane) perpendicular to the floor and aligned with the bottom arm (i.e., from top to bottom—wrist, elbow, shoulder, shoulder, elbow).
4. While bracing the core, lift the top leg slightly up and off the bottom leg while simultaneously flexing the top leg's hip and drawing the knee toward the chest. (Do *not* move the chest to the knee; maintain straight body alignment throughout the action.)
5. Return to the start position.

Specific Benefits **⑤** **⑫** **⑬**

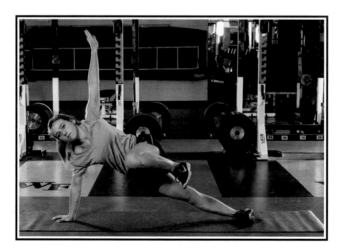

■ LATERAL ELBOW PLANK ■
BALL TOSS

Modifications

1. In the lateral elbow plank position, hold a ball (e.g., tennis ball, basketball, football) with the top hand.
2. While bracing the core and with straight body alignment, toss the ball to a partner. The partner tosses the ball back.
3. Continue tossing back and forth for a predetermined number of repetitions or time interval; repeat on opposite side.

Specific Benefits **⑤** **⑫** **⑬** **⑭** **⑮**

■ LATERAL STRAIGHT-ARM PLANK ■
BALL TOSS

Modifications

1. Lying on one side, position the bottom hand on the floor directly under the shoulder with the arm perpendicular to the floor.
2. Lift the body so the only contact points are the lateral side of the bottom foot and the bottom hand on the floor. Hold a ball with the top hand.

3. While bracing the core and with straight body alignment, toss the ball to a partner. The partner tosses the ball back.
4. Continue tossing back and forth for a predetermined number of repetitions or time interval; repeat on opposite side.

Specific Benefits

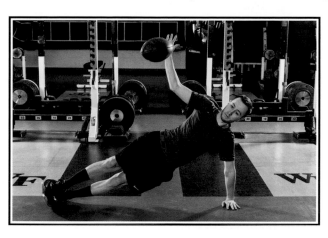

■ LATERAL ELBOW PLANK ■
BALL TOSS, FEET ELEVATED

Modifications

1. In the lateral elbow plank position, stack the feet on a raised platform (box, bench, stair step, etc.).
2. Lift the body so the only contact points are the lateral side of the bottom foot on the raised platform and the bottom elbow and forearm on the floor. Hold a ball with the top hand.
3. While bracing the core and with straight body alignment, toss the ball to a partner. The partner tosses the ball back.
4. Continue tossing back and forth for a predetermined number of repetitions or time interval; repeat on opposite side.

Specific Benefits

■ LATERAL STRAIGHT-ARM PLANK ■
BALL TOSS, FEET ELEVATED

Modifications

1. Lying on one side, position the bottom hand on the floor directly under the shoulder with the arm perpendicular to the floor. Place the feet on a raised platform.
2. Lift the body so the only contact points are the lateral side of the bottom foot on the raised platform and the bottom hand on the floor. Hold a ball with the top hand.
3. The action is identical to Lateral Elbow Plank Ball Toss, Feet Elevated.

Specific Benefits

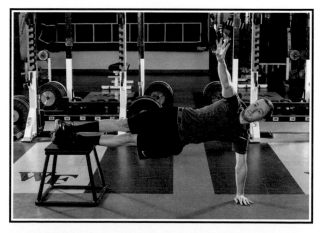

▪ LATERAL ELBOW PLANK ▪
BALL TOSS, UNSTABLE UPPER

Modifications

1. Assume the lateral elbow plank position with the bottom elbow and forearm on a moderately unstable apparatus.
2. Lift the body so the only contact points are the elbow and forearm on the unstable apparatus and the lateral side of the bottom foot on the floor. Hold a ball with the top hand.

3. While bracing the core and with straight body alignment, toss the ball to a partner. The partner tosses the ball back.
4. Continue tossing back and forth for a predetermined number of repetitions or time interval; repeat on opposite side.

Specific Benefits **❶ ❺ ⓬ ⓭ ⓮ ⓯**

▪ LATERAL STRAIGHT-ARM PLANK ▪
BALL TOSS, UNSTABLE UPPER

Modifications

1. Lying on one side, position the bottom hand on a moderately unstable apparatus directly under the shoulder with the arm perpendicular to the floor.
2. Lift the body so the only contact points are the hand on the unstable apparatus and the lateral side of the bottom foot on the floor. Hold a ball with the top hand.

3. While bracing the core and with straight body alignment, toss the ball to a partner. The partner tosses the ball back.
4. Continue tossing back and forth for a predetermined number of repetitions or time interval; repeat on opposite side.

Specific Benefits **❶ ❺ ⓬ ⓭ ⓮ ⓯**

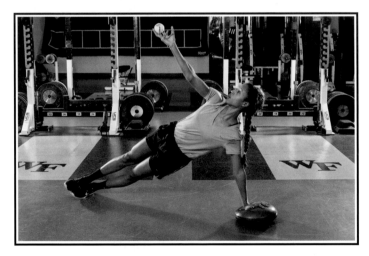

▪ LATERAL ELBOW PLANK ▪
BALL TOSS, UNSTABLE LOWER, ARM ELEVATED

Modifications

1. In the lateral elbow plank position, place the bottom elbow and forearm on a raised platform. Stack the feet on a moderately unstable apparatus so that only the lateral side of the bottom foot is on the apparatus.
2. Lift the body so the only contact points are the elbow and forearm on the raised surface and the lateral side of the bottom foot on the unstable apparatus. Hold a ball with the top hand.

3. While bracing the core and with straight body alignment, toss the ball to a partner. The partner tosses the ball back.
4. Continue tossing back and forth for a predetermined number of repetitions or time interval; repeat on opposite side.

Specific Benefits **❶ ❷ ❺ ⓬ ⓭ ⓮ ⓯**

■ LATERAL STRAIGHT-ARM PLANK ■
BALL TOSS, UNSTABLE LOWER, ARM ELEVATED

Modifications

1. Lying on one side, position the bottom hand on a raised platform. The hand is directly under the shoulder with the arm perpendicular to the floor. Stack the feet on a moderately unstable apparatus so that only the lateral side of the bottom foot is on the apparatus.

2. Lift the body so the only contact points are the hand on the raised surface and the lateral side of the bottom foot on the unstable apparatus. Hold a ball with the top hand.

3. While bracing the core and with straight body alignment, toss the ball to a partner. The partner tosses the ball back.

4. Continue tossing back and forth for a predetermined number of repetitions or time interval; repeat on opposite side.

Specific Benefits ❶ ❷ ❺ ⑫ ⑬ ⑭ ⑮

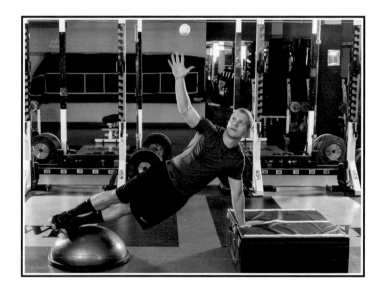

Approach the following exercises with caution. Complete support of the leg, from near the hip (groin) to the foot and ankle, provides the greatest degree of structural support and joint protection. However, the greater the support, the less core involvement. The further the support from the axis point (located within the core), the more challenging the effort, but with an increased stress on the unsupported joints of the lower leg.

LATERAL ELBOW PLANK

TOP LEG SUPPORT, BOTTOM LEG ADDUCTION

MOVEMENTS

1. Lie on one side with the legs straight and the top leg supported on a solid raised structure, such as a box, a weight room utility bench, or even a stack of mats (support is anywhere from the ankle to the hip depending on strength and comfort level).

2. Place the bottom elbow and forearm on a soft surface, such as a gym mat or folded towel. The upper arm is perpendicular to the floor; the forearm is perpendicular to the body. The majority of the upper-body weight is supported by the bottom arm, so correct positioning is critical.

3. The medial side of the top leg (from the hip to the foot and any point along this distance) is on the support structure; the bottom elbow and forearm are on the floor; the bottom leg is straight and resting on the floor.

4. While bracing the core and with straight body alignment, lift (adduct) the lower leg to the top leg (midline of the body position).

5. Lower the leg down to the start position with control; do not let the leg simply drop back to the floor. Lightly tap the floor and immediately repeat the action for a predetermined number of repetitions.

6. Repeat on opposite side.

CONSIDERATIONS

1. The top hand can be placed on the top hip, or the top arm can simply lie on top of the body. The top hand can also be placed on the floor in front of the athlete to assist with balance and lessen load.

2. Review the considerations for the lateral elbow plank at the beginning of the chapter with regard to additional support and proper body alignment.

3. Ideal body alignment would be parallel to the ground. But this depends on the height of the support structure. Regardless, avoid sagging the body.

4. If joint pain or general discomfort is felt at any point, discontinue the exercise immediately.

SPECIFIC BENEFITS

■ LATERAL STRAIGHT-ARM PLANK ■
TOP LEG SUPPORT, BOTTOM LEG ADDUCTION

Modifications

1. Lie on one side with the legs straight and the top leg supported on a solid raised structure, such as a box, a weight room utility bench, or even a stack of mats (support is anywhere from the ankle to the hip depending on strength and comfort level).

2. Position the bottom hand on the floor directly under the shoulder with the arm perpendicular to the floor.

3. The only contact points throughout the exercise are the medial side of the top leg (from the hip to the foot and any point along this distance) on the support structure and the bottom hand on the floor.

4. While bracing the core and with straight body alignment, lift (adduct) the lower leg to the top leg (midline of the body position).

5. Lower the leg down to the start position with control; do not let the leg simply drop back to the floor. Lightly tap the floor and immediately repeat the action.

6. Repeat on opposite side.

Specific Benefits

Note As noted in the elbow plank version of this exercise, the top hand can be placed on the top hip, or the top arm can simply lie on top of the body. You can also abduct the top arm as shown for an additional degree of difficulty.

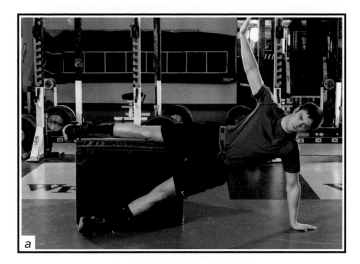

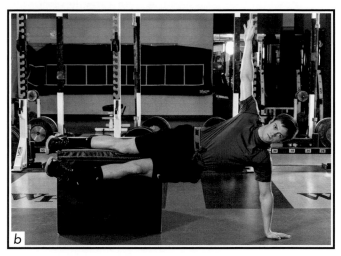

▪ LATERAL ELBOW PLANK ▪
TOP LEG SUPPORT, BOTTOM LEG ADDUCTION, STABILITY BALL

Modifications

1. Lie on one side with the legs straight and the top leg supported on a stability ball (anywhere from the ankle to the hip depending on strength and comfort level).
2. The only contact points throughout the exercise are the medial side of the top leg (from the hip to the foot and any point along this distance) on the stability ball and the bottom elbow and forearm on the floor.
3. The action is the same as for the Lateral Elbow Plank, Top Leg Support, Bottom Leg Adduction.

Specific Benefits ❶ ❺ ⓬ ⓭

▪ LATERAL STRAIGHT-ARM PLANK ▪
TOP LEG SUPPORT, BOTTOM LEG ADDUCTION, STABILITY BALL

Modifications

1. Lie on one side with the legs straight and the top leg supported on a stability ball (anywhere from the ankle to the hip depending on strength and comfort level).
2. Position the bottom hand on the floor directly under the shoulder with the arm perpendicular to the floor.
3. The only contact points throughout the exercise are the medial side of the top leg (from the hip to the foot and any point along this distance) on the stability ball and the bottom hand on the floor.
4. The action is the same as for the Lateral Straight-Arm Plank, Top Leg Support, Bottom Leg Adduction.

Specific Benefits ❶ ❺ ⓬ ⓭

PRONE ROTARY STABILITY
PROGRESSION 1: SINGLE-LEG HIP EXTENSION

MOVEMENTS

1. Position the hands on the floor directly under the shoulders with the arms straight and perpendicular to the floor and the feet about shoulder-width apart.
2. Keeping one foot on the floor, lift the body so the only contact points are the hands on the floor and the ball of one foot and that foot's toes on the floor.
3. Brace the core, maintain a straight spine, engage the glutes, and extend the hip (raise the straight leg off the floor). Avoid extension of the lumbar spine
4. Lower the leg and repeat on the opposite side.
5. Continue the exercise in a rhythmic fashion for a predetermined number of repetitions.

CONSIDERATIONS

1. Maintain straight body alignment (ears, shoulders, hips, knees, and ankles are in a straight line, with no arching or sagging of the midsection). Do not sag hips (do not drop pelvis toward the floor). Do not pike hips (do not arch pelvis and butt toward ceiling).
2. Keep the chin pushed back (think double chin) and avoid dropping the head (cervical vertebrae are straight, with the head tilted neither forward or back).
3. Do not allow any rotational movement at the hips.

SPECIFIC BENEFITS

④ ⑫

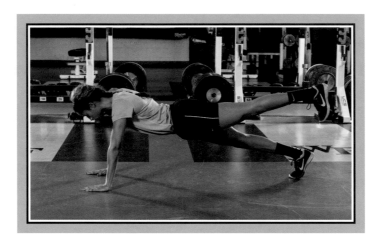

▪ PRONE ROTARY STABILITY ▪
PROGRESSION 2: SINGLE-LEG FULL FLEXION

Modifications

Specific Benefits ⑨ ⑫

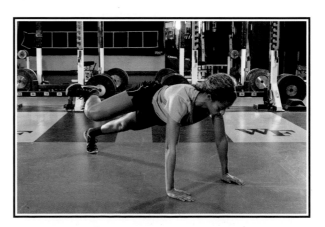

1. Position the hands on the floor directly under the shoulders with the arms straight and perpendicular to the floor and the feet about shoulder-width apart.
2. Brace the core, maintain a straight spine, engage the glutes, and extend one hip off the floor.
3. Flex the hip and the knee. Move the flexed knee toward the chest.
4. Engage the glute complex and rotate the leg outward to a point at which the inner thigh is parallel to the floor.
5. Return the leg back to neutral (midline of parallel to the ground thigh).
6. Lower the leg to the start position.

■ PRONE ROTARY STABILITY ■
PROGRESSION 3: SINGLE-LEG HIP INTERNAL ROTATION AND TAP

Modifications

1. Position the hands on the floor directly under the shoulders with the arms straight and perpendicular to the floor and the feet about shoulder-width apart.
2. Brace the core, maintain a straight spine, engage the glutes, and extend one hip off the floor.
3. Flex at the hip and knee and tuck the leg under the torso.
4. Tap the floor with the foot below the opposite hip (i.e., right foot taps under the left hip; left foot taps under the right hip).

5. Return the leg to neutral (midline of parallel to the ground thigh).
6. Lower the leg to the start position.

Specific Benefits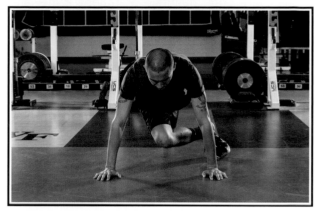

For the following prone upper-body exercises, foot position can have a significant impact on total body stabilization. A wider stance creates more stability; a narrow stance makes for slightly less stability. As proprioceptive awareness improves, strive to use a more narrow stance, but never sacrifice technique or risk injury to create an additional challenge of intensified stress.

■ PRONE ROTARY STABILITY ■
PROGRESSION 4: SINGLE-ARM FULL FLEXION TO TAP

Modifications

1. Position the hands on the floor directly under the shoulders with the arms straight and perpendicular to the floor and the feet about shoulder-width apart.
2. Brace the core, maintain a straight spine, and simply lift one hand off the floor and reach across to tap the opposite shoulder.

3. Avoid rolling in opposition to the removal of one point in the base of support in an effort to reposition body weight and thereby counterbalancing the movement.
4. Maintain straight body alignment throughout.
5. Return the hand to the start position. Either continue with the same arm or alternate arms.

Specific Benefits

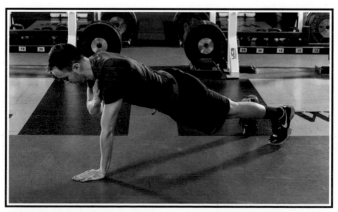

▪ PRONE ROTARY STABILITY ▪
PROGRESSION 5: SINGLE-ARM OVERHEAD SHOULDER FLEHION

Modifications

1. Position the hands on the floor directly under the shoulders with the arms straight and perpendicular to the floor and the feet about shoulder-width apart.
2. Brace the core, maintain a straight spine, and simply lift one hand off the floor and extend that arm (shoulder, elbow, wrist, fingers) directly overhead. The arm should align with the rest of the body (fingers, wrist, elbow, ear, shoulder, hip, knee, ankle all in a straight line).
3. Return the hand to the start position.

Specific Benefits **9** **12**

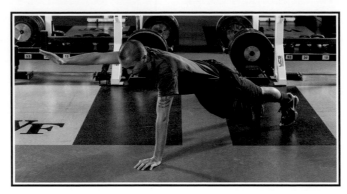

▪ PRONE ROTARY STABILITY ▪
PROGRESSION 6: SINGLE-ARM SHOULDER EHTENSION TO HIP TAP

Modifications

1. Position the hands on the floor directly under the shoulders with the arms straight and perpendicular to the floor and the feet about shoulder-width apart.
2. Brace the core, maintain a straight spine, and simply lift one hand off the floor and reach down to tap the ipsilateral hip.
3. Avoid rolling in opposition to the removal of one point in the base of support in an effort to reposition the body weight and thereby counterbalancing the movement.
4. Maintain straight body alignment throughout.
5. Return the hand to the start position. Either continue with the same arm or alternate arms.

Specific Benefits **9** **12**

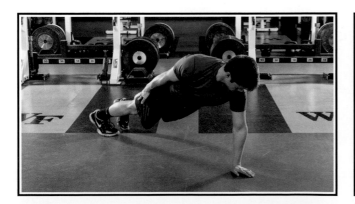

▪ PRONE ROTARY STABILITY ▪
PROGRESSION 7: CONTRALATERAL HIP AND SHOULDER EHTENSION

Modifications

1. Position the hands on the floor directly under the shoulders with the arms straight and perpendicular to the floor and the feet about shoulder-width apart.
2. Brace the core, maintain a straight spine, engage the glutes, extend one hip, and lift that straight leg off the floor.
3. Simultaneously lift the opposite (contralateral) hand off the floor and extend that arm (shoulder, elbow, wrist, fingers) overhead.
4. In the full extension position both the raised leg and the raised arm should be in alignment and parallel to the floor.
5. Return the hand and foot to the start position. Either continue with the same contralateral limbs or alternate sides.

Specific Benefits **4** **11** **12**

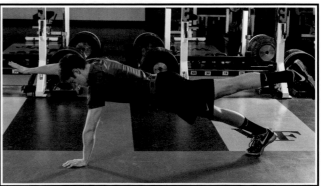

▪ PRONE ROTARY STABILITY ▪
PROGRESSION 8: CONTRALATERAL FOOT TO OPPOSITE HAND

Modifications

1. Position the hands on the floor directly under the shoulders with the arms straight and perpendicular to the floor and the feet about shoulder-width apart.
2. Brace the core, maintain a straight spine, engage the glutes, and extend one hip off the floor.
3. Flex at the hip and knee and tuck the leg under the torso. Tap the floor with the foot as close to the opposite hand (contralateral side) as possible (e.g., right foot taps near the left hand).
4. Return the leg to neutral (midline of parallel to the ground thigh).
5. Lower the leg and foot to the start position. Either continue with the same contralateral limbs or alternate sides.

Specific Benefits

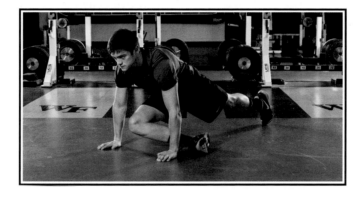

▪ PRONE ROTARY STABILITY ▪
PROGRESSION 9: CONTRALATERAL KNEE TO OPPOSITE ELBOW

Modifications

1. Position the hands on the floor directly under the shoulders with the arms straight and perpendicular to the floor and the feet about shoulder-width apart.
2. Brace the core, maintain a straight spine, engage the glutes, and extend one hip off the floor.
3. Flex at the hip and knee and tuck the leg under the torso. Simultaneously lift the opposite (contralateral) hand off the floor and reach back and under the body with a bent elbow and touch the knee to the elbow underneath the body.
4. Return the arm and leg to the original start position and repeat.

Specific Benefits

▪ PRONE ROTARY STABILITY ▪
PROGRESSION 10: IPSILATERAL ELBOW TO KNEE

Modifications

1. Position the hands on the floor directly under the shoulders with the arms straight and perpendicular to the floor and the feet about shoulder-width apart.
2. Brace the core, engage the glutes, and lift one leg off the floor while simultaneously lifting the same-side (ipsilateral) hand off the floor.
3. Flex the hip and knee and tuck the leg under the torso.
4. In unison, move the up elbow back toward the up knee.
5. Tap at the midpoint and return to the start position. Continue with the same ipsilateral limbs or alternate sides.

Specific Benefits

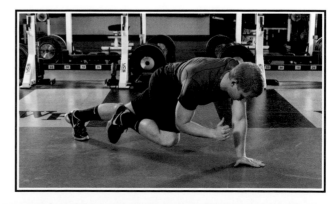

PROGRESSION 1: LOWER BODY ABDUCTION AND ADDUCTION WALK

MOVEMENTS

1. Lie face down in a prone position with the feet together. Place the hands on the floor directly under the shoulders with the arms perpendicular to the floor.
2. Brace the core and lift the body so the only contact points are the hands and the balls of the feet and toes on the floor.
3. In a controlled manner, extend the left hip, lift the left foot up, and place it on the floor lateral and further to the left (abduction).
4. Repeat the same action with the right foot.
5. Return to the start position by reversing the action. Lift the left foot up and move it back medially to the neutral position (adduction), followed by the same action with the right foot.
6. Perform for a predetermined set of repetitions or time interval.

CONSIDERATIONS

1. Lock the knees, engage the glutes, and brace the core.
2. Maintain a solid core throughout (when appropriate, shoulders, hips, knees, and ankles are all in alignment with no arching, sagging, or rolling of the midsection).
3. Move only as fast and step only as far as the body can control without sacrificing technique.

SPECIFIC BENEFITS

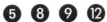

5 8 9 12

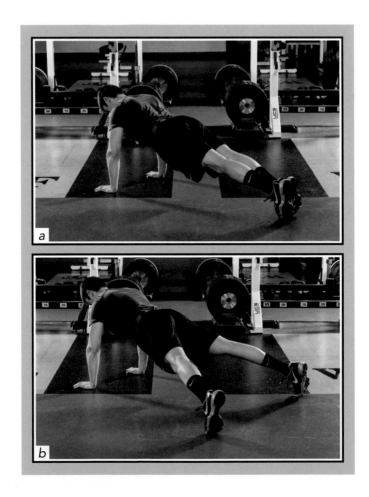

■ STRAIGHT-ARM PLANK DISPLACEMENT SERIES ■
PROGRESSION 2: UPPER BODY ABDUCTION AND ADDUCTION WALK

Modifications

1. Assume the straight-arm plank start position as described for Progression 1. The only difference might be a slightly wider foot placement for additional stabilization, if necessary. Remember to always brace the core and maintain proper body alignment.

2. In a controlled manner, raise the left hand and place it back on the floor lateral and further to the left (abduction).

3. Repeat the same action with the right hand.

4. Return to the start position by reversing the action. Lift the left hand up and move it back medially to the neutral position (adduction), followed by the same action with the right hand.

Specific Benefits

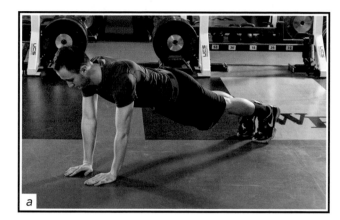

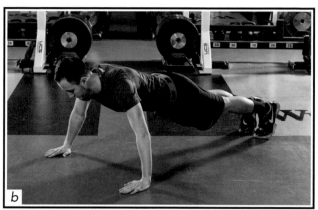

■ STRAIGHT-ARM PLANK DISPLACEMENT SERIES ■
PROGRESSION 3: UPPER AND LOWER BODY ABDUCTION AND ADDUCTION WALK

Modifications

1. Assume the straight-arm plank start position as described for Progression 1. The only difference might be a slightly wider foot placement for additional stabilization, if necessary. Remember to always brace the core and maintain proper body alignment.

2. In a controlled manner, lift the left hand and the right leg simultaneously. Move both laterally and place them back on the floor further to the left and to the right, respectively (abduction).

3. Repeat the action with the right hand and left leg.

4. Return to the start position by reversing the action. The left hand and right leg move back to neutral, followed by the right hand and left leg.

Specific Benefits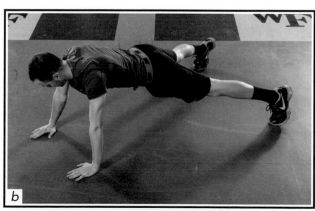

Note Try these variations:

- Left hand simultaneous with left foot; right hand simultaneous with right foot
- Left hand; right hand; left foot; right foot
- Left hand; right foot, right hand; left foot
- Right and left double-hand jump; right and left double-foot jump (be cautious; perform on a soft surface)

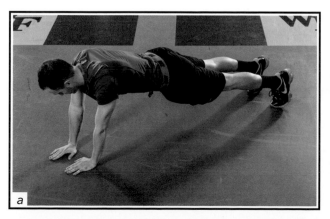

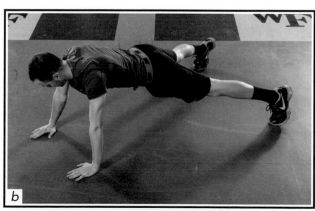

▪ STRAIGHT-ARM PLANK DISPLACEMENT SERIES ▪
PROGRESSION 4: UPPER AND LOWER BODY ABDUCTION AND ADDUCTION CRAB WALK

Modifications

1. Assume the straight-arm plank start position as described for Progression 1. The only difference might be a slightly wider foot placement for additional stabilization, if necessary. Remember to always brace the core and maintain proper body alignment.

2. In a controlled manner, lift the left hand and left leg simultaneously. Move both laterally and place them back on the floor further to the left (abduction).

3. Lift the right hand and right leg and move them also to the left. (Yes, to the left.)

4. Repeat with the left extremities followed by the right extremities.

5. Perform for a predetermined number of repetitions or time interval, or for a set distance. Be sure to train the other direction to avoid creating imbalances.

Specific Benefits ❺ ❼ ❽ ❾ ❿ ⓬

Note There are many varieties of the crab walk. Some variations follow. Assume that movement in a set is always in one direction. Here all instructions for movement will be to the left, but be sure to work both directions.

- Left hand simultaneous with right leg; right hand simultaneous with left leg
- Left hand; right hand; left leg; right leg
- Crab walk forward
- Crab walk backward
- Crab walk diagonal
- Crab walk combination movements (on command)
- Crab walk from a low position (elbows flexed under 90 degrees—crazy hard, even for a crab)

▪ STRAIGHT-ARM PLANK DISPLACEMENT SERIES ▪
PROGRESSION 5: UPPER AND LOWER BODY CIRCLE PIVOT WALK

Modifications

1. Assume the straight-arm plank start position as described for Progression 1. The only difference might be a slightly wider foot placement for additional stabilization, if necessary. Remember to always brace the core and maintain proper body alignment.

2. In a controlled manner, lift the left hand and left leg simultaneously. Move both laterally and place them back on the floor further to the left (abduction), but be sure to move the lower body further than the upper body (because the goal of the exercise is to walk in a circle).

3. Continuing, lift the right hand and right leg and move them also to the left.

4. Repeat with the left extremities, followed by the right extremities.

5. Continue for a predetermined length of time or number of revolutions. Train both clockwise and counterclockwise.

Specific Benefits ❺ ❼ ❽ ❾ ❿ ⓬

Note Some variations are as follows:

- Straight-arm plank with hands on a medicine ball
- Straight-arm plank with hands on a stability ball
- Straight-arm plank with hands on a plyometric box
- This is a great drill for some perturbation activity

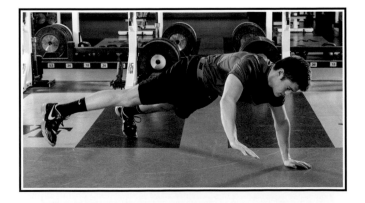

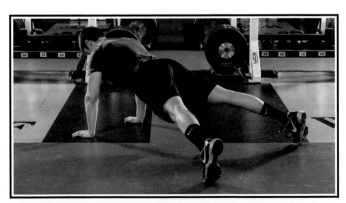

LOW PRONE PLANK SPIDER-MAN

MOVEMENTS

1. Position the hands on the floor directly under the shoulders with the arms perpendicular to the floor. Feet are approximately shoulder-width apart.

2. Lower the body to a position that is challenging yet comfortable enough to complete the exercise without sacrificing technique. At the highest point, the arms are straight. At the lowest point, the elbows are bent below 90 degrees with the chest merely inches from the floor.

3. Only the balls of the feet, toes, and the hands contact the floor. Maintain straight body alignment (ears, shoulders, hips, knees, and ankles are in a straight line). Do not sag or pike the hips.

4. Lift one foot off the floor and drive the knee toward the elbow. The goal is to touch the knee to the same-side elbow. During the movement, the entire leg remains low, to the side (lateral), and parallel to the floor.

5. Return the leg and foot to the start position. Immediately repeat with the opposite leg.

6. Perform for a predetermined number of repetitions or time interval.

CONSIDERATIONS

1. Until strength improves, elbows might progressively move from straight arm to greater than 90 degrees, to 90 degrees, to less than 90 degrees.

2. The exercise resembles and feels like a floating army crawl.

3. As strength improves, try this exercise with both hands on an unstable surface.

SPECIFIC BENEFITS

 5 **9** **12**

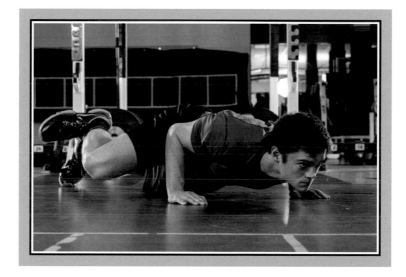

▪ LOW PRONE PLANK SPIDER-MAN PUSH-UP ▪

Modifications

Note: This is the same exercise as the Low Prone Plank Spider-Man with the simple addition of a push-up after each bilateral movement (i.e., left leg, right leg, push-up, repeat).

1. Position the hands on the floor directly under the shoulders with the arms perpendicular to the floor.

2. Only the balls of the feet, toes, and the hands contact the floor.

3. From a straight-arm plank, lower to a push-up plank position. (Because a straight body alignment is critical, strength level will dictate the level of elbow flexion in the push-up position.)

4. Move the right knee to the right elbow, return, the left knee to the left elbow, and return.

5. Press back to the straight-arm start position

Specific Benefits   ⑫

Note As strength improves, try this exercise with both hands on an unstable surface.

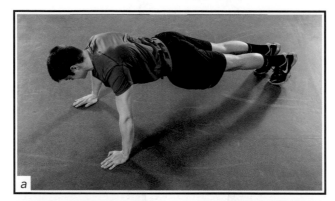

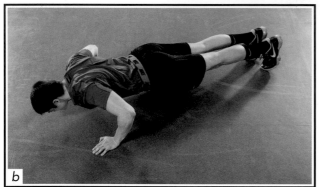

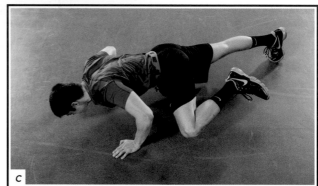

CONDITIONING TO THE CORE

Scapulothoracic Exercises

To understand why scapular stability is so important you must first understand how the scapula moves. The scapulae have the capacity to negotiate every possible direction due to their unique placement and attachment to the posterior of the rib cage. They essentially can function in three dimensions, allowing for both anterior tipping as well as posterior tipping. In a more rotational fashion, the scapulae move inward and outward and upward and downward. Finally through force couple and synergistic relationships with 17 other muscles, the scapulae can both elevate and depress.

Considering how much free movement is available to the scapula, it is amazing that its only true boney attachment points are the acromioclavicular (AC) joint and a few ligaments. Due to these attachment points and anatomical location, however, the scapula makes up half of the glenohumeral joint and becomes the foundation for the shoulder. Therefore, any distorted scapula function or inability to stabilize the scapula in an appropriate position (appropriate to the task at hand) results in a direct effect on the shoulder joint with severe consequences. There are a plethora of problems that stem from

glenohumeral instability, the biggest of which include arthritis, impingement, rotator cuff tendinitis or tendinosis, or tears as well as a variety of labral damage.

Knowing that the scapulae must be able to freely move into correct positions and when there stabilize quickly and adequately makes the exercises in this chapter all the more important. Remember, stability is not just about the ability to hold static positions but also the ability for a joint system to control itself in the presence of change. All of the following exercises may involve larger muscles such as the deltoids driving the movement, but at all times appropriate scapulae positioning and the ability to stabilize in those positions is vital to each activity. Once again this concept works with our continuum planning of local stabilizer training prior to global mobilizer training as well as stability gains coming before strength and finally power.

The following exercise finder lists the benefits, difficulty level, and equipment needed for every exercise that appears in this chapter. Primary exercises are highlighted in beige, with their progressions in blue. The primary exercises are also noted in the text with a blue title bar.

Scapulothoracic Stability Exercise Finder

Exercise Name	Specific Benefits (see chapter 5)	Difficulty Level			Equipment
		Easy	Medium	Hard	
Prone Scaption (Y), Floor	❺	X			
Prone Scaption (Y), Incline Bench	❷ ❺	X			Bench
Prone Scaption (Y), Stability Ball	❶ ❺		X		Stability ball
Prone Shoulder Abduction (T), Floor	❺	X			
Prone Shoulder Abduction (T), Incline Bench	❷ ❺	X			Bench
Prone Shoulder Abduction (T), Stability Ball	❶ ❺		X		Stability ball
Prone Scapular Retraction and Depression (A), Floor	❺	X			
Prone Scapular Retraction and Depression (A), Incline Bench	❷ ❺	X			Bench
Prone Scapular Retraction and Depression (A), Stability Ball	❶ ❺		X		Stability ball
Prone Scapulothoracic Combination (YTA), Floor	❺ ⑱	X			
Prone Scapulothoracic Combination (YTA), Incline Bench	❷ ❺ ⑱	X			Bench
Prone Scapulothoracic Combination (YTA), Stability Ball	❶ ❺ ⑱		X		Stability ball

MOVEMENTS

1. Lie face down on the floor (prone position) with the feet together.
2. Outstretch the arms to form a Y position. The hands must be in a neutral (thumbs-up) position. This is critically important.
3. Throughout the exercise, keep the chin pushed back (think double chin) and avoid dropping the head (cervical vertebrae are straight, with the head tilted neither forward or back), keep the chest on the floor, and depress and retract the scapulae.
4. From the floor, raise the arms up to a Y position.
5. Lower the arms to the start position.
6. Perform a predetermined number of repetitions.

CONSIDERATIONS

1. The shoulder blades remain depressed and retracted throughout the exercise.
2. Avoid the chicken head. Do not lift and then extend the head and neck in opposition to the arm raise.
3. Raise the arms as high as comfortably possible without additional body compensation.

SPECIFIC BENEFITS

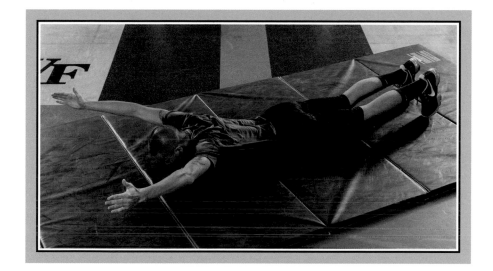

▪ PRONE SCAPTION (Y) ▪
INCLINE BENCH

Modifications

1. Lie face down on an incline bench. The legs are straight with the feet securely on the floor.
2. Throughout the exercise, keep the chin pushed back (think double chin) and avoid dropping the head (cervical vertebrae are straight, with the head tilted neither forward or back), keep the chest on the bench, and depress and retract the scapulae.

3. From the incline bench, raise the arms up to a Y position.
4. Lower the arms to the start position.

Specific Benefits

▪ PRONE SCAPTION (Y) ▪
STABILITY BALL

Modifications

1. Lie face down on a stability ball. The legs are straight with the feet securely on the floor.
2. Throughout the exercise, keep the chin pushed back (think double chin) and avoid dropping the head (cervical vertebrae are straight, with the head tilted neither forward or back), keep the chest on the ball, and depress and retract the scapulae.

3. From the stability ball, raise the arms up to a Y position.
4. Lower the arms to the start position.

Specific Benefits

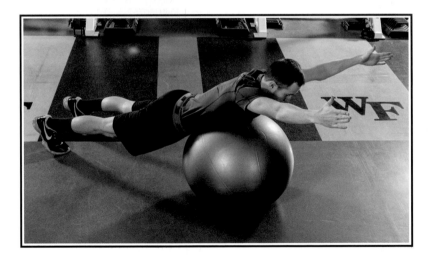

PRONE SHOULDER ABDUCTION (T)

FLOOR

MOVEMENTS

1. Lie face down on the floor (prone position) with the feet together.
2. Outstretch the arms to form a T position (90-degree angle to the body, palms down). The hand position is critically important.
3. Throughout the exercise, keep the chin pushed back (think double chin) and avoid dropping the head (cervical vertebrae are straight, with the head tilted neither forward or back), keep the chest on the floor, and depress and retract the scapulae.
4. From the floor, raise the arms up to a T position.
5. Lower the arms to the start position.
6. Perform a predetermined number of repetitions.

CONSIDERATIONS

1. The shoulder blades remain depressed and retracted throughout the exercise.
2. With arms raised and outstretched, draw arms inward (squeeze shoulder blades together).
3. Avoid the chicken head. Do not lift and then extend the head and neck in opposition to the arm raise.
4. Raise the arms as high as comfortably possible without additional body compensation.

SPECIFIC BENEFITS

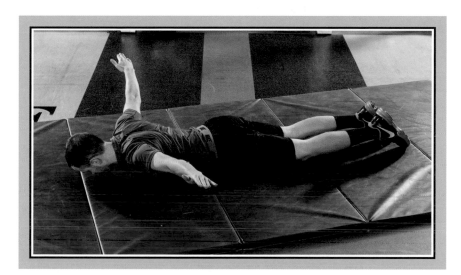

■ PRONE SHOULDER ABDUCTION (T) ■

INCLINE BENCH

Modifications

1. Lie face down on an incline bench. The legs are straight with the feet securely on the floor.
2. Throughout the exercise, keep the chin pushed back (think double chin) and avoid dropping the head (cervical vertebrae are straight, with the head tilted neither forward or back), keep the chest on the bench, and depress and retract the scapulae.

3. From the incline bench, raise the arms up to a T position.
4. Lower the arms to the start position

Specific Benefits

■ PRONE SHOULDER ABDUCTION (T) ■
STABILITY BALL

Modifications

1. Lie face down on a stability ball. The legs are straight with the feet securely on the floor.
2. Throughout the exercise, keep the chin pushed back (think double chin) and avoid dropping the head (cervical vertebrae are straight, with the head tilted neither forward or back), keep the chest on the ball, and depress and retract the scapulae.

3. From the stability ball, raise the arms up to a T position.
4. Lower the arms to the start position.

Specific Benefits

PRONE SCAPULAR RETRACTION AND DEPRESSION (A)
FLOOR

MOVEMENTS

1. Lie face down on the floor (prone position) with the feet together.
2. The arms are straight and close to the sides of the body, resembling the letter A. The palms are down at the start of the exercise.
3. Throughout the exercise, keep the chin pushed back (think double chin) and avoid dropping the head (cervical vertebrae are straight, with the head tilted neither forward or back), keep the chest on the floor, and depress and retract the scapulae.
4. Raise the arms up from the floor. During the lift, externally rotate the straight arms from the shoulder so that the thumbs point up and out.

5. Lower the arms to the start position.
6. Perform a predetermined number of repetitions.

CONSIDERATIONS

1. The shoulder blades remain depressed and retracted throughout the exercise.
2. Raise the arms as high as comfortably possible without additional body compensation.

SPECIFIC BENEFITS

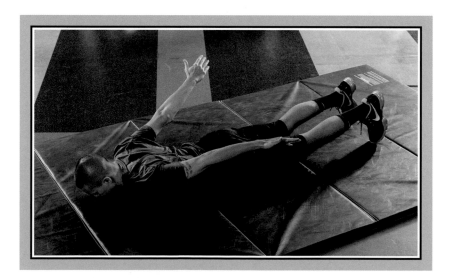

■ PRONE SCAPULAR RETRACTION AND DEPRESSION (A) ■
INCLINE BENCH

Modifications

1. Lie face down on an incline bench. The legs are straight with the feet securely on the floor.
2. Throughout the exercise, keep the chin pushed back (think double chin) and avoid dropping the head (cervical vertebrae are straight, with the head tilted neither forward or back), keep the chest on the bench, and depress and retract the scapulae.

3. Raise the arms up from the bench. During the lift, externally rotate the straight-arms from the shoulder so that the thumbs point up and out.
4. Lower the arms to the start position.

Specific Benefits ❷ ❺

■ PRONE SCAPULAR RETRACTION AND DEPRESSION (A) ■
STABILITY BALL

Modifications

1. Lie face down on a stability ball. The legs are straight with the feet securely on the floor.
2. Throughout the exercise, keep the chin pushed back (think double chin) and avoid dropping the head (cervical vertebrae are straight, with the head tilted neither forward or back), keep the chest on the ball, and depress and retract the scapulae.

3. Raise the arms up from the stability ball. During the lift, externally rotate the straight arms from the shoulder so that the thumbs point up and out.
4. Lower the arms to the start position.

Specific Benefits   ❺

PRONE SCAPULOTHORACIC COMBINATION (YTA)
FLOOR

MOVEMENTS

1. Lie face down on the floor (prone position) with the feet together.
2. Outstretch the arms to form a Y position. The hands must be in a neutral (thumbs-up) position. This is critically important.
3. Throughout the exercise, keep the chin pushed back (think double chin) and avoid dropping the head (cervical vertebrae are straight, with the head tilted neither forward or back), keep the chest on the floor, and depress and retract the scapulae.
4. To start this three-part action, first, from the floor, raise the arms up to a Y position. Lower the arms to the start position.
5. Now immediately reposition the arms to form a T (90-degree angle to the body, palms down). From the floor, raise the arms up to a T position. Lower the arms to the start position.

6. Again, immediately reposition the arms to form an A (arms straight and close to the sides of the body, palms down). Raise the arms up from the floor keeping the arms outstretched and scapula drawn inward. During the lift, externally rotate the straight arms from the shoulder so that the thumbs point up and out. Return the hands to the floor and rotate the palms down.
7. Move to the original start (Y) position.
8. Perform a predetermined number of repetitions.

CONSIDERATIONS

1. The shoulder blades remain depressed and retracted throughout the exercise.
2. Raise the arms as high as comfortably possible without additional body compensation

SPECIFIC BENEFITS

▪ PRONE SCAPULOTHORACIC COMBINATION (YTA) ▪
INCLINE BENCH

Modifications

1. Lie face down on an incline bench. The legs are straight with the feet securely on the floor.
2. Throughout the exercise, keep the chin pushed back (think double chin) and avoid dropping the head (cervical vertebrae are straight, with the head tilted neither forward or back), keep the chest on the bench, and depress and retract the scapulae.

3. Perform the same movements as described for the Prone Scapulothoracic Combination (YTA), Floor.

Specific Benefits ❷ ❺ ⓲

▪ PRONE SCAPULOTHORACIC COMBINATION (YTA) ▪
STABILITY BALL

Modifications

1. Lie face down on a stability ball. The legs are straight with the feet securely on the floor.
2. Throughout the exercise, keep the chin pushed back (think double chin) and avoid dropping the head (cervical vertebrae are straight, with the head tilted neither forward or back), keep the chest on the ball, and depress and retract the scapulae.

3. Perform the same movements as described for the Prone Scapulothoracic Combination (YTA), Floor.

Specific Benefits ❶ ❺ ⓲

Lumbo-Pelvic Hip Exercises

You would be hard pressed to find a coach, trainer, or physical therapist who does not generalize the lumbo-pelvic hip complex (LPHC) as simply "the core." With 29 muscles attached in the area, the core's importance, from a stabilization and mobilizing perspective, has been well documented. Effective functional kinematics would not be possible without the efficient length–tension relationship and force couple characteristics associated with the synergistic relationship between the deep stabilizers and outer mobilizers of the LPHC.

Assuming a positive functional assessment outcome (to be discussed further in chapter 18) and that the athlete is free of significant inhibitions that might result from muscle imbalance or back pain, he or she may begin the LPHC exercise program. Establishing and maintaining dynamic control from a neutral pelvis through a neutral spine right up to, and including, a neutral head is of critical importance. Any instability along the core chain will decrease functional performance. Likewise, because the core stabilizers are primarily type I oxidative fibers, all training must be relatively specific to the predominant system being stressed. Thus, time-under-tension has been prominently considered in the ensuing program design. Muscle endurance, and ultimately prolonged core equilibrium, will facilitate spinal stability for a prolonged duration, allowing for high-level performance without the fear of structural breakdown caused by fatigue. This structural breakdown can certainly contribute to less than effective performance and possibly compensation injury.

When performing the exercises described in this program (or any other exercises you choose to do), always train specific to the associated physiology and the movement requirements inherent to the structure being addressed. Your exercise program should be integrated and progressively demanding from simple bracing techniques necessary to establish spinal neutrality and dynamic postural control, to complex and proprioceptively challenging, multiplanar, load-bearing patterns. Always stress quality over quantity; never sacrifice form and function for additional load, sets, or repetitions.

The following exercise finder lists the benefits, difficulty level, and equipment needed for every exercise that appears in this chapter. Primary exercises are highlighted in beige, with their progressions in blue. The primary exercises are also noted in the text with a blue title bar.

Lumbo-Pelvic Hip Stability Exercise Finder

Exercise Name	Specific Benefits (see chapter 5)	Difficulty Level			Equipment
		Easy	Medium	Hard	
Bridge on Floor	⑫	X			
Bridge on Floor With Resistance Band	❺ ⑰	X			Mini-band
Bridge on Floor With Medicine Ball	❺ ⑰	X			Medicine ball
Unilateral Bridge	❾		X		Tennis ball
Bridge on Stability Ball	❶	X			Stability ball
Bridge on Stability Ball With Resistance Band	❶ ❺ ⑰	X			Stability ball, mini-band
Bridge on Stability Ball With Medicine Ball	❶ ❺ ⑰	X			Stability ball, medicine ball
Single-Leg Bridge on Stability Ball	❶ ❾		X		Stability ball
Hip Lift on Stability Ball	❶ ❸	X			Stability ball
Single-Leg Hip Lift on Stability Ball	❶ ❸ ❾		X		Stability ball
Foundational Core Squat Series Progression 1: Prisoner Squat	⑫	X			
Foundational Core Squat Series Progression 2: Overhead Squat	⑫	X			Broomstick, PVC pipe
Single-Leg Balance	❾	X			
Single-Leg Balance and Reach	❹ ❺ ❾ ⑫ ⑱ ㉔	X			

MOVEMENTS

1. Lie face up (supine) on the floor with the knees bent. Feet are flat on the floor and the toes are pointing slightly in. Hands are on the hips.
2. Simultaneously contract the glutes and brace the core.
3. Smoothly raise the hips off the floor until fully extended, but not hyperextended (avoid extreme lumbar arch).
4. All contact points, including both feet (slightly toed in), shoulders, and the back of the head, are on the floor.
5. Return to the start position by slowly lowering the hips back to the floor.
6. Perform for a predetermined number of repetitions or time interval.

CONSIDERATIONS

1. Avoid excessive pressure on the head and neck. Maintain most of the load on the shoulders.
2. If excessive tightening of the upper hamstrings or lower back is felt, return to the starting point, reposition and try again. Discontinue this and all other drills if excessive tightness or pain persists.

SPECIFIC BENEFITS

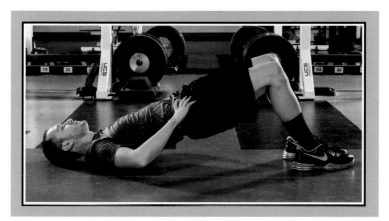

■ BRIDGE ON FLOOR ■
WITH RESISTANCE BAND

Modifications

1. Lie face up on the floor with a rubber resistance band positioned slightly above the knees.
2. Follow the steps as described for Bridge on Floor with the addition of a co-contraction of the hip abductors, forcing the knees lateral against the band resistance.

Specific Benefits ❺ ⓱

Note

- Ensure the knees do not collapse inward into a valgus (knock-kneed) position.
- Select a resistance that is appropriate for your present strength level. Never sacrifice technique for added resistance. Progressive overload is exactly that—progressive.

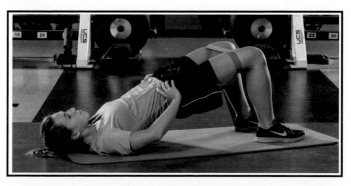

▪ BRIDGE ON FLOOR ▪
WITH MEDICINE BALL

Modifications

1. Lie face up on the floor and place a medicine ball between the knees.
2. Follow the steps as described for Bridge on Floor, with the addition of a co-contraction of the hip adductors, firmly squeezing inward against the ball.

Specific Benefits ⑤ ⑰

Note

• Ensure the knees do not collapse inward into a valgus (knock-kneed) position.
• Select a resistance that is appropriate for your present strength level. Never sacrifice technique for added resistance. Progressive overload is exactly that—progressive.

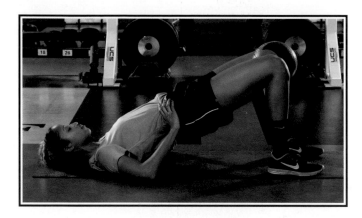

▪ UNILATERAL BRIDGE ▪

Modifications

1. Lie face up on the floor with one knee drawn toward the chest.
2. Hold onto the bent knee with both hands below the knee; maintain this position throughout the exercise. If you feel any discomfort or have a history of knee problems (specifically patellar tendon issues), rather than pulling from on top of the knee as shown, alternatively place the hands under the knee thereby pulling against the upper hamstring as opposed to pulling from the top of the knee itself.
3. Perform for a predetermined number of repetitions or time interval and repeat on the opposite side.

Specific Benefits ⑨

Note In the photo we show a tennis ball between the thigh and ribcage, which provides a gauge for maintaining appropriate body mechanics, but the exercise can be done without the ball. Be sure to focus on proper alignment and positioning throughout.

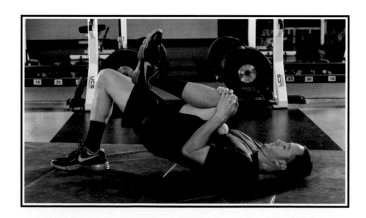

Along with influencing the common variations of load, repetitions, sets, and drill duration, the following bridge exercises with a stability ball can be additionally intensified through the manipulation of the body's orientation. For example, the position of the arms or legs will shift the center of mass, which will then further challenge the adaptive qualities of this, or any other, exercise. For example, with the hands on hips, the drill is fairly straightforward. However, when the limbs are moved to various positions away from the body's centerline, this unassuming modification can make a simple drill progressively more difficult. The following alternatives will progressively make a relatively uncomplicated drill more challenging.

1. Arms abducted in the various planes
2. Symmetrical and asymmetrical arm position
3. Holding onto weighted devices
4. Catching tossed balls
5. Pulling or pressing rubber power bands
6. Partner assisted perturbation techniques.

▪ BRIDGE ON STABILITY BALL ▪

Modifications

1. Lie face up on a stability ball with the shoulders and head supported by the ball and the low back and hips hanging toward the floor (but not touching the floor).
2. The only contact points are both feet flat on the floor (slightly toed in) and the shoulders and back of the head on the stability ball.

3. Smoothly raise the hips off the floor until fully extended, but not hyperextended (avoid extreme lumbar arch). In the up position, the knees should be bent at about 90 degrees and the torso parallel to floor.

Specific Benefits ❶

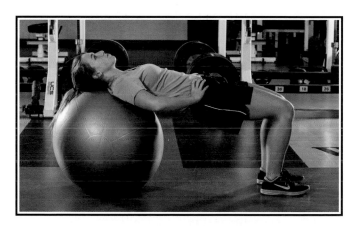

▪ BRIDGE ON STABILITY BALL ▪
WITH RESISTANCE BAND

Modifications

1. Begin in a standing position; place a rubber resistance band slightly above and around both knees.
2. Follow the steps as described for Bridge on Stability ball; with the addition of a co-contraction of the hip abductors, forcing knees lateral against band resistance.

Specific Benefits ❶ ❺ ⓱

Note Ensure the knees do not collapse inward into a valgus (knock-kneed) position.

Select a resistance that is appropriate for your present strength level. Never sacrifice technique for added resistance. Progressive overload is exactly that—progressive.

■ BRIDGE ON STABILITY BALL ■
WITH MEDICINE BALL

Modifications

1. Lie face up on a stability ball with the shoulders and head supported by the ball and the low back and hips hanging toward the floor (but not touching the floor) and place a medicine ball between the knees.

2. Follow the steps as described for Bridge on Stability Ball, with the addition of a co-contraction of the hip adductors, firmly squeezing inward against the ball.

Specific Benefits **1** **5** **17**

■ SINGLE-LEG BRIDGE ON STABILITY BALL ■

Modifications

1. Lie face up (supine) on a stability ball with the shoulders and head supported by the ball and the low back and hips hanging toward the floor (but not touching the floor).

2. Smoothly raise the hips off the floor until fully extended, but not hyperextended (avoid extreme lumbar arch). In the up position, the knees should be bent at about 90 degrees and the torso parallel to the floor.

3. While in the up position, extend one leg until it is approximately parallel to the floor. In this position, the only contact points are one foot flat on floor and the shoulders and back of the head on the stability ball.

4. Return that leg to the floor and either continue with the same leg or perform the action with alternating legs.

Specific Benefits **1** **9**

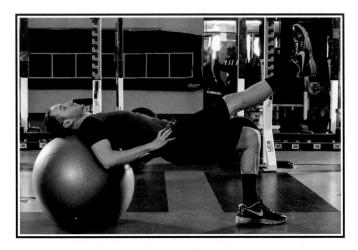

CONDITIONING TO THE CORE

HIP LIFT ON STABILITY BALL

MOVEMENTS

1. Lie face up on the floor with the knees bent, heels directly on top of the stability ball, toes pointing to the ceiling (foot dorsiflexed), and the hands on the hips.
2. Contract the glutes and brace the core.
3. Smoothly raise the hips off the floor until fully extended, but not hyperextended (avoid extreme lumbar arch). The knees, hips, and shoulders are in a straight line. While in the up position, the knees should be bent about 90 degrees.
4. In the up position, the knees should be bent about 90 degrees, and the contact points are the heels of both feet on the top of the stability ball and the shoulders and back of the head on the floor.
5. Return to the start position by slowly lowering the hips back to the floor.
6. Perform for a predetermined number of repetitions or time interval.

CONSIDERATIONS

1. Avoid excessive pressure on the head and neck. Maintain most of the load on the shoulders.
2. If excessive tightening of the upper hamstrings or lower back is felt, return to the starting point, reposition, and try again. If the tightness does not dissipate, discontinue the drill.
3. For the novice, this is a challenging drill. Arm position can have a tremendous influence on total body balance and ultimately the success of the drill. The following are a few examples of progressively demanding stabilization techniques.

   a. For greatest stability, extend the arms perpendicular to the body with the palms down.
   b. For a lesser degree of stability, place the arms next to the sides of the body with palms down and eventually, palms up.
   c. For an even greater challenge, hold the arms completely off the floor.

SPECIFIC BENEFITS

 ❶ ❸

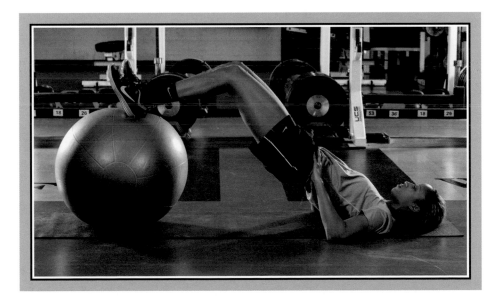

Modifications

1. Start in the same position as Hip Lift on Stability Ball. Lift one leg completely off the ball. This leg will remain flexed at the hip throughout the exercise.

2. Smoothly raise the hips off the floor until fully extended, but not hyperextended (avoid extreme lumbar arch). The knee (of the foot that is on the ball), hip, and shoulder are in a straight line. While in the up position, the knee (of the foot on the ball) should be bent at about 90 degrees.

3. In the up position, the contact points are one foot on top of the stability ball and the shoulders and back of the head on the floor. The noncontact knee remains floating, flexed at the hip.

Specific Benefits ❶ ❸ ❾

Note The extremely unstable complexity of this drill will greatly challenge the athlete's kinesthesis and more fully develop their proprioceptive responsiveness. All balance suggestions mentioned in Hip Lift on Stability Ball apply.

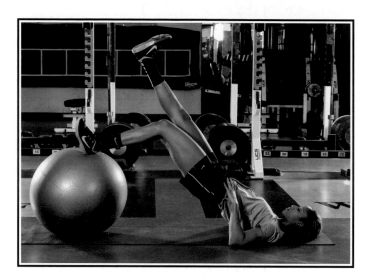

PROGRESSION 1: PRISONER SQUAT

MOVEMENTS

1. Stand erect with the shoulders retracted. Feet are slightly wider than shoulder width, parallel, and pointing forward.
2. Place hands behind the head. Pull elbows backward with the chest out.
3. Maintain a neutral or slightly anterior pelvic tilt throughout. Avoid extreme anterior pelvic tilt.
4. Brace the core and sit down and back into a squat. Co-contract the low back, glutes, quads, hamstrings, and calves, all the while maintaining a neutral or slightly anterior pelvic tilt. The body moves as one complete unit.
5. Return to the start position; perform a predetermined number of repetitions.

CONSIDERATIONS

1. With appropriate technique and supervision, the squat can be a safe and effective total-body strength developer. Also, research strongly suggests the squat can be a significant deterrent to serial distortion patterns, specifically knee injury and chronic back pain. As with any new training, always be aware of variables (e.g., fatigue, improper technique, preexisting structural abnormalities) that can affect the effectiveness and safety of this multijoint, total body exercise.

2. When the thighs reach parallel to the floor, or just below, stop the downward movement.
3. The butt should be comfortably at or behind heels, which places the knees over the midpoint of the foot
4. When returning to the start position, the body moves as a single unit. Don't let the lower body get ahead of the upper body or vice versa.
5. To ensure proper weight distribution during the drop phase, try lifting your big toes slightly (but avoid rocking back completely onto the heels).

SPECIFIC BENEFITS

 12

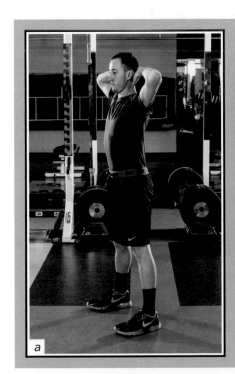
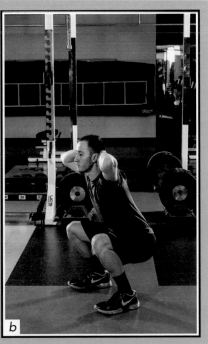

Modifications

1. Stand erect with the shoulders retracted. Feet are slightly wider than shoulder width, parallel, and pointing forward.
2. With an overhand grip, grasp a light bar (or a broomstick or PVC pipe) and raise the bar directly overhead. If possible, hold the bar slightly behind the head. Hands should be positioned comfortably at least "Y" distance apart (slightly wider if possible).
3. Brace the core and sit down and back into a squat. Keep the elbows locked with the bar overhead throughout the exercise.

Specific Benefits

SINGLE-LEG BALANCE

MOVEMENTS

1. Stand erect with the shoulders retracted. Feet are parallel and flat on floor, pointing forward. Hands are on the hips.
2. Brace the core; flex the hips and knees to a squat of about three-quarter depth. Actual squat depth will be dictated by athlete strength and joint range of motion.
3. Lift one foot off the floor and shift the center of mass over the base of support (the foot on the ground).
4. Maintain the squat position, balance, and body control for a predetermined amount of time.
5. Return to the start position; repeat on opposite leg.

CONSIDERATIONS

1. Keep the chin pushed back (think double chin) and avoid dropping the head (cervical vertebrae are straight, with the head tilted neither forward or back).
2. Keep the toe of the raised foot pointed upward (dorsiflexed) throughout the duration of the drill.

SPECIFIC BENEFITS

9

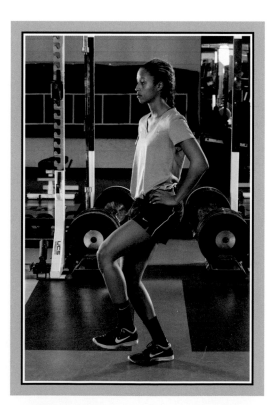

Modifications

1. Begin in a neutral three-quarter squat, single-leg position as described for the primary exercise, Single-Leg Balance.
2. Maintaining balance, reach forward with the up leg and tap the floor with that foot.
3. Return back to the neutral position.
4. Maintaining balance, reach out laterally with same up foot as far as possible without losing balance or compromising form. Tap the floor.
5. Return back to the neutral position.

6. Finally, open your hip and reach to the side and behind you (transverse plane). Tap the floor and return to the neutral start position. (Note that this movement can cause torque stress to the joints of the support leg, so caution is warranted.) Continue with the same leg for a predetermined number of repetitions or time interval.
7. Repeat on the opposite leg.

Specific Benefits ❹ ❺ ❾ ⓬ ⓲ ㉔

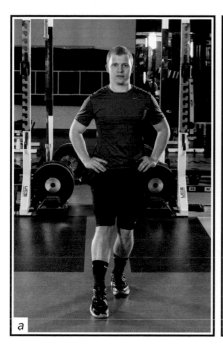
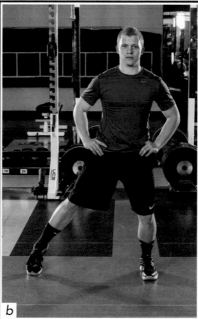
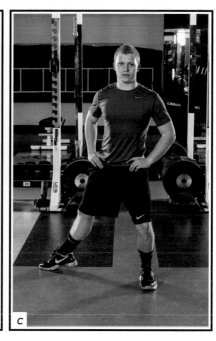

III

CORE STRENGTH TRAINING

There should be no doubt that core stabilization is a critical building block to athletic aptitude. That said, the ability to overcome greater external resistance, such as that encountered in sport, becomes progressively more important once a stable foundation has been established.

As we mentioned in the introduction and chapter 3, the body's capacity for athletic output is affected by each level of a performance-training paradigm—one in which high levels of stability, strength, and power are sequentially realized. None of these qualities occurs alone; rather, each works synergistically with the others. Thus the distinction is not in their individual contribution but in the effective functioning of their combination. Each of these variables is as important as the other, and so must be trained accordingly and with equal attention respective to individual needs. The body will be only as strong as it is stable and will allow a high power output only from a platform of strength. If one area lacks equivalent development or is neglected entirely, performance capability will never reach its full potential.

This is often the missing link with many athletes. They have phenomenal individual skills, such as a killer forehand, a 16-foot jump shot, or great hands for catching a football. But if an athlete can't get to the ball no one will see her great forehand, if an athlete can't elude the defender he won't get off the jumper, and if the receiver is unable to shake the cornerback the pass will be intercepted. To fully develop your athleticism, a total training concept must include all variables of physicality. While you can give less emphasis to areas of greater aptitude, greater importance should be placed on your limitations. However, just because you possess superior skills with one specific component doesn't mean that it should be ignored entirely. Continued development of your strengths will in fact take place as other, less robust, capacities play catch up.

THE RELATIONSHIP BETWEEN STRENGTH AND FORCE

Nearly every situation in athletics requires an athlete to cope with external forces that can either positively or negatively affect performance. These events can be as obvious as two wrestlers grappling or as subtle as a swimmer fighting the drag forces created by water.

Collision sports such as rugby are excellent for visualizing the need for core strength, primarily from a force-production and force-reduction perspective and, in many cases, from a safety standpoint (force absorption). Over the course of a contest, the main function of the core is to deal constantly with the task of effectively redistributing ground reaction forces. Inevitably, the ferocity of an open-field tackle will occur, requiring the core to alter its function in a matter of milliseconds. At the moment of contact, the velocity of the external forces impacting the body can be dangerously overwhelming. The body must be not only incredibly stable to endure this violent collision but also strong enough to withstand the hit, arrest the force, and, ideally, shrug off the tackler.

Strength is pervasive in all sports and can be quickly influenced without a necessary gain in muscle size. The latter of these two points is critical to sports such as cross-country or marathon running, which require great strength of endurance while demanding a low body mass. To clarify this point, strength can be understood in two ways: muscular strength and muscular endurance:

1. *Muscular strength* is determined by the maximal amount of force that a muscle or group of muscles can exert against resistance.

2. *Muscular endurance* is the capacity of a muscle or group of muscles to contract and exert force repeatedly over an extended period of time.

As we have tried to demonstrate, functional strength can be defined in many ways. But as we continue to discuss the important role strength plays in sport performance, we should never lose sight of the fact that, in terms of core strength, we are commenting principally on the ability to resist movement against differing quantities of external force, particularly throughout the spine. This approach tends to be in opposition to the fundamental purpose when training the limbs and extremities, in which increased strength is typically displayed through the causation of movement. This principle is important and merits repeating.

PROGRESSIVE OVERLOAD

Strength is gained through adaptation of the body's physiological systems. For positive adaptation to occur, these systems must be increasingly challenged. Progressive overload is a concept that has been around for years, and rightly so; it should be the definitive goal of every strength and conditioning program. As defined by the American College of Sports Medicine, progressive overload is "the gradual increase of stress placed upon the body during exercise training."

The stability exercises in part II are designed to progress the athlete from simple foundational activities to more challenging actions by manipulating such variables as increasing the duration of an isometrically held movement or by changing the position of the body to increase overall pattern difficulty. Although this is effective as a baseline, holding positions statically for an extended time is not overly athletic; thus once the spine is stabilized, movement must be deliberately integrated. This progressive approach promotes a balanced functional development of the core musculature and, over time, auxiliary development throughout the kinetic chain. One major training mistake is adding too much time to stability exercises in an attempt to make them more challenging. If a situation is unrealistic in your athletic event, it should likewise not be part of your approach to training. There is typically little to no time in sport to consciously react and respond—everything happens quickly. Training should be specific to the energy system and movement patterns inherent to your sport and, preferably, to your specific position in your sport.

The idea of progressive overload holds true to core training, in which not only your body's position is altered and the angles of equipment manipulated, but the actual weight involved is systematically increased to further challenge you in an attempt to achieve a desired goal. The exercises in part III are characterized by controlled movement and working against external resistance.

MANUALLY APPLIED EXTERNAL RESISTANCE

Applying external resistance can be as obvious as loading 300 pounds (136 kg) on a bar to perform a squat or as subtle as placing a resistance band around the ankles to execute a slide-step. In situations where equipment is limited, or if you simply want to change the routine with regard to external stimulus, exercises with perturbation techniques can provide a remarkably demanding alternative to customary load. Manual perturbation has been used in rehabilitation situations for years. For our purposes, it is the instinctive reaction to a sudden disturbance of action, divergent to the original action's intended objective.

Perturbation can be any unexpected outside force or movement that challenges or alters homeostasis, balance, or body control. For example, over time a straight-arm plank, even with both the upper and lower body on unstable surfaces, will eventually seem less difficult, and you might start to question continuing to perform the exercise. Even with the unstable surfaces, you will quickly adapt, discover the balance point, and likely be able to maintain a rock-solid, straight-line plank for an extended period of time. At this point, if a coach or teammate were to simply nudge, tap, or tug as they moved around, you will instinctively make subtle adjustments in order to maintain balance (figure 1). Depending on the intensity of the nudge, the adjustment might be as simple as absorbing the tap with minimal effort or as vigorous as shifting your center of mass.

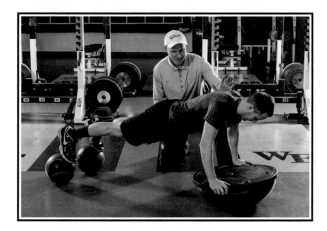

Figure 1 Plank with perturbation.

Research shows that exercises involving perturbation techniques can augment the proprioceptive signals to the joints and muscles. These simple techniques will amplify the acute responsiveness to your body's spatial awareness, enhance coordination, and increase total body control, which in turn will bolster your confidence, boost your performance, and likely reduce the possible incidence or severity of injury.

Closely associated with perturbation techniques and their intended neural corrective response is the enhanced quality of reaction time and subsequent mobilizing response—an extremely important element in all major sport performance. The ability to recognize a stimulus, consciously or not, and effectively and rapidly respond to that stimulus is the single-most important characteristic of high-level performance. "He's lost a step." "She's slow to react." "He keeps getting blown by." These are common criticisms of athletes by outside observers. I have often had players who could react with the best athletes in the world, but the neural transmission to do something about that reaction was lacking. In other words, you know that the player you are defending is going to drive to your right, but you

just cannot get your body to move in that direction fast enough to turn him back.

Reaction can involve all senses, including audio (such as instinctively reacting to a shouting coach's command from the sideline) and visual (such as staying down on a shot fake and then beating a defender over a screen). We have employed perturbation and other task-complexity, reaction-type techniques to all facets of training—everything from performing a hanging knee-up while being poked with a stick to shooting a free-throw while standing on a Bosu ball with a coach nudging from behind. Perturbation can be safely added to nearly any training modality, including to all exercises presented in part II and most in part III.

Often confused with perturbation are complex moves. The difference between these two is that with perturbation the action is unexpected and the resulting response is to retain overall body control, whereas in a complex move, the action is preestablished and usually consistent in its force, load, and line of pull. For example, an athlete in the weight room might be performing a straight-arm plank variation while a coach pulls a large resistance band placed around the athlete's waist (figure 2). The action for the plank is constant; the difference is that the coach is pulling laterally on the band. The athlete, using the informed feedback and knowing the line of pull, must engage the rotary stabilizers of the core to counter this pull and attempt to keep the body in line with the original intended action (straight-arm plank). Thus a relatively simple task of performing an unstable plank has been made more challenging by creating a complex action,

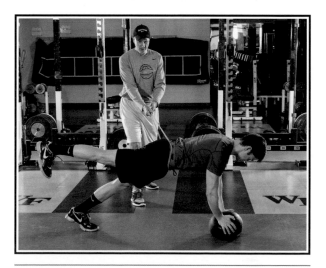

Figure 2 Straight-arm plank complex move.

again training globally and avoiding muscle isolation. This type of training, while posing slightly more risk, has the potential for greater adaptive qualities and can thereby accomplish more in the same amount of time.

In younger or relatively untrained individuals, the ability to increase strength levels feels almost limitless at times. This is because of the large window of adaptation available to those with low training age. The rapid rise on the strength curve is also aided by a direct increase in the neurological linking to the muscular system, making for a much more efficient system overall. For those who are more highly trained and have a longer history, the window for adaptation tends to be slightly smaller. The aforementioned newbies can do almost anything in any order at any time and still realize positive gains. Veterans of training must be much more methodical and precise in their exercise choices and rep and set selections.

As an athlete, you must understand where your training history lies on this sliding scale and then challenge yourself appropriately. Use the tests in chapter 18 to guide you. A clear understanding of your current abilities allows you to create a core-training regimen and optimize your foundational strength.

Anti-Extension Exercises

One of the great fallacies that manual therapists champion is the misguided belief that simply manipulating the body through a unique pattern of movement will automatically result in the adoption and precise utilization of that pattern on the court or the pitch. This could not be further from the truth. Cognition plays a critical role in the retention and application of any new learned motor pattern. If athletes have a full understanding of a new pattern, as well as its purpose, methodology, and application, with practice they will be able to apply the new movement within their sport. Athletes must demonstrate a baseline of skill development before advancing to more demanding and comprehensive movement techniques. In other words, you must learn to walk before you run. A common characteristic among great athletes is the uncanny ability to move with great fluidity and efficient purpose. This quality is only possible if the athlete maintains the dynamic postural stabilization necessary to apply strength and power in a meaningful way.

Assuming that postural distortion patterns are in check, the athlete's exercise program should now shift toward the application of strength upon the base of structural core stability. All too often, well-meaning therapists and fitness specialists, in an attempt to expedite measurable results, implement a strength or power philosophy into an athlete's regimen without first establishing the foundation needed to support that strength. In the following chapters we address these performance-reliant, indispensable strength variables from a core functionality precept.

This chapter introduces the complex exercise. A complex is a multifaceted exercise that typically involves a variety of movement patterns within a variety of planes of motion encompassing a variety of velocity and load options.

The following exercise finder lists the benefits, difficulty level, and equipment needed for every exercise that appears in this chapter. Primary exercises are highlighted in blue with their progressions in red. The primary exercises are also noted in the text with a red title bar.

Anti-Extension Strength Exercise Finder

Exercise Name	Specific Benefits (see chapter 5)	Easy	Medium	Hard	Equipment
Elbow Plank With Resistance: Band Walk	❼ ⑪ ⑫ ⑰		X		Resistance band/cable tubing
Straight-Arm Plank With Resistance: Horizontal Shoulder Press	❾ ⑫ ⑰		X		Resistance band/cable tubing
Straight-Arm Plank With Resistance: Horizontal Shoulder Press With Hip Flexion	❾ ⑪ ⑫ ⑰		X		Resistance band/cable tubing
Straight-Arm Plank With Resistance: Horizontal Shoulder Press With Hip Extension	❹ ❾ ⑪ ⑫ ⑰		X		Resistance band/cable tubing
Rollout: Stability Ball, Kneeling	❶ ❷ ❼ ⑫		X		Stability ball
Rollout: Dolly, Kneeling	❶ ❼ ⑫		X		Dolly
Rollout: Ab Wheel, Kneeling	❶ ❼ ⑫			X	Ab wheel
Rollout: Suspended Upper, Kneeling	❷ ❻ ❼ ⑫			X	Suspension trainer
Rollout: Slideboard, Kneeling	❶ ❼ ⑫ ⑲			X	Slideboard
Rollout: Barbell, Kneeling	❼ ⑫ ⑰			X	Barbell
Rollout: Dolly, Legs Extended	❶ ⑫			X	Dolly
Rollout: Ab Wheel, Legs Extended	❶ ⑫			X	Ab wheel
Rollout: Suspended Upper, Legs Extended	❷ ❻ ⑫			X	Suspension trainer
Rollout: Slideboard, Legs Extended	❶ ⑫ ⑲			X	Slideboard
Rollout: Barbell, Legs Extended	⑫ ⑰			X	Barbell
Dolly Walks	❶ ❼ ❾		X		Dolly
Elbow Plank on Stability Ball: Rock the Cradle	❶ ❷ ❼ ⑫ ㉔		X		Stability ball
Straight-Arm Plank on Stability Ball: Rock the Cradle	❶ ❷ ❼ ⑫ ㉔		X		Stability ball
Elbow Plank on Stability Ball: Stir the Pot	❶ ❷ ❼ ⑫ ㉔		X		Stability ball
Straight-Arm Plank on Stability Ball: Stir the Pot	❶ ❷ ❼ ⑫ ㉔		X		Stability ball
Slideboard Feet: Elbow Bodysaw	❶ ❽ ⑫ ⑲		X		Slideboard
Slideboard Feet: Straight-Arm Bodysaw	❶ ❽ ⑫ ⑲		X		Slideboard
Mountain Climber: Slideboard	❶ ❹ ❽ ❾ ⑫ ⑲		X		Slideboard
Mountain Climber: Slideboard, Unstable Upper	❶ ❷ ❹ ❽ ❾ ⑫ ⑲			X	Unstable apparatus*, slideboard
Mountain Climber: Slideboard, Double-Leg Knee Tuck	❶ ❽ ⑫ ⑲			X	Slideboard
Mountain Climber: Slideboard, Circular Double-Leg Knee Tuck	❶ ❽ ⑫ ⑲ ㉔			X	Slideboard

* Many options are available for the unstable apparatus, including a thick foam pad, wobble board, balance disc, pillows, or stability ball.
** Many options are available for the raised platform, including a box, bench, stair, or step.

Exercise Name	Specific Benefits (see chapter 5)	Difficulty Level Easy	Medium	Hard	Equipment
Mountain Climber: Slideboard, Single-Leg	❶❹❽⑫⑲			X	Slideboard
Mountain Climber: Slideboard, Double-Leg Pike	❶❽⑫⑲			X	Slideboard
Mountain Climber: Slideboard, Double-Leg Pike, Left and Right	❶❽⑫⑲㉔			X	Slideboard
Mountain Climber: Slideboard Complex: Pike, Mountain Climber, Push-Up	❶❽⑫⑲㉔			X	Slideboard
Mountain Climber: Stability Ball, Elastic Band Resistance	❶❷❹❽⑫ ⑰			X	Stability ball, band
Mountain Climber: Suspended Lower	❹❻❽⑫			X	Suspension trainer
Mountain Climber: Suspended Lower, Double-Leg Knee Tuck	❻❽⑫			X	Suspension trainer
Mountain Climber: Suspended Lower, Double-Leg Knee Tuck: Middle, Right, Middle, Left, Middle	❻❽⑫㉔			X	Suspension trainer
Mountain Climber: Unstable Upper, Suspended Lower, Double-Leg Knee Tuck	❶❷❻❽⑫			X	Suspension trainer, unstable apparatus
Mountain Climber: Unstable Upper on Stability Ball, Suspended Lower, Double-Leg Knee Tuck	❶❷❻❽⑫			X	Suspension trainer, stability ball
Mountain Climber: Slideboard, Simultaneous Abduction and Adduction	❶❺⑫⑲			X	Slideboard
Mountain Climber: Slideboard, Alternating Abduction and Adduction	❶❺⑫⑲			X	Slideboard
Mountain Climber: Slideboard, Simultaneous Abduction and Adduction With Push-Up	❶❺⑫⑱⑲ ㉔			X	Slideboard
Mountain Climber: Slideboard Complex: Abduction and Adduction With Pike and Push-Up	❶❺❽⑫⑱ ⑲㉔			X	Slideboard
Push-Up	⑫	X			
Push-Up With Hip Extension	❹⑫	X			
Push-Up With Alternating Abduction and Adduction	❺⑫	X			
Push-Up With Box, Asymmetrical	⑫	X			Raised platform**
Push-Up, Unstable Upper With Medicine Ball, Asymmetrical	❶⑫		X		Medicine ball
Push-Up, Unstable Upper With Medicine Ball, Roll Across	❶❼❾⑫⑭ ⑰⑱		X		Medicine ball
Push-Up, Unstable Upper With Medicine Ball, Walk Across	❶❼⑫		X		Medicine ball
Push-Up, Unstable Lower With Medicine Ball	❶❸⑫		X		Medicine ball

(continued)

135

Exercise Name	Specific Benefits (see chapter 5)	Difficulty Level			Equipment
		Easy	Medium	Hard	
Push-up, Unstable Upper and Lower With Medicine Balls	❶ ⓬			X	Three medicine balls
Push-Up, Unstable Lower, Narrow Grip With Medicine Ball	❶ ⓬			X	Medicine ball, unstable apparatus
Push-Up, Unstable Lower, Complex	❶ ❷ ❼ ⓬ ⓲			X	Raised platform, unstable apparatus
Push-Up, Arms Elevated, Pike Complex	❷ ❽ ⓬ ⓲		X		Raised platform
Push-Up, Suspended Upper	❷ ❻ ⓬		X		Suspension trainer
Push-Up, Suspended Lower	❸ ❻ ⓬		X		Suspension trainer
Push-Up, Suspended Lower, Box Walk-Up	❸ ❻ ❼ ⓬ ⓲			X	Raised platform, suspension trainer
Push-Up, Suspended Upper and Unstable Lower	❶ ❷ ❸ ❻ ⓬			X	Unstable apparatus, suspension trainer
Push-Up, Suspended Lower, Complex	❶ ❸ ❻ ⓬ ⓱ ⓲			X	Suspension trainer, two dumbbells
Hanging Knee-Up (Rock Back)	⓬ ⓰ ⓱			X	Chin-up bar
Hanging Inverted Bent Knee to Straight Leg	⓬ ⓰ ⓱			X	Chin-up bar
Hanging Shin Tap	⓬ ⓰ ⓱			X	Chin-up bar
Hanging Pike Pull-Up	⓬ ⓰ ⓱			X	Chin-upbar
Hanging Straight Leg to Bent Knee	⓬ ⓰ ⓱			X	Chin-up bar
Hanging Straight Leg to Bent Knee, Medicine Ball Between Knees	⓬ ⓰ ⓱			X	Chin-up bar, medicine ball
Hanging Straight Leg to Bent Knee, Medicine Ball Between Ankles	⓬ ⓰ ⓱			X	Chin-up bar, medicine ball
Hanging Straight Leg to Bent Knee, Posterior Resistance Band	⓬ ⓰ ⓱			X	Chin-up bar, resistance band
Hanging L Series: Alternating Straight Leg to L	❹ ⓫ ⓬ ⓰ ⓱			X	Chin-up bar
Hanging L Series: Straight Legs to L and Return	⓬ ⓰ ⓱			X	Chin-up bar
Hanging L Series: L to Knee Tuck and Back to L	⓬ ⓰ ⓱			X	Chin-up bar
Hanging L Series: L to Ankle Tap and Back to L	⓬ ⓰ ⓱			X	Chin-up bar
Hanging L Series: Abduction and Adduction	❺ ⓬ ⓰ ⓱			X	Chin-up bar
Hanging L Series: Isometric L Pull-Up	⓬ ⓰ ⓱ ⓲			X	Chin-up bar

ELBOW PLANK WITH RESISTANCE

BAND WALK

MOVEMENTS

1. Lie prone (face down) on the floor with the feet together. (A slightly wider foot placement provides additional stabilization if needed.)
2. Attach some sort of resistance (rubber bands, cable, tubing, or other resistance apparatus) securely behind you, 1 to 2 feet (.3-.6 m) off the floor.
3. Hold one band (or cable or tubing, etc.) in each hand. Place upper-body weight on the forearms and dorsiflex the feet and toes toward the shins.
4. Lock the knees, tighten the glutes, and brace the core. Lift the body so the only contact points are the balls of the feet and toes, along with the elbows and forearms, on the floor.
5. Continuing to brace the core and maintaining proper body alignment, "walk" forward on the elbow and forearm against the resistance. The distance walked might be two "steps" or several, depending on the strength of the athlete, type of resistance used, and tensile concentration of that resistance.
6. Maintaining the same controlled dynamic posture, "walk" back to the start position. Perform for a predetermined number of repetitions or time interval.

CONSIDERATIONS

1. Maintain a solid core throughout (ears, shoulders, hips, knees, and ankles are in a straight line, with no arching, sagging, or rolling of the midsection).
2. Move only as fast and "step" only as far as your body can control without sacrificing technique.

SPECIFIC BENEFITS

7 **11** **12** **17**

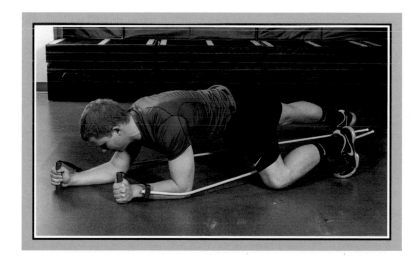

▪ STRAIGHT-ARM PLANK WITH RESISTANCE ▪
HORIZONTAL SHOULDER PRESS

Modifications

1. To begin, position one hand on the floor directly under the shoulder with the floor arm perpendicular to the floor.

2. Attach some sort of resistance (rubber bands, cable, tubing, or other resistance apparatus) securely behind you 1 to 2 feet (.3-.6 m) off the floor. Grasp the band or handle with the "up" hand.

3. Lock the knees, engage the glutes, and brace the core. Lift the body so the only contact points are the balls of the feet and toes and one hand on the floor. Maintain a solid core throughout (ears, shoulders, hips, knees, and ankles are in a straight line, with no arching, sagging, or rolling of the midsection).

4. Lift the "up" hand and the resistance to a palm-up position directly under that hand's shoulder.

5. Press overhead; in doing so, the hand turns to a palm-down position. The press is an overhead press but is in fact parallel to the ground (because of the body's plank position).

6. Return to the start position.

Specific Benefits ❾ ⓬ ⓱

Note Be sure to maintain proper body alignment. When the body has a three-point base of support, the tendency is to roll or rotate in opposition as a counterbalance. Avoid this and make every attempt to retain level hips throughout the exercise.

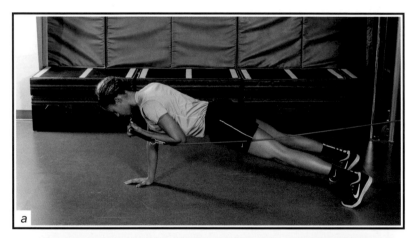

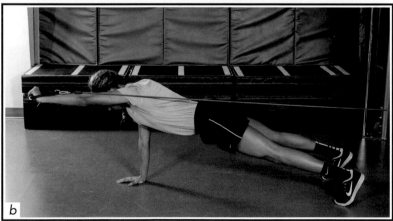

■ STRAIGHT-ARM PLANK WITH RESISTANCE ■
HORIZONTAL SHOULDER PRESS WITH HIP FLEXION

Modifications

1. Position the left hand on the floor directly under the shoulder with that arm perpendicular to the floor.

2. Attach some sort of resistance (rubber bands, cable, tubing, or other resistance apparatus) securely behind you 1 to 2 feet (.3-.6 m) off the floor. Grasp the band or handle with your right hand.

3. Lock the knees, engage the glutes, and brace the core. Lift the body so the only contact points are the balls of the feet and toes and the left hand on floor. Maintain a solid core throughout (ears, shoulders, hips, knees, and ankles are in a straight line, with no arching, sagging, or rolling of the midsection).

4. Extend the left (contralateral) hip and lift that leg off the floor.

5. Lift the right hand and resistance to a palm-up position directly under the right shoulder.

6. Flex the left hip and drive the left knee under the torso toward the chest while simultaneously pressing the right hand overhead (parallel to the floor). During the overhead press, the hand turns to a palm-down position.

7. Maintain proper body alignment. Avoid hunching in an attempt to assist the knee drive.

8. Return to the start position.

Specific Benefits **9** **11** **12** **17**

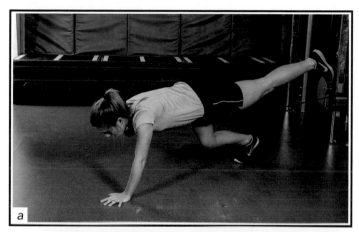

a

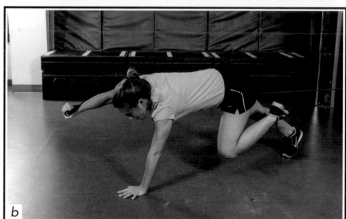

b

Modifications

1. Assume the body posture and start position as described in the previous exercise, except in these photos, the left hand is the up hand and the right leg drives first.

2. Tuck the right (contralateral) leg under the torso toward the chest. Lift the left hand and resistance to a palm-up position directly under the left shoulder.

3. Extend the right (contralateral) hip back and up while simultaneously pressing the left hand overhead (parallel to the floor). Both the right leg and the left arm are now parallel to the floor.

4. During the overhead press, the hand turns to a palm-down position.

5. Maintain proper body alignment. Avoid hunching in an attempt to assist the knee return back to the start position.

6. Return to the start position

Specific Benefits

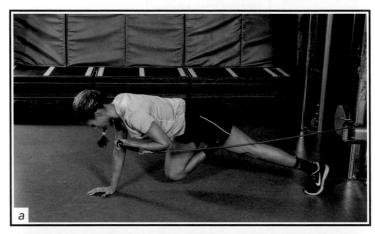

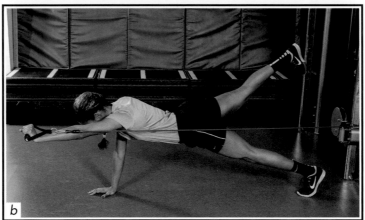

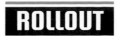

ROLLOUT

STABILITY BALL, KNEELING

MOVEMENTS

1. Kneel on the floor with the stability ball directly in front of your body.
2. Place the hands and forearms on top of the ball.
3. Lift the body so the only contact points are the knees, balls of the feet, and toes on the floor and the elbows and forearms on the ball. Brace the core for spinal stability.
4. Smoothly extend forward at the elbows, shoulders, hips, and knees. The forearms should roll across the top of the ball as the ball moves forward.
5. Push out as far forward as possible while maintaining a stable, relatively straight spine with a neutral pelvic angle.
6. Reverse the action and pull (roll) the ball backward to the start position.
7. Perform a predetermined number of repetitions.

CONSIDERATIONS

1. Brace your abdomen and contract your glutes for the duration of the drill.
2. Maintain a solid core throughout (ears, shoulders, hips, knees, and ankles are in a straight line, with no arching, sagging, or rolling of the midsection).
3. Avoid extreme anterior pelvic tilt (arched or hyperextended lumbar). Maintain a neutral pelvic alignment throughout.

SPECIFIC BENEFITS

1 **2** **7** **12**

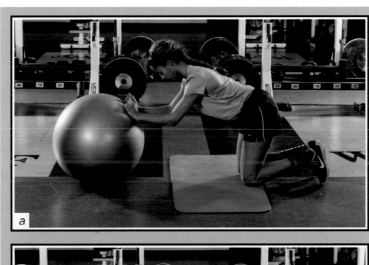

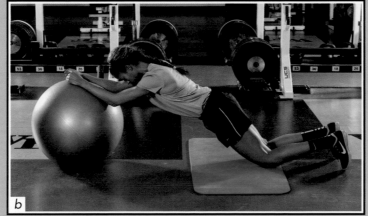

◾ ROLLOUT ◾
DOLLY, KNEELING

Modifications

1. Assume the body posture and start position described for Rollout: Stability Ball, Kneeling. The action is the same; the only difference is the use of a dolly apparatus instead of a stability ball.

Specific Benefits

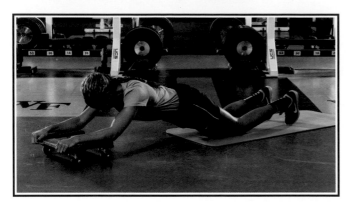

◾ ROLLOUT ◾
AB WHEEL, KNEELING

Modifications

1. Assume the body posture and start position described for Rollout: Dolly, Kneeling. The action is the same; the only difference is the use of an ab wheel instead of a dolly.

Specific Benefits

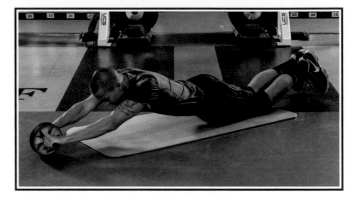

◾ ROLLOUT ◾
SUSPENDED UPPER, KNEELING

Modifications

1. Kneel on the floor with the straps (or grips) of a suspension device hanging in front of you. The height of the handles and foot placement determine load demand and exercise difficulty.

2. With the hands in the grips, support the body so that only the knees, balls of the feet, and toes are on the floor. The spine is stabilized in a relatively straight position with a neutral pelvic angle.

3. Push out forward as far as possible while maintaining a relatively straight spine.

4. Reverse the action and pull back to the start position.

Specific Benefits

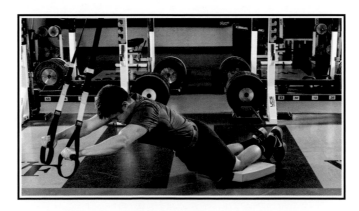

▪ ROLLOUT ▪
SLIDEBOARD, KNEELING

Modifications

1. In a kneeling position, carefully place your hands on the slideboard directly under the shoulders with the arms perpendicular to the floor. The only contact points are the knees, balls of the feet, and toes on the floor.

2. Smoothly extend forward at the shoulders, hips, and knees. Push out forward as far as possible, maintaining a braced and relatively straight spine.

3. Reverse the action and pull back to the start position.

Specific Benefits ❶ ❼ ⓬ ⓭

▪ ROLLOUT ▪
BARBELL, KNEELING

Modifications

1. Assume the body posture and start position described for the Rollout: Ab Wheel, Kneeling. The action is the same; the only difference is the use of a barbell instead of an ab wheel. Grip the bar with the hands placed a little wider than shoulder width.

Specific Benefits ❼ ⓬ ⓱

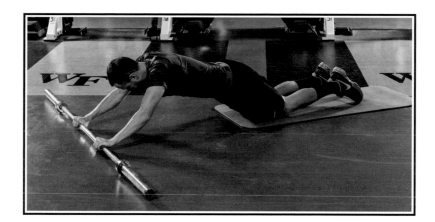

▪ ROLLOUT ▪
DOLLY, LEGS EHTENDED

Modifications

1. Position yourself on all fours with the dolly in front of your body. Place the forearms on the dolly.

2. Extend the legs. Only the balls of the feet and toes are on the floor.

3. Push out forward as far as possible. The spine is stabilized; maintain a relatively straight position with a neutral pelvic angle throughout the action.

4. Reverse the action and pull back to the start position.

Specific Benefits ❶ ⓬

■ ROLLOUT ■
AB WHEEL, LEGS EXTENDED

Modifications

1. Assume the body posture and start position described for Rollout: Dolly, Legs Extended. The action is the same; the only difference is the use of an ab wheel instead of a dolly.

Specific Benefits

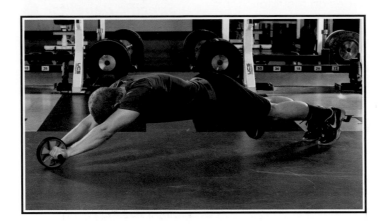

■ ROLLOUT ■
SUSPENDED UPPER, LEGS EXTENDED

Modifications

1. Kneel on the floor with the straps (or grips) of a suspension device hanging in front of you. The height of the handles and foot placement determine load demand and exercise difficulty.
2. Extend the legs. Only the balls of the feet and toes are on the floor.

3. Push out forward as far as possible. The spine is stabilized; maintain a relatively straight position with a neutral pelvic angle throughout the action.

Specific Benefits

■ ROLLOUT ■
SLIDEBOARD, LEGS EXTENDED

Modifications

1. Position yourself on all fours. Place the hands on the slideboard directly under the shoulders with the arms perpendicular to the floor.
2. Extend the legs. Only the balls of the feet and toes are on the floor.

3. Push out forward as far as possible. The spine is stabilized; maintain a relatively straight position with a neutral pelvic angle throughout the action.
4. Reverse the action and pull back to the start position.

Specific Benefits

▪ ROLLOUT ▪
BARBELL, LEGS EXTENDED

Modifications

1. Assume the body posture and start position as described for Rollout: Ab Wheel, Legs Extended.

2. The action is the same; the only difference is the use of a barbell instead of an ab wheel. Grip the bar with the hands placed a little wider than shoulder width.

Specific Benefits ⓬ ⓱

▪ DOLLY WALKS ▪

Modifications

1. Place the feet on top of a dolly and kneel on the floor.
2. Place your upper-body weight on straight arms and pull the toes toward the shins.
3. In a controlled manner, lift the left hand and place it firmly out in front of you.
4. Repeat the movement with the right hand, thereby dragging yourself forward.
5. Continue "walking" forward for desired distance.

Specific Benefits ❶ ❼ ❾

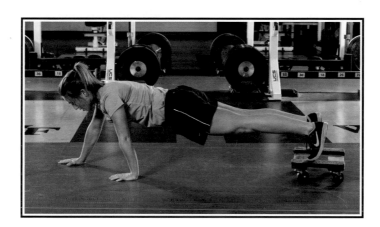

ROCK THE CRADLE

MOVEMENTS

1. Lie prone (face down) on a stability ball with the elbows on the ball. The feet are together, ankles dorsiflexed.

2. Lift the body so the only contact points are the balls of the feet and the toes on the floor and the wrists and forearms positioned on the "near" side of the ball. Place upper-body weight on the forearms.

3. Brace the core, maintaining a straight-line plank position (ear, shoulder, hip, knee, and ankle in alignment) throughout the duration of the exercise.

4. With movement originating at shoulders, smoothly extend (push) forward as far as possible without sacrificing body alignment or mechanics. Extension distance depends on the athlete's strength, stability, and comfort levels.

5. Maintaining spinal stabilization, pull the ball back to the start position. Most of the action is at the shoulder girdle.

6. Continue for a predetermined number of repetitions or time interval.

CONSIDERATIONS

1. Stabilization requirements greatly depend on foot placement. Maintaining stabilization during the exercise with the feet together (or a single foot on the floor) is far more difficult than with the feet spread, which provides a wider base of support.

2. The height of the stability ball, and thus the angle of the body, can also affect drill difficulty.

SPECIFIC BENEFITS

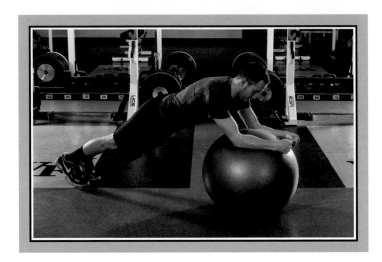

■ STRAIGHT-ARM PLANK ON STABILITY BALL ■
ROCK THE CRADLE

Modifications

1. Straighten the arms with the hands on a stability ball. The hands are directly under the shoulders with the arms perpendicular to the floor.

2. Lift the body so the only contact points are the balls of the feet and toes on the floor and the hands on the ball.

3. Follow the action as described for Elbow Plank on Stability Ball: Rock the Cradle.

Specific Benefits

▪ ELBOW PLANK ON STABILITY BALL ▪
STIR THE POT

Modifications

1. Assume the start position described for Elbow Plank on Stability Ball: Rock the Cradle.
2. With movement originating at shoulders and without sacrificing body alignment, smoothly push forward as far as possible and make circular motions.

3. Maintaining spinal stability, continue to rotate the ball in one circular direction with the majority of the action at the shoulder girdle. Circle size will depend on the athlete's strength, stability, and comfort levels.
4. Continue in one direction for a predetermined number of revolutions before repeating immediately in the opposite direction.

Specific Benefits ❶ ❷ ❼ ⑫ ㉔

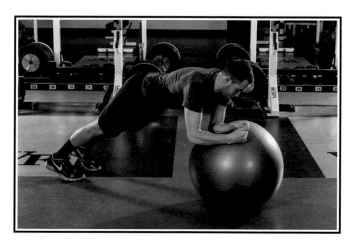

▪ STRAIGHT-ARM PLANK ON STABILITY BALL ▪
STIR THE POT

Modifications

1. Assume the start position described for Straight-Arm Plank on Stability Ball: Rock the Cradle.
2. Lift the body so the only contact points are the balls of the feet and toes on the floor and the hands on the ball.
3. Follow the action as described for Elbow Plank on Stability Ball: Stir the Pot.

Specific Benefits ❶ ❷ ❼ ⑫ ㉔

Note Try different hand positions for additional control or difficulty. For example, point fingers forward for greater difficulty or lateral toward the floor for greater control. Be conscious of your individual stability and control and never place a joint or body part into a position that could lead to injury.

ELBOW BODYSAW

MOVEMENTS

1. Kneel on the slideboard. Place your forearms on the floor just in front of the outside edge of the slideboard.
2. Lift the body and pull your toes toward your shins.
3. Push backward, allowing the toes to slide along the board, extending at the shoulders and hips.
4. Extend backward as far as you can while maintaining a completely straight spine.
5. Pull forward back to the start position.
6. Perform a predetermined number of repetitions.

CONSIDERATIONS

1. Brace the core and contract the glutes throughout.
2. Maintain a solid core with no arching, sagging, or rolling of the midsection.

SPECIFIC BENEFITS

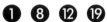

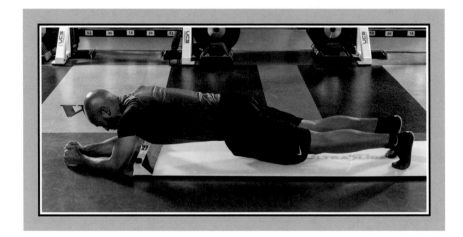

■ SLIDEBOARD FEET ■
STRAIGHT-ARM BODYSAW

Modifications

1. Place the hands on the floor close to one end of the slideboard with the arms perpendicular to floor.

2. With the arms straight, lift the body and pull your toes toward your shins. Follow the action as described for the Slideboard Feet: Elbow Bodysaw.

Specific Benefits   ❶ ❽ ⑫ ⑲

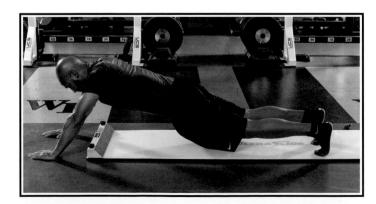

MOUNTAIN CLIMBER

SLIDEBOARD

MOVEMENTS

1. Place the hands on the floor close to one end of the slideboard with the arms perpendicular to the floor.
2. Position the feet on the slideboard and pull the balls of the feet and toes toward your shins.
3. The body is in a straight-line plank position (ears, shoulders, hips, knees, and ankles are in alignment).
4. Maintaining a relatively straight spine and neutral pelvis, slide one foot up and under the torso. The knee moves toward the chest while the opposite knee remains straight.

5. Extend the bent knee and hip back to the start position while simultaneously sliding the opposite straight leg up and under the torso (knee toward the chest).
6. Continue, alternating legs, for a predetermined number of repetitions or time interval.

CONSIDERATIONS

1. Brace the core and avoid hunching.
2. Maintain a solid core with no arching, sagging, or rolling of the midsection.

SPECIFIC BENEFITS

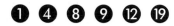

1 **4** **8** **9** **12** **19**

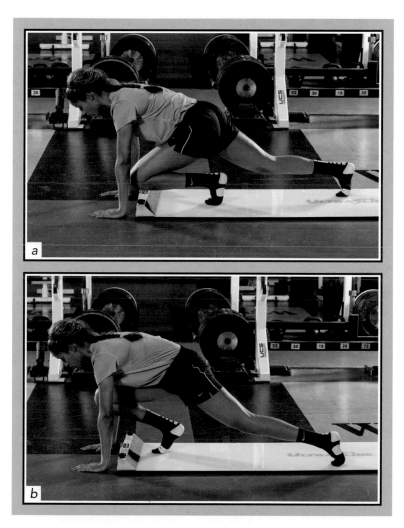

▪ MOUNTAIN CLIMBER ▪
SLIDEBOARD, UNSTABLE UPPER

Modifications

1. Place the hands on a stability ball (or similar object) positioned close to one end of the slideboard. The arms are straight and close to perpendicular to the floor (the degree of perpendicularity is dependent on the size of the stability ball).
2. Position the balls of the feet and toes on the slideboard.
3. Follow the action as described for the Mountain Climber: Slideboard.

Specific Benefits ❶ ❷ ④ ⑧ ⑨ ⑫ ⑲

Note Try different hand positions for additional control or difficulty. For example, point the fingers forward for greater difficulty or lateral toward the floor for greater control. Be conscious of your individual stability and control and never place a joint or body part into a position that could lead to injury.

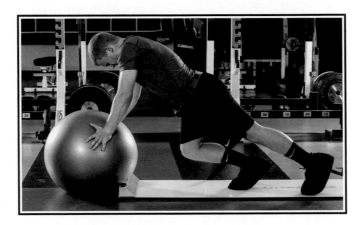

▪ MOUNTAIN CLIMBER ▪
SLIDEBOARD, DOUBLE-LEG KNEE TUCK

Modifications

1. Assume the straight-arm plank start position described for Mountain Climber: Slideboard.
2. Maintaining a relatively straight spine and neutral pelvis, slide both feet up and under the torso. Both knees will synchronously tuck toward the chest.
3. Extend both knees and hips back to the start position.

Specific Benefits ❶ ⑧ ⑫ ⑲

Note A natural lift of the hips will occur to accommodate the knee tuck, but try to keep the hips as low as possible. This maintains lumbar alignment and stability while challenging hip, knee, and ankle range of motion.

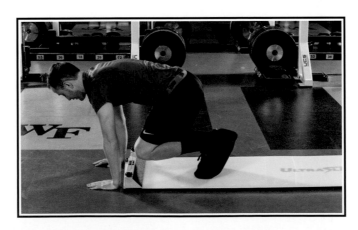

■ MOUNTAIN CLIMBER ■
SLIDEBOARD, CIRCULAR DOUBLE-LEG KNEE TUCK

Modifications

1. Assume the straight-arm plank start position described for Mountain Climber: Slideboard. Position the feet on the slideboard.

2. The action is identical to the Mountain Climber: Slideboard, Double-Leg Knee Tuck but with the addition of a slight circular motion with the lower body, specifically the feet.

3. Continue the movement clockwise for a pre-determined number of repetitions or time interval, then repeat counterclockwise.

Specific Benefits

■ MOUNTAIN CLIMBER ■
SLIDEBOARD, SINGLE LEG

Modifications

1. Assume the straight-arm plank start position described for Mountain Climber, Slideboard. Position the feet on the slideboard.

2. The action is identical to the Mountain Climber: Slideboard, Double-Leg Knee Tuck drill except you are using a single leg.

3. Hold the opposite leg off slideboard with the knee and hip flexed ("up" knee tucked to chest).

4. Continue the movement for a predetermined number of repetitions or length of time; then repeat with the opposite leg.

Specific Benefits

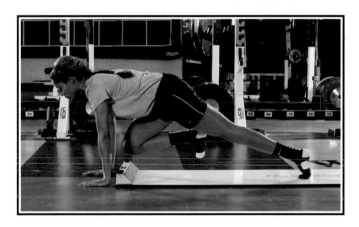

▪ MOUNTAIN CLIMBER ▪
SLIDEBOARD, DOUBLE-LEG PIKE

Modifications

1. Assume the straight-arm plank start position described for Mountain Climber: Slideboard. Position the feet on the slideboard.

2. Maintaining a relatively straight spine and locked knees, brace the core, flex the hips, and slide both feet toward the hands (pike).

3. Once maximum flexion has been reached (pike height will differ among athletes), in a controlled manner push the feet back to the start position.

Specific Benefits **❶ ❽ ⑫ ⑲**

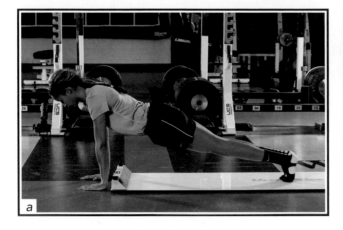

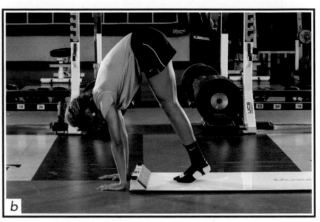

▪ MOUNTAIN CLIMBER ▪
SLIDEBOARD, DOUBLE-LEG PIKE, LEFT AND RIGHT

Modifications

1. Assume the straight-arm plank start position described for Mountain Climber: Slideboard. Position the feet on the slideboard.

2. The action is identical to the Mountain Climber: Slideboard, Double-Leg Pike with the addition of an altered movement pattern.

3. Slide the feet from the far left side of the slideboard to the pike position. Rather than return to the start position on the left side of the slideboard, return to the *right* side.

4. Repeat the action with a maximum flexion from the right side (pike height will differ among athletes); then, in a controlled manner push the feet back to the original (left) start position.

Specific Benefits **❶ ❽ ⑫ ⑲ ㉔**

▪ MOUNTAIN CLIMBER ▪
SLIDEBOARD COMPLEX: PIKE, MOUNTAIN CLIMBER, PUSH-UP

Modifications

1. Assume the straight-arm plank start position described for Mountain Climber: Slideboard. Position the feet on the slideboard.

2. The complex action is as follows:
   a. Pike and return from pike to start position.
   b. Mountain climber left, then right.
   c. While in the starting (neutral) position, perform a push-up.

Specific Benefits **❶ ❽ ⑫ ⑲ ㉔**

Note This is just one example of the many complex movement options you might employ. Be creative and develop your own routines.

▪ MOUNTAIN CLIMBER ▪
STABILITY BALL, ELASTIC BAND RESISTANCE

Modifications

1. Attach two elastic bands to an immovable object; attach the other ends of the bands around the ankles or feet. Place your hands on a stability ball (or similar unstable object) with the arms straight and close to perpendicular to the floor (depending on size of stability ball).

2. With the body is in a straight-line plank position (ears, shoulders, hips, knees, and ankles are in alignment) and a neutral pelvis, drive one foot up and under the torso. The knee moves toward the chest while the opposite knee remains straight.

3. Extend the bent knee and hip back to the start position. Continue, alternating legs.

Specific Benefits   ❶ ❷ ❹ ❽ ⑫ ⑰

Note Try different hand positions for additional control or difficulty. For example, point the fingers forward for greater difficulty or lateral toward the floor for greater control. Be conscious of your individual stability and control and never place a joint or body part into a position that could lead to injury.

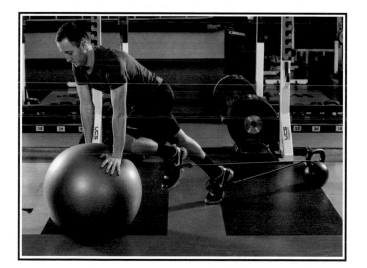

▪ MOUNTAIN CLIMBER ▪
SUSPENDED LOWER

Modifications

1. Position yourself on all fours with the straps (or grips) of a suspension device hanging behind you.

2. Place the feet securely in the straps (this might require assistance from a partner). The height of the handles along with hand and foot placement determine load demand and thus exercise difficulty.

3. Assume a straight body alignment (ears, shoulders, hips, knees, ankles in a straight line, with no arching or sagging of the midsection). Do not sag the hips (pelvis should not drop toward floor) or pike the hips (pelvis and buttocks should not arch toward ceiling).

4. Brace the core and drive one knee up and under the torso. The knee moves toward the chest while the opposite knee remains straight.

5. Simultaneously extend the bent knee and hip back to the start position while the straight leg drives up and under the torso (knee toward the chest).

6. Continue, alternating legs.

Specific Benefits   ❹ ❻ ❽ ⑫

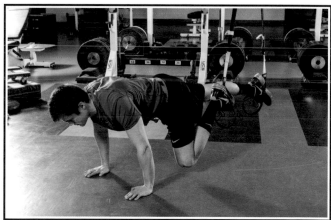

■ MOUNTAIN CLIMBER ■
SUSPENDED LOWER, DOUBLE-LEG KNEE TUCK

Modifications

1. Assume the start position described for Mountain Climber: Suspended Lower.
2. Maintaining a relatively straight spine and neutral pelvis, pull both knees up and under the torso. Both knees will synchronously tuck toward the chest.
3. Extend both bent knees and hips back to the start position, reestablishing ear, shoulder, hip, knee, and ankle alignment.

Specific Benefits 6 8 12

Note A natural lift of the hips will occur to accommodate the knee tuck, but try to keep the hips as low as possible. This maintains lumbar alignment and stability while challenging hip, knee, and ankle range of motion.

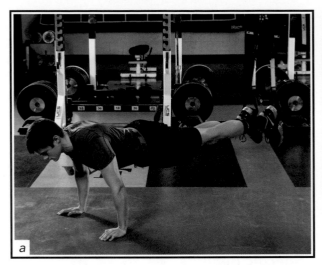

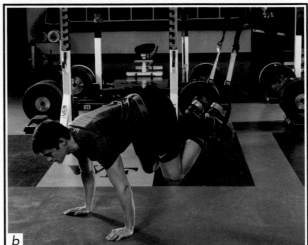

■ MOUNTAIN CLIMBER ■
SUSPENDED LOWER, DOUBLE-LEG KNEE TUCK: MIDDLE, RIGHT, MIDDLE, LEFT, MIDDLE

Modifications

1. Assume the start position described for Mountain Climber: Suspended Lower.
2. Maintaining a relatively straight spine and neutral pelvis, pull both knees up and under the torso. Both knees synchronously tuck toward the chest.
3. Perform the following movement pattern:
   a. Up to the middle
   b. Back to the right
   c. Up to the middle
   d. Back to the middle
   e. Up to the middle
   f. Back to the left
   g. Up to the middle
   h. Back to the middle (start position)

Specific Benefits 6 8 12 24

Note A natural lift of the hips will occur to accommodate the knee tuck, but try to keep the hips as low as possible. This maintains lumbar alignment and stability while challenging hip, knee, and ankle range of motion.

▪ MOUNTAIN CLIMBER ▪

UNSTABLE UPPER, SUSPENDED LOWER, DOUBLE-LEG KNEE TUCK

Modifications

1. Position the hands on the floor directly under the shoulders to provide stability while placing the feet securely in the perpendicular hanging straps. This might require assistance from a partner.
2. Once the feet are fixed in the straps, with assistance, place the hands on an unstable apparatus (bosu ball, balance board, etc.) positioned the appropriate distance from the straps (which should be perpendicular to the floor). This distance will be determined by the height of the athlete and should be exactly the distance necessary to accommodate perpendicular arms. Arms should be as straight and as close to perpendicular to the floor as possible (depending on the size of the unstable device and the length of the straps).
3. Do not sag the hips (pelvis should not drop toward the floor) or pike the hips (pelvis and buttocks should not arch toward the ceiling).
4. Maintaining a relatively straight spine and neutral pelvis, pull both knees up and under the torso. Both knees synchronously tuck toward the chest.

Specific Benefits [1] [2] [6] [8] [12]

Note Be aware of your individual stability and control and never place a joint or body part into a position that could lead to injury.

▪ MOUNTAIN CLIMBER ▪

UNSTABLE UPPER ON STABILITY BALL, SUSPENDED LOWER, DOUBLE-LEG KNEE TUCK

Modifications

1. Assume the start position described for the previous exercise, Mountain Climber: Unstable Upper, Suspended Lower, Double-Leg Knee Tuck.
2. The action is identical to the previous exercise.

Specific Benefits [1] [2] [6] [8] [12]

Note Try different hand positions for additional control or difficulty. For example, point the fingers forward for greater difficulty or lateral toward the floor for greater control. Be conscious of your individual stability and control and never place a joint or body part into a position that could lead to injury.

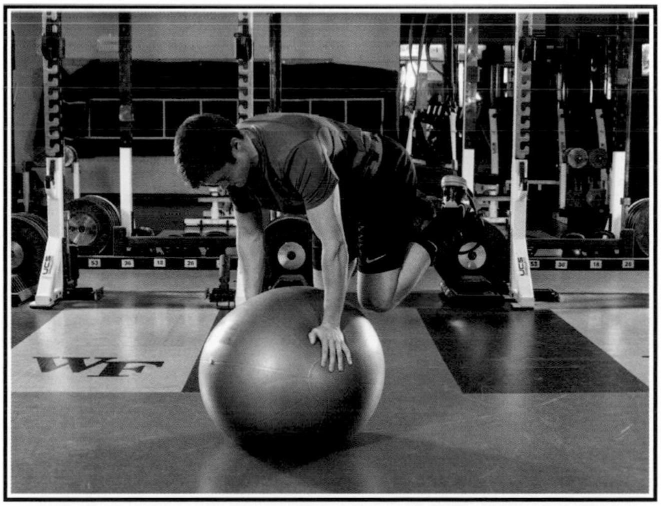

MOUNTAIN CLIMBER

SLIDEBOARD, SIMULTANEOUS ABDUCTION AND ADDUCTION

MOVEMENTS

1. Position the hands on the floor perpendicular to the long side of the slideboard with the arms perpendicular to the floor. The distance from the hands to the slideboard is determined by the length from the athlete's feet to his shoulders.
2. To begin, the feet are together and positioned on the middle part of the slideboard with the toes tucked toward the shins.
3. The core is braced and the body is in a straight-line plank position (ears, shoulders, hips, knees, and ankles are in alignment).
4. Maintaining a straight spine and neutral pelvis, slide the feet a comfortable distance apart (abduction).

5. Simultaneously draw the feet back to the start position at the midline of the body (adduction).
6. Continue for a predetermined number of repetitions or time interval.

CONSIDERATIONS

1. Maintain a solid, braced core (no arching, sagging, or rolling of the midsection). Do not sag the hips (pelvis should not drop toward the floor) or pike the hips (pelvis and buttocks should not arch toward the ceiling).

SPECIFIC BENEFITS

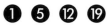 ❶ ❺ ⓬ ⓭

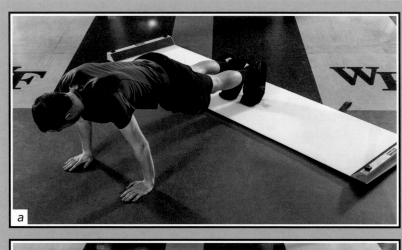

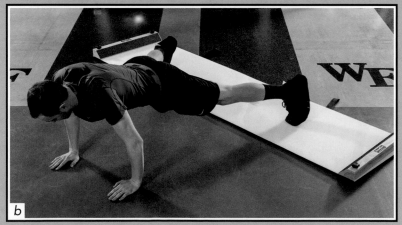

■ MOUNTAIN CLIMBER ■
SLIDEBOARD, ALTERNATING ABDUCTION AND ADDUCTION

Modifications

1. Assume the start position described for Mountain Climber: Slideboard, Simultaneous Abduction and Adduction
2. Abduct the right leg and return (adduction) to neutral with the feet together at the middle of the slideboard.
3. Abduct the left leg and return (adduction) back to neutral with the feet together at the middle of the slideboard.

Specific Benefits

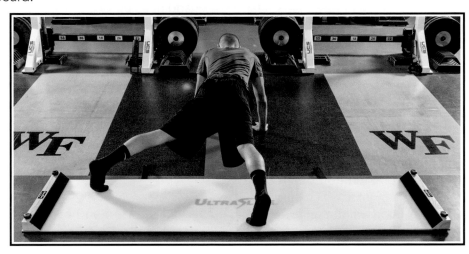

■ MOUNTAIN CLIMBER ■
SLIDEBOARD, SIMULTANEOUS ABDUCTION AND ADDUCTION WITH PUSH-UP

Modifications

1. Assume the start position described for Mountain Climber: Slideboard, Simultaneous Abduction and Adduction
2. Follow the steps for Mountain Climber: Simultaneous Abduction and Adduction, but now add a push-up each time the body adducts back to the neutral (start) position.

Specific Benefits

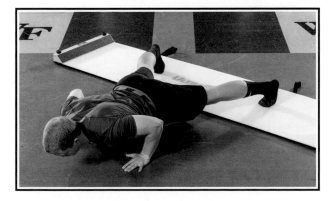

■ MOUNTAIN CLIMBER ■
SLIDEBOARD COMPLEX: ABDUCTION AND ADDUCTION WITH PIKE AND PUSH-UP

Modifications

1. Assume the start position described for Mountain Climber: Slideboard, Simultaneous Abduction and Adduction
2. Brace the core; the complex action is as follows:
   a. Spread the straight legs out (abduction), then bring the straight legs back to neutral (adduction).
   b. Pike and return from the pike to the start position.
   c. While in the neutral (start) position, perform a push-up.

Specific Benefits

Note This is just one example of the many movements you might employ. Be creative and develop your own routines.

MOVEMENTS

1. In the prone position (face down), place the hands on the floor directly under the shoulders. The feet are together, but if additional balance is needed the feet can be spread for comfort and stability (especially for the advanced push-up variations to follow).

2. Lift the body so the only contact points are the balls of the feet, toes, and hands on the floor. Brace the core and maintain straight body alignment (ears, shoulders, hips, knees, and ankles are in alignment). The start (neutral) position is arms perpendicular to the floor.

3. In a controlled manner, lower the body to a point in which you are in complete control of your spine (down position). For some individuals, a slight elbow flexion might lead to a breakdown in postural control; others can comfortably lower to a point at which the chest nearly touches the floor while maintaining a completely stable spine. A 90-degree elbow bend is usually sufficient.

4. Press back up to the start (neutral) position.

5. Perform a predetermined number of repetitions.

CONSIDERATIONS

1. The position of the hands relative to the shoulders can have a tremendously positive adaptive quality. Narrow grip push-ups with the hands close together, to the point that they sometimes touch, have the added benefit of maximizing triceps usage. On the other hand, a wider hand position will necessitate more motor unit recruitment of the total chest and shoulders (deltoids). Similarly, the hand placement can also influence the effectiveness of the push-up. However, this variable is much more individualized and primarily based on personal comfort. Some athletes like to keep the fingers pointed in slightly while others like to have the fingers angled out. As long as the joints of the wrist, elbow, and shoulder are not compromised, hand placement is a personal preference.

2. Avoid excessive shoulder protraction.

3. Avoid the chicken head. Do not extend the head and neck in opposition to scapular retraction.

4. Maintain straight body alignment. Do not sag the hips (pelvis should not drop toward the floor) or pike the hips (pelvis and buttocks should not arch toward the ceiling).

SPECIFIC BENEFITS

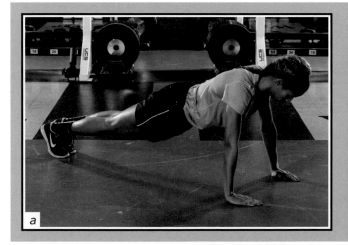

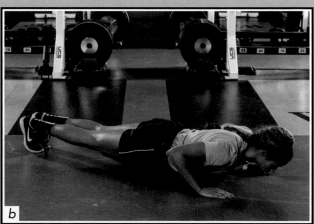

▪ PUSH-UP ▪
WITH HIP EXTENSION

Modifications

1. Assume the Push-Up start (neutral) position. Extend the hip of one leg; do not hyperextend the hip. Maintain straight body alignment of the ground leg with the rest of the body (ears, shoulders, hips, knees, and ankles in a straight line).

2. Lower to the down position; press back to the start position, maintaining hip extension throughout.

3. Continue with the same leg, hip extended, for the duration of the set, or switch and alternate legs during each rep.

Specific Benefits

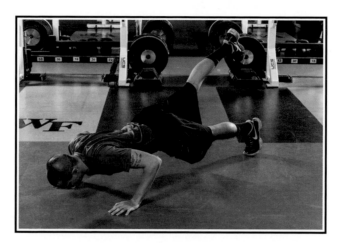

▪ PUSH-UP ▪
WITH ALTERNATING ABDUCTION AND ADDUCTION

Modifications

1. Assume the Push-Up start (neutral) position.

2. Brace the core and lower to the down position. Abduct the right leg. Press back up to the straight-arm position.

3. Adduct the right leg back to the start position.

4. Repeat with the opposite leg: Lower to the down position, abduct the left leg, press back up to the straight-arm position; and adduct the left leg back to the start position).

Specific Benefits

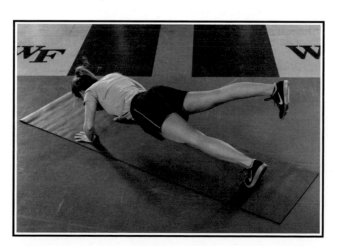

▪ PUSH-UP ▪
WITH BOX, ASYMMETRICAL

Modifications

1. Position the body next to a box or other raised, stable apparatus.
2. Assume the Push-Up neutral start position, but put the right hand on the box and the left hand on the floor.
3. Lift the body so the only contact points are the balls of feet, toes, and left hand on the floor and the right hand on the box.

4. The action is a simple push-up with one hand on the box and the other hand on the floor. All other variables remain constant.

Specific Benefits ⓬

Note Be vigilant in assessing joint stability and comfort, especially in the wrist. The wrist on the box may be highly stressed. Use good judgment.

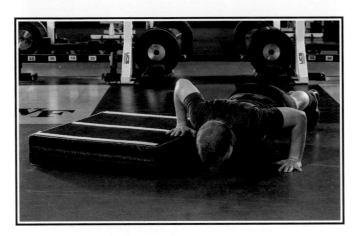

▪ PUSH-UP ▪
UNSTABLE UPPER WITH MEDICINE BALL, ASYMMETRICAL

Modifications

1. Position the body next to a relatively solid medicine ball. The weight of the ball helps to control the exercise. Place the right hand on the ball and the left hand on the floor.
2. Lift the body so the only contact points are the balls of feet, toes, and the left hand on the floor and the right hand on the ball.

3. The action is a simple push-up with one hand on the medicine ball and the other hand on the floor.

Special Benefits ❶ ⓬

Note Be aware of the unstable nature of the medicine ball; attempt the exercise only if confident in proprioceptive abilities. A training partner might be needed to prevent uncontrolled ball movement.

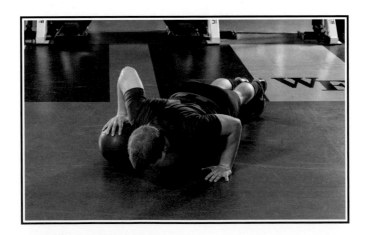

▪ PUSH-UP ▪
UNSTABLE UPPER WITH MEDICINE BALL, ROLL ACROSS

Modifications

1. Assume the same start (neutral) position and body alignment described for Push-Up, Unstable Upper With Medicine Ball, Asymmetrical.

2. Lift the body so the only contact points are the balls of the feet, toes, and the left hand on the floor and the right hand on the ball.

3. Brace the core and maintain straight body alignment; lower the body to the down position.

4. Press back to the start position, at which point the athlete's weight shifts to the left (ground) hand and arm. Simultaneously roll the ball from the right hand to the left hand. As the ball is rolling from right to left, place the right hand on the floor; the body weight shifts from left to right, and the left hand comes off the floor to stop the ball. Place the left hand on top of the ball and do another push-up rep.

5. Repeat back to the start position (the ball rolls back from the left hand to the right hand).

Specific Benefits ❶ ❼ ❾ ⓬ ⓮ ⓱ ⓲

Note This can be a challenging drill. A training partner is advised.

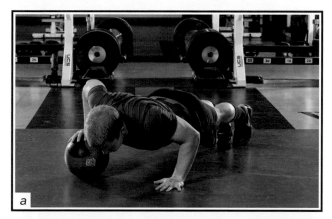

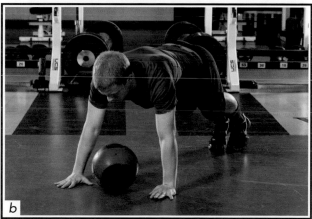

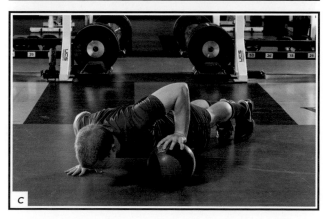

▪ PUSH-UP ▪
UNSTABLE UPPER WITH MEDICINE BALL, WALK ACROSS

Modifications

1. Assume the same start (neutral) position and body alignment described for Push-up, Unstable Upper With Medicine Ball, Roll Across.
2. Brace the core and maintain straight body alignment; lower the body to the down position.
3. Press back to the start position. Remove the left hand from the floor and place it next to the right hand on the ball. Then carefully lift the right hand off the ball and place it onto the floor to the right of the ball; simultaneously shift the body to the right and immediately do another push-up.
4. Reverse the action by removing the right hand from the floor and placing it next to the left hand on the ball. Then move the left hand from the ball to the floor to the left of the ball while shifting the body weight to the left.

Specific Benefits ❶ ❼ ⑫

Note This can be a challenging drill. A training partner is advised.

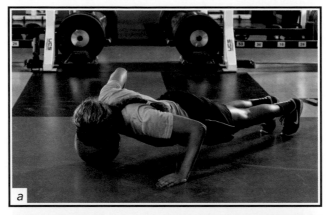

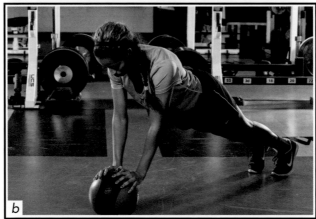

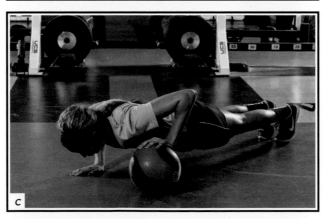

▪ PUSH-UP ▪
UNSTABLE LOWER WITH MEDICINE BALL

Modifications

1. Lie face down on the floor and position a medicine ball on the floor at about shin level. Assume the neutral straight-arm plank start position described for the Push-Up.

2. From this position, either wriggle onto the ball on your own or have a partner assist with positioning. The ball should start at shin level. "Walk" forward with the arms so the ball is either at the ankles or the toes are on the ball. The contact points are the shins, ankles, or balls of the feet and toes on the ball and the hands on the floor.

3. Perform a push-up while maintaining balance on the ball. Do not sag at the knees or hips. Avoid extreme scapular retraction.

Specific Benefits

Note The difficulty progression might look something like this:

1. Shins on the ball
2. Ankles on the ball
3. Balls of the feet and toes on the ball

Additionally, you can use another unstable apparatus instead of a medicine ball.

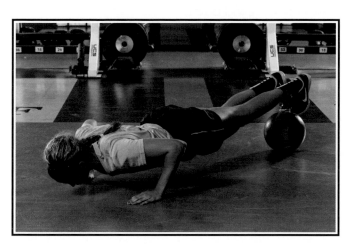

▪ PUSH-UP ▪
UNSTABLE UPPER AND LOWER WITH MEDICINE BALLS

Modifications

1. Place a medicine ball on the floor at about shin level. Place one additional ball by each hand. Assume the neutral straight-arm plank start position described for the Push-Up.

2. Techniques can vary for getting onto the medicine balls. We have found that partner assistance is the best way to get into the start position. If this is not possible, try getting the lower-body ball into position (with the shins, ankles, or balls of the feet and toes on the ball) and then "walk" onto the balls with the hands. The contact points are the lower body (shins, ankles, or balls of the feet and toes) and both hands all on medicine balls.

3. Perform a push-up, maintaining balance on all three balls. Limiting the down position might be warranted until strength and comfort levels improve.

4. Do not sag at the knees or hips. Avoid extreme scapular retraction.

Specific Benefits

Note This is a difficult exercise that initially requires additional stability techniques or precautions. Try one of the following, or a combination:

- Use a somewhat mushy ball. These balls will not roll around as much and thus provide more stability.
- One hand on a ball and the other hand on the floor.
- One foot on a ball and the other foot on the floor
- Both hands on balls and the feet on a relatively stable surface (though not entirely stable).

Using a medicine ball, the difficulty progression might look something like this:

1. Shins on the ball
2. Ankles on the ball
3. Balls of the feet and toes on the ball

Additionally, you can use another unstable apparatus instead of a medicine ball.

Once again, this is a challenging exercise and should be approached with the utmost care. Do not attempt if your strength and proprioceptive abilities are less than stellar.

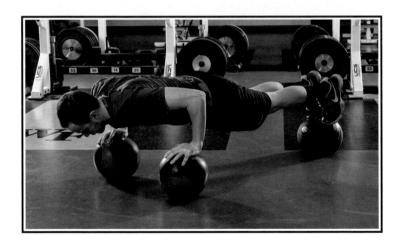

■ PUSH-UP ■
UNSTABLE LOWER, NARROW GRIP WITH MEDICINE BALL

Modifications

1. Place both hands on a medicine ball. The feet are together and placed on a moderately unstable apparatus (e.g., thick foam pad, wobble board, pillows, etc.). If this proves too challenging, for increased stability, try spreading the legs and placing each foot on its own unstable apparatus.

2. Press up to straight-arm plank position; the only contact points are the balls of the feet and toes on the apparatus and both hands on the medicine ball.

3. Brace and maintain extreme dynamic stabilization; perform a narrow-grip unstable push-up. Do not sag or hunch during the action.

Specific Benefits ❶ ⓬

Notes Try different hand positions for additional control or difficulty. For example, point the fingers forward for greater difficulty or lateral toward the floor for greater control. Be conscious of your individual stability and control and never place a joint or body part into a position that could lead to injury.

Initially, the athlete might simply balance in the start position and only progress to a full push-up as proprioceptive comfort develops.

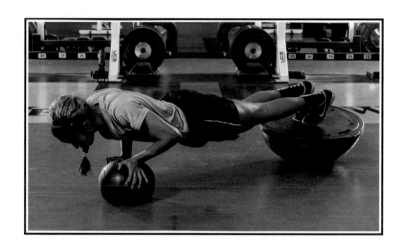

▪ PUSH-UP ▪
UNSTABLE LOWER, COMPLEX

Modifications

1. Lie face down (prone) on the floor and position the upper body close to a raised platform (box, bench, or stair step). Upper-body weight is on the elbows and forearms, and the upper arms are perpendicular to the floor.

2. Brace the core, lock the knees, tighten the glutes, dorsiflex the feet, and place the shins, ankles, or balls of the feet and toes on an unstable apparatus.

3. Lift the body so the only contact points are the shins, ankles, or the balls of the feet and toes on the unstable apparatus and the elbows and forearms on the floor.

4. The complex action is as follows:

   a. Perform an elbow push-up; move into a straight-arm plank position.

   b. Perform a normal push-up; "walk" up onto the raised platform.

   c. Perform a box push-up; "walk" back down off the raised platform and onto the floor.

   d. Perform a normal push-up; then slowly drop back down to the forearm start position.

   e. Perform an elbow push-up.

   f. Maintain a completely straight line in the body (ears, shoulders, hips, knees, and ankles are in alignment) for a predetermined number of round trips. Up and back equals one round trip or repetition.

Specific Benefits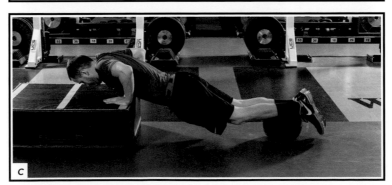

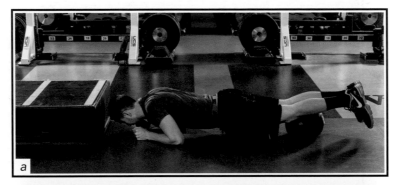

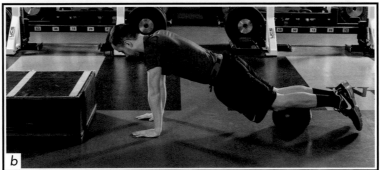

■ PUSH-UP
ARMS ELEVATED, PIKE COMPLEX

Modifications

1. Lie face down (prone) with the hands on or close to the edge of a raised platform. Position the hands directly under the shoulders with the arms perpendicular to the floor.

2. Brace the core, lock the knees, and tighten the glutes. Lift the body so the only contact points are the balls of the feet and toes on the floor and the hands on the raised surface.

3. The complex action is as follows:

   a. Perform a box push-up.

   b. In a straight-arm plank position (hands on the raised surface), walk the hands backward, flexing at the hips and ankles (knees remain as straight as possible).

   c. Perform a pike push-up. Carefully lower the upper body to the raised platform, nearly touching the top of the head to the surface before pressing back to the locked-arm position.

   d. Walk the arms back out to the start position.

   e. Up and back equals one round trip or repetition.

Specific Benefits ❷ ❽ ⓬ ⓲

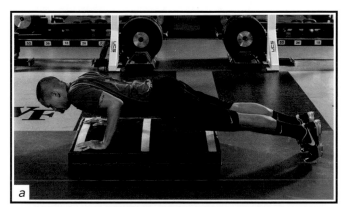

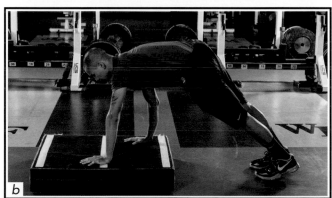

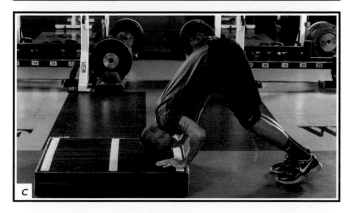

■ PUSH-UP ■
SUSPENDED UPPER

Modifications

1. Place hands in the grips or straps. The arms are straight with a relatively rigid elbow.
2. With a firmly braced abdomen, assume a straight body alignment (ears, shoulders, hips, knees, and ankles are aligned with no arching or sagging of the midsection). Only the balls of the feet and toes are in contact with the floor. Maintain this position throughout.
3. With focused control, drop the body to the down position.
4. Press back up to the start position.

Specific Benefits

Note The depth of the drop is determined by total body strength and the ability to dynamically stabilize the body. Likewise, how far the hands spread is directly dependent upon the athlete's ability to stabilize the shoulder girdle. This will vary from person to person. In most cases a wider grip is more difficult, but not always.

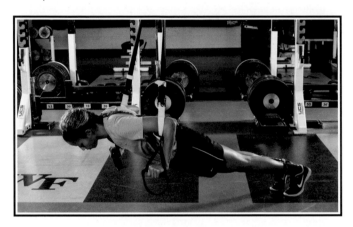

■ PUSH-UP ■
SUSPENDED LOWER

Modifications

1. Position the hands on the floor directly under the shoulders with the arms straight and perpendicular to the floor.
2. Place the feet securely in the grips or straps. Initially, this might require assistance from a training partner.
3. With a firmly braced abdomen, assume a straight body alignment (ears, shoulders, hips, knees, and ankles are aligned with no arching or sagging of the midsection). Maintain this position throughout. Only the hands contact the floor.

4. Maintaining a braced and rigid body alignment, slowly lower the body to the down position.
5. Press back up to the start position.

Specific Benefits

CONDITIONING TO THE CORE

▪ PUSH-UP ▪
SUSPENDED LOWER, BOX WALK-UP

Modifications

1. Position the hands on the floor directly under the shoulders and close to the edge of a box. Assume the start position described for Push-Up, Suspended Lower.

2. Maintaining a braced and rigid body alignment (no sagging or hunching), lift one hand off the floor and place it onto the box. Then lift the other hand off the floor and place it on the box.

3. Hold the up position for a count or two, then reverse the action and "walk" off the box one hand at a time, returning to the start position.

4. Up and return equals one repetition.

Specific Benefits

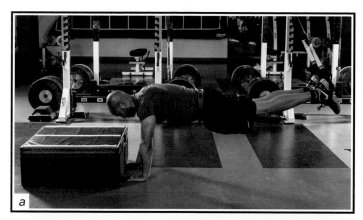

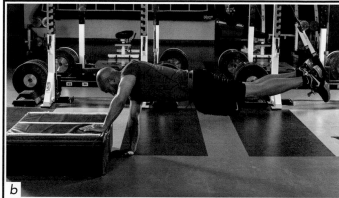

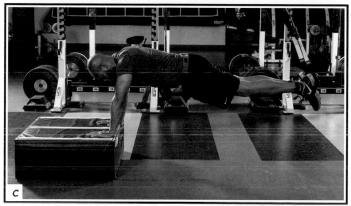

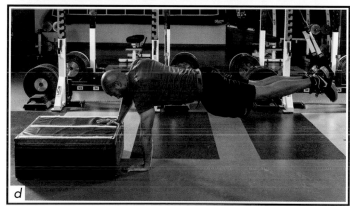

■ PUSH-UP ■
SUSPENDED UPPER AND UNSTABLE LOWER

Modifications

1. Place the hands in the grips or straps. The arms are straight with a relatively rigid elbow.

2. Place the feet on a stability ball or a moderately unstable apparatus, such as a thick foam pad, wobble board, or pillows. Note that if using a stability ball, the height of the handles should be adjusted based on your strength and size of the ball. As a rule for push-ups, the higher the handles, the easier the exercise. Low handles and elevated feet make the exercise very challenging.

3. With a firmly braced abdomen, assume a straight body alignment (ears, shoulders, hips, knees, and ankles are aligned with no arching or sagging of the midsection). Maintain this position throughout. The only contact points are the balls of the feet and toes on the unstable apparatus and the hands on the grips or straps.

4. In a controlled fashion, lower the body to the down position.

5. Press back to the start position.

Specific Benefits ❶ ❷ ❸ ❻ ⓬

■ PUSH-UP ■
SUSPENDED LOWER, COMPLEX

Modifications

1. Assume the start position as described for Push-Up, Suspended Lower. The height of the handles should be such that when the feet are secured and the arms extended and perpendicular to the body, the body is parallel to the floor.

2. Grip a dumbbell in each hand; position the hands (with dumbbells) on the floor, directly under the shoulders.

3. Brace the core, lock the knees, tighten the glutes, dorsiflex the feet; avoid sagging or hunching. The contact points are the balls of the feet and toes in the straps and the hands gripping the dumbbells on the floor.

4. The complex action is as follows:
   a. Perform a normal push-up.
   b. While in a straight-arm position, perform an alternate arm rear pull. First, pull the right hand and dumbbell from the floor to the armpit. Return the right hand and dumbbell to the floor; repeat with the left hand and dumbbell. Attempt to counter the rotational forces that will challenge your equilibrium created through the elimination of the symmetrical base of support by simply lifting of one hand off floor.
   c. Maintaining a relatively straight spine and neutral pelvis, pull both feet up and under the torso. The knees will tuck toward the chest; a natural lift of the hips will occur to accommodate the knee tuck, but try to keep the hips as low as possible. This will help to maintain osteoarticular and specifically lumbar alignment and dynamic stability while challenging hip, knee, and ankle range of motion.
   d. Hold the up position for a count or two; under control, extend both bent knees and hips back to the start position.
   e. Repeat steps a through d for a predetermined number of repetitions.

Specific Benefits ❶ ❸ ❻ ⓬ ⓱ ⓲

HANGING KNEE-UP (ROCK BACK)

MOVEMENTS

1. Grip the chin-up bar. Retract the scapulae and maintain this position throughout the exercise. Avoid the chicken head!
2. Lift the knees to a 90-90 lower-body position (in 90-90 position both the hip and knee joints are flexed to 90 degrees). The upper legs (thighs) are parallel to the ground and never drop below this position throughout the exercise.
3. To begin, the pelvis is in neutral position with a *slight* anterior tilt. In a controlled manner, tilt the pelvis posteriorly, lifting the 90-90 legs up and back.
4. Slowly lower the legs back to the start position, not allowing the upper legs to drop below parallel. Note, you should also be back to the neutral pelvis position with a *slight* anterior tilt.
5. Perform a predetermined number of repetitions.
6. Upon completion of the set, carefully return to a straight-body hang and drop to floor.

CONSIDERATIONS

1. It is important to avoid an extreme kyphotic lumbar curve during this and all exercises.
2. Grip choices vary from wide to narrow, underhand to overhand, and elbow flexed to elbow straight. However, one constant is retraction and thus stabilization of the scapula.

SPECIFIC BENEFITS

12 **16** **17**

NOTE

All precautions and suggestions listed here apply to all of the following hanging exercises.

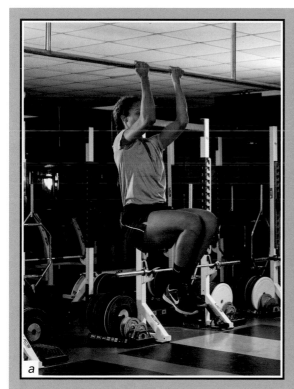
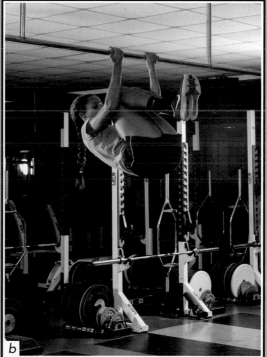

■ HANGING INVERTED BENT KNEE TO STRAIGHT LEG ■

Modifications

1. Grip the bar and lift the legs up and back. This is the start position.

2. Straighten the legs and shoot them toward the ceiling. This action is similar to a pole vaulter shooting his legs toward the bar while in an inverted (almost upside down) position.

3. In a slow, controlled manner, bend the knees and lower the legs back to the start position.

Specific Benefits ⑫ ⑯ ⑰

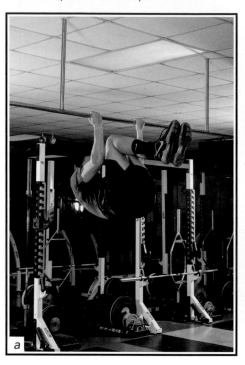

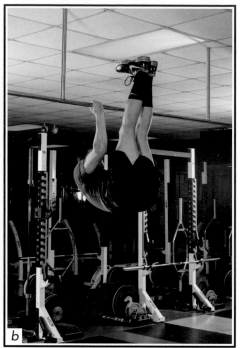

■ HANGING SHIN TAP ■

Modifications

1. Grip the bar and lift slightly into a scapular retraction position.
2. Brace the core, contract the abdominals and hip flexors, and lift the straight legs toward the ceiling.
3. Tap the shins to the bar.
4. In a slow, controlled manner, lower the straight legs down to the hanging start position.

Specific Benefits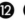

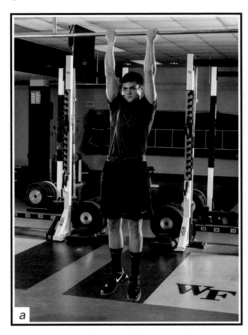
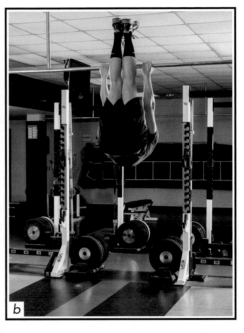

■ HANGING PIKE PULL-UP ■

Modifications

1. Assume the starting position and initial action as described for the Hanging Shin Tap.
2. Maintain the pike position in which the shins are at the bar.
3. While in the pike position perform an inverted pull-up, lifting the chest toward the bar (scapulae retraction).
4. Slowly lower to the start position.

Specific Benefits

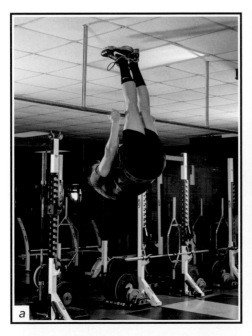
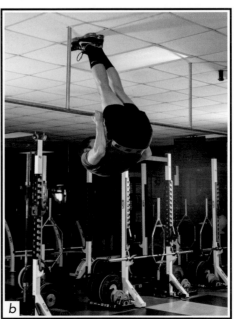

MOVEMENTS

1. Grip the chin-up bar with the legs hanging straight to the floor (the entire body is perpendicular to the floor). Retract the scapulae and maintain this position throughout the exercise. Avoid the chicken head!

2. Lift the knees to a 90-90 lower-body position (in a 90-90 position both the hip and knee joints are flexed to 90 degrees). The upper legs (thighs) are parallel to the ground and never drop below this position throughout the exercise. The pelvis is in neutral position with a *slight* anterior tilt.

3. Slowly lower the legs back to the hanging start position.

4. Perform a predetermined number of repetitions.

CONSIDERATIONS

1. It's important to avoid an extreme kyphotic lumbar curve during this and all exercises.

2. Grip choices vary from wide to narrow, underhand to overhand, and elbow flexed to elbow straight. However, one constant is retraction and thus stabilization of the scapula.

SPECIFIC BENEFITS

12 **16** **17**

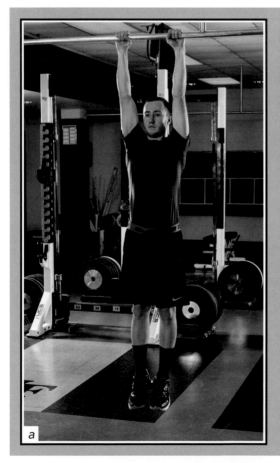
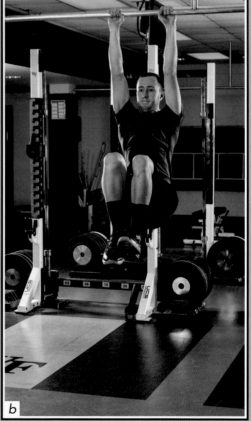

■ HANGING STRAIGHT LEG TO BENT KNEE ■
MEDICINE BALL BETWEEN KNEES

Modifications

1. Assume the same start position described for Hanging Straight Leg to Bent Knee.
2. Place a medicine ball (or similar resistance) between the knees. Engage the hip adductors to maintain secure control of the ball. (Note Unless you are a member of Cirque du Soleil, it will probably be necessary for a partner to position the medicine ball while you are in the hanging position.)

3. Brace the core, flex the hips and knees, and lift the legs to the 90-90 position. The medicine ball remains secure between the knees.
4. Lower the legs back to the start position. Do not lose control of the medicine ball throughout the exercise. If the ball starts to slip, have your training partner reposition it and continue with the remainder of the set.

Specific Benefits **12** **16** **17**

■ HANGING STRAIGHT LEG TO BENT KNEE ■
MEDICINE BALL BETWEEN ANKLES

Modifications

1. Assume the same start position described for Hanging Straight Leg to Bent Knee, Medicine Ball Between Knees, but this time hold the ball firmly between the ankles and perform the same action.

Specific Benefits **12** **16** **17**

Note Adding resistance (a medicine ball or similar) further from the axis point (the hips) places more ancillary stress on the joint, increasing the risk factors of this exercise.

■ HANGING STRAIGHT LEG TO BENT KNEE ■
POSTERIOR RESISTANCE BAND

Modifications

1. Assume the same start position described for Hanging Straight Leg to Bent Knee.
2. A partner places a resistance band around your dorsiflexed feet. A rubber band works best, but a jump rope, stretch strap, or something similar can also work; however, your training partner will need to constantly monitor the uniformity of resistance throughout range of motion.
3. Brace the core, flex the hips and knees, and lift the legs to the 90-90 position.

4. Throughout the exercise, the training partner applies resistance from behind, constantly adjusting band tension based on observation and physical feedback.
5. Carefully lower the legs to the start position.

Specific Benefits **12** **16** **17**

Note For some individuals, the resistance band might need to be double wrapped around the ankles to stay secure. However, a strong dorsiflexion should not necessitate the need to double wrap.

ALTERNATING STRAIGHT LEG TO L

MOVEMENTS

1. Grip the chin-up bar or place your arms in the straps as shown. The legs hang straight to the floor (the entire body is perpendicular to the floor).

2. Retract the scapulae and maintain throughout the exercise. Avoid the chicken head! The pelvis is in neutral position with a *slight* anterior tilt.

3. Brace the entire core and raise the right leg to parallel. The left leg remains hanging directly to the floor. Maintain straight body alignment between the ear, shoulder, hip, left knee, and left ankle.

4. Slowly lower the right leg back to the start position; repeat the action with the left leg.

5. Continue alternating legs for a predetermined number of repetitions or length of time.

CONSIDERATIONS

1. The height of the leg raise depends on your level of flexibility. If you lack the necessary lumbar and pelvic mobility and attempt to raise the leg higher than you are capable, you will compensate with a contraindicated posterior pelvic tilt.

2. If you grip the chin-up bar itself rather than using the straps, grip choices vary from wide to narrow, underhand to overhand, and elbow flexed to elbow straight. However, one constant is retraction and thus stabilization of the scapula.

SPECIFIC BENEFITS

4 11 12 16 17

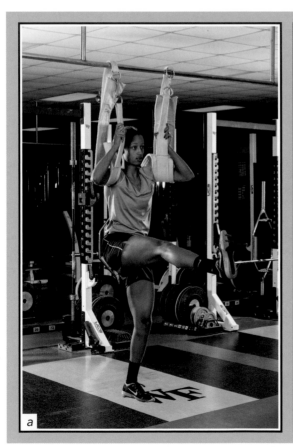
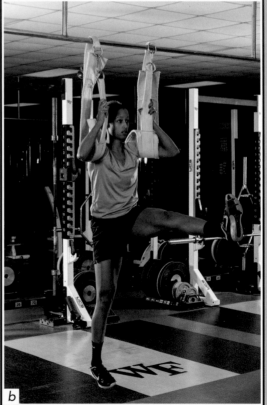

Modifications

1. Assume the same start position and posture described for Hanging L Series: Alternating Straight Leg to L.
2. Brace the core and flex both hips, raising both straight legs from perpendicular to the floor to parallel to the floor to the L position.
3. Slowly lower the legs back to the start position.

Specific Benefits ⑫ ⑯ ⑰

Note Controlling anterior and posterior tilt of the pelvis can help to constrain the "swinging" action often associated with hanging exercises.

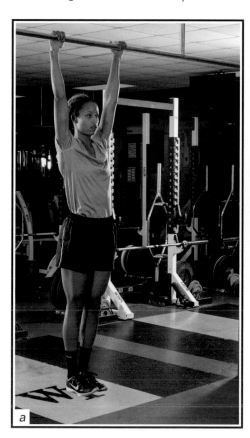

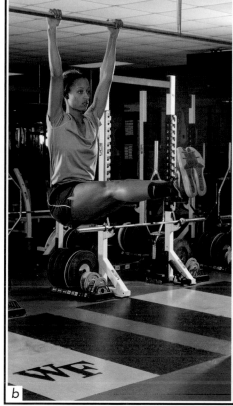

Modifications

1. Assume the same start position and posture described for Hanging L Series: Alternating Straight Leg to L. The pelvis is in neutral position with a *slight* anterior tilt.

2. Brace the core and raise the legs to the L position. Maintain the L position throughout the exercise (do not let the legs drop back to the hanging position at any point during the action).

3. From the L position, draw the knees to the body. The knees are flexed; the pelvis has slight posterior tilt. Extend the knees and return back to the starting L position.

4. L to knee tuck and back to L counts as one repetition.

Specific Benefits **12** **16** **17**

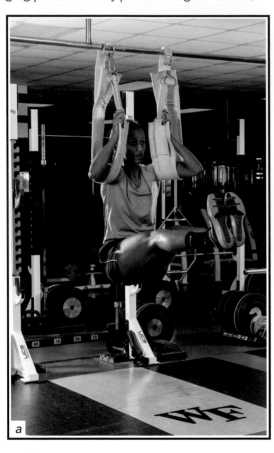

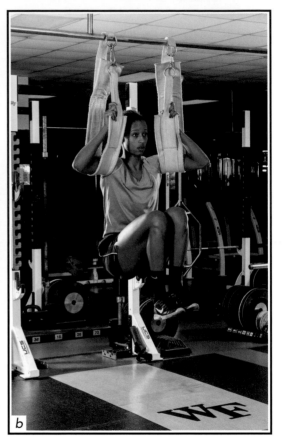

▪ HANGING L SERIES ▪
L TO ANKLE TAP AND BACK TO L

Modifications

1. Assume the same start position posture described for Hanging L Series: L to Knee Tuck and Back to L.

2. Brace the core and raise the legs to the L position. Maintain the L position throughout the exercise (do not let the legs drop back to the hanging position at any point during the action).

3. From the L position, flex the hips and raise the straight legs to a point at which the ankles touch the bar.

4. Slowly lower the straight legs back to the L position.

5. L to ankle tap and back to L counts as one repetition.

Specific Benefits   **17**

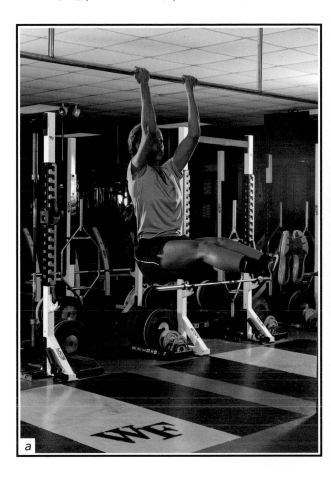

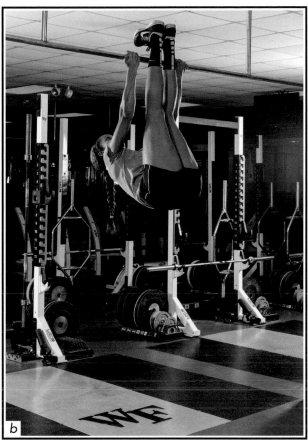

▪ HANGING L SERIES ▪
ABDUCTION AND ADDUCTION

Modifications

1. Assume the same start position and posture described for Hanging L Series: Alternating Straight Leg to L.

2. From the L position, brace the core and spread the legs (abduction) as wide as possible while maintaining the hanging L position.

3. Adduct the straight legs back to the L position.

Specific Benefits **5**

Modifications

1. Assume the same start position and posture described for Hanging L Series: Alternating Straight Leg to L.

2. The arms are relatively straight while maintaining a retracted scapulae. (Note: A slight elbow flexion might be necessary; the degree of flexion depends on your strength level.)

3. From the L position, brace the core and perform a pull-up if you are gripping the chin-up bar. If using straps as in the photo, pull yourself into the straps and maintain good posture.

Specific Benefits ⑫ ⑯ ⑰ ⑱

Note While in the straight-arm position, avoid subluxation of the shoulder. A slight elbow flexion might be necessary to avoid dropping too deep into the shoulder.

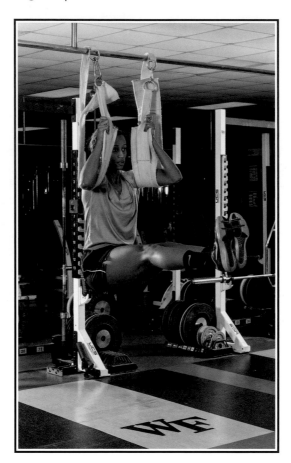

Anti-Rotation
Exercises

If you are reading these opening paragraphs, then you feel comfortable with your foundation of dynamic stabilization and are ready to continue toward further integrated strengthening of musculature. An argument has been made about the importance of postural control and dynamic equilibrium during application of enhanced performance variables. Without first laying a foundation of osteoarticular stabilization, many athletes make the mistake of simply incorporating excessive levels of concentric flexion, extension, and rotation activities that promote recruitment of the prime movers but often at the sacrifice of desensitizing the deep stabilizers. This can lead to a whole host of issues, including submaximal performance and increased potential for injury. Decisions to move from stabilization

to strength and eventually strength to power are the result of functional progress, not that of pain tolerance or the illusion of accomplishment associated with the appearance of six-pack abs.

Any core program worth its salt should consider, at the very least, the following training parameters: frequency, intensity, duration, balance, proprioception, load considerations, movement tempo, range of motion, and planes of motion. Movement can be generalized as taking place within one or any combination of three planes of movement (see figure 11.1).

Frontal plane movement occurs on an anterior-posterior axis and hypothetically divides the body into front and back halves and can be characterized by adduction/abduction, lateral flexion, and eversion/inversion motions (e.g., side lunges). Sagittal

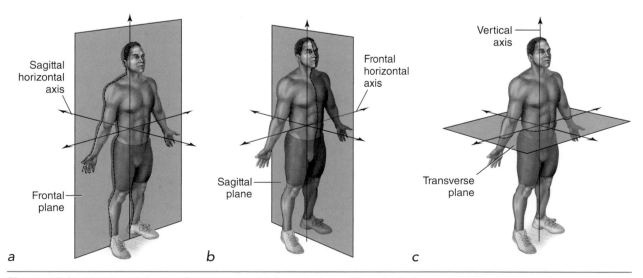

Figure 11.1   The three planes of movement. (*a*) frontal plane, (*b*) sagittal plane, and (*c*) transverse plane.

plane movement occurs on a coronal axis and divide the body into left and right halves and is typified by flexion/extension actions (e.g., squats). Finally, transverse plane activities, the most pertinent to this chapter, are on a longitudinal axis and dissect the body into top and bottom halves and are expressed during internal/external rotation, left/right rotation, and horizontal abduction/adduction.

Typically, when we look at planes of motion we are discussing gross motor patterns of the body; however when examining the reason behind anti-rotation training we are moving from large, sweeping movements to the organization of finite joint actions. Always look at the body in a complete sense, but remember that anti-rotation training is principally about not rotating through L1 to L5 but instead training the body to rotate at T1-T12. This fits into our innate anatomical model as well as enabling the separation between shoulders and hips and thereby initiating the stretch-shortening cycle and increasing our ability to express force appropriately.

When thoracic strength is built upon a foundation of lumbar stabilization, the athlete can now move functionally closer to his or her athletic potential. The Empire State Building was not built upon a foundation of sand. Without the underlying bedrock, the enormity of the structure could not have possibly been realized. From an athletic perspective, the height of your potential is directly related to your foundational bedrock.

As in chapter 9, this chapter also includes complex exercises. A "complex" is a multifaceted exercise that typically involves a variety of movement patterns within a variety of planes of motion encompassing a variety of velocity and load options.

The following exercise finder lists the benefits, difficulty level, and equipment needed for every exercise that appears in this chapter. Primary exercises are highlighted in blue, with their progressions in red. The primary exercises are also noted in the text with a red title bar.

Anti-Rotation Strength Exercise Finder

Exercise Name	Specific Benefits (see chapter 5)	Easy	Medium	Hard	Equipment
Windshield Wiper	(12)		X		
Windshield Wiper Variation	(5) (12)		X		
Windshield Wiper With Flutter Kick	(5) (12)		X		
Straight-Arm Plank Complex 1: Overhead Pull	(9) (12) (17)		X		Cable machine or resistance band/cable
Straight-Arm Plank Complex 2: Front Raise (Sagittal Flexion)	(5) (9) (12) (17)		X		Cable machine or resistance band/cable
Straight-Arm Plank Complex 3: Lateral Pull	(9) (12) (17)		X		Cable machine or resistance band/cable
Straight-Arm Plank Complex 4: Lateral Pull, Elbow Extension	(9) (12) (17)		X		Cable machine or resistance band/cable
Straight-Arm Plank Complex 5: Lateral Rear Deltoid Fly	(9) (12) (17)		X		Cable machine or resistance band/cable
Push-Up Complex, Rear Deltoid	(5) (9) (12) (13) (17) (18) (24)		X		Two dumbbells
Slideboard Hands Single-Arm Overhead Reach	(7) (9) (12) (19) (24)	X			Slideboard
Slideboard Hands Full-Body Extension, Alternating Wax On/Wax Off	(12) (19) (24)			X	Slideboard
Slideboard Hands Full-Body Extension, Simultaneous Wax On/Wax Off	(12) (19) (24)			X	Slideboard
Slideboard Hands Abduction and Adduction	(5) (12) (19) (24)			X	Slideboard
Slideboard Feet Lateral Cross	(4) (9) (12) (19) (24)		X		Slideboard
Slideboard Feet Lateral Cross With Push-Up	(4) (9) (12) (18) (19) (24)		X		Slideboard
Slideboard Feet Sandbag Pull	(5) (9) (12) (17) (18) (19)			X	Slideboard, sandbag
Slideboard Feet Sandbag Pull, Abduction and Adduction	(5) (9) (12) (17) (18) (19)			X	Slideboard, sandbag
Slideboard Feet Sandbag Pull, Mountain Climber	(4) (5) (9) (12) (17) (18) (19)			X	Slideboard, sandbag
Lateral Elbow Plank Cable Row	(9) (12) (13) (17)		X		Cable section with handle
Lateral Straight-Arm Plank Cable Row	(9) (12) (13) (17)		X		Cable section with handle
Lateral Elbow Plank Cable Row, Feet Elevated	(3) (9) (12) (13) (17)		X		Cable section with handle, raised platform**
Lateral Straight-Arm Plank Cable Row, Feet Elevated	(3) (9) (12) (13) (17)		X		Cable section with handle, raised platform

* Many options are available for the unstable apparatus, including a thick foam pad, wobble board, balance disc, pillows, or stability ball.

** Many options are available for the raised platform, including a box, bench, stair, or step.

(continued)

Exercise Name	Specific Benefits (see chapter 5)	Difficulty Level Easy	Difficulty Level Medium	Difficulty Level Hard	Equipment
Lateral Elbow Plank Cable Row, Unstable Upper	1 9 12 13 17		X		Cable section with handle, unstable apparatus*
Lateral Straight-Arm Plank Cable Row, Unstable Upper	1 9 12 13 17		X		Cable section with handle, unstable apparatus
Lateral Elbow Plank Cable Row, Unstable Lower	1 9 12 13 17 (and 3 if using stability ball)		X		Cable section with handle, unstable apparatus
Lateral Straight-Arm Plank Cable Row, Unstable Lower	1 9 12 13 17 (and 3 if using stability ball)		X		Cable section with handle, unstable apparatus
Pallof Isometric Press Progression 1: Half-Kneeling	12 17 24		X		Cable section with rope or handle, or core bar
Pallof Isometric Press Progression 2: Tall Kneeling	12 17 24		X		Cable section with rope or handle, or core bar
Pallof Isometric Press Progression 3: Standing	12 17 24		X		Cable section with rope or handle, or core bar
Pallof Isometric Press Progression 4: Staggered Stance	12 17 18 24			X	Cable section with rope or handle, or core bar
Pallof Isometric Press Progression 5: Lunge Stance	12 17 18 24			X	Cable section with rope or handle, or core bar
Pallof Horizontal Press Progression 1: Half-Kneeling	12 17 24		X		Cable section with rope or handle, or core bar
Pallof Horizontal Press Progression 2: Tall Kneeling	12 17 24		X		Cable section with rope or handle, or core bar
Pallof Horizontal Press Progression 3: Standing	12 17 24		X		Cable section with rope or handle, or core bar
Pallof Horizontal Press Progression 4: Staggered Stance	12 17 18 24			X	Cable section with rope or handle, or core bar
Pallof Horizontal Press Progression 5: Lunge Stance	12 17 18 24			X	Cable section with rope or handle, or core bar
Cable Chop Progression 1: Half-Kneeling	12 17 24		X		Cable section with rope or handle, or core bar
Cable Chop Progression 2: Tall Kneeling	12 17 24		X		Cable section with rope or handle, or core bar
Cable Chop Progression 3: Standing	12 17 24		X		Cable section with rope or handle, or core bar
Cable Chop Progression 4: Staggered Stance	12 17 18 24			X	Cable section with rope or handle, or core bar
Cable Chop Progression 5: Lunge Stance	12 17 18 24			X	Cable section with rope or handle, or core bar
Cable Lift Progression 1: Half-Kneeling	12 17 24		X		Cable section with rope or handle, or core bar
Cable Lift Progression 2: Tall Kneeling	12 17 24		X		Cable section with rope or handle, or core bar
Cable Lift Progression 3: Standing	12 17 24		X		Cable section with rope or handle, or core bar
Cable Lift Progression 4: Staggered Stance	12 17 18 24			X	Cable section with rope or handle, or core bar

Exercise Name	Specific Benefits (see chapter 5)	Easy	Medium	Hard	Equipment
Cable Lift Progression 5: Lunge Stance	⑫ ⑰ ⑱ ㉔			X	Cable section with rope or handle, or core bar
Anti-Rotation Press Progression 1: Half-Kneeling	⑫ ⑰ ㉔		X		Cable section with rope or handle, or core bar
Anti-Rotation Press Progression 2: Tall Kneeling	⑫ ⑰ ㉔		X		Cable section with rope or handle, or core bar
Anti-Rotation Press Progression 3: Standing	⑫ ⑰ ㉔		X		Cable section with rope or handle, or core bar
Anti-Rotation Press Progression 4: Staggered Stance	⑫ ⑰ ⑱ ㉔			X	Cable section with rope or handle, or core bar
Anti-Rotation Press Progression 5: Lunge Stance	⑫ ⑰ ⑱ ㉔			X	Cable section with rope or handle, or core bar
Pull and Press Progression 1: Half-Kneeling	⑨ ⑫ ⑰ ㉔		X		Cable sections with handles
Pull and Press Progression 2: Tall Kneeling	⑨ ⑫ ⑰ ㉔		X		Cable sections with handles
Pull and Press Progression 3: Standing	⑨ ⑫ ⑰ ㉔		X		Cable sections with handles
Pull and Press Progression 4: Staggered Stance	⑨ ⑫ ⑰ ⑱ ㉔			X	Cable sections with handles
Pull and Press Progression 5: Lunge Stance	⑨ ⑫ ⑰ ⑱ ㉔			X	Cable sections with handles
Landmine Rotation	⑫ ⑰ ㉔		X		Plate, barbell
Landmine Rotation With Handle	⑫ ⑰ ㉔		X		Plate, barbell with handle
Landmine Rotation With Handle and Load	⑫ ⑰ ㉔			X	Plates, barbell with handle
Cable Rotation With Stability Ball, Standing	⑫ ⑰		X		Two cable sections with handles, stability ball
Hanging Knee Tuck	⑫ ⑯ ⑰			X	Chin-up bar
Hanging Knee Tuck, Extended L	⑫ ⑯ ⑰			X	Chin-up bar
Hanging Knee Tuck, Extended L Twist	⑫ ⑯ ⑰ ⑱ ㉔			X	Chin-up bar
Hanging Knee Tuck, Up and Twist	⑫ ⑯ ⑰ ⑱ ㉔			X	Chin-up bar
Hanging Knee Tuck, Bent Knee Windshield Wiper	⑫ ⑯ ⑰ ⑱ ㉔			X	Chin-up bar
Hanging Knee Tuck, Bent Knee Windshield Wiper for Speed	⑫ ⑯ ⑰ ⑱ ㉒ ㉓ ㉔			X	Chin-up bar
Hanging Inverted Pike, Double-Leg Windshield Wiper	⑫ ⑯ ⑰ ⑱ ㉒ ㉔			X	Chin-up bar
Hanging Inverted Pike, Windshield Wiper Abduction and Adduction	⑤ ⑨ ⑫ ⑯ ⑰ ⑱ ㉒ ㉔			X	Chin-up bar
Hanging Inverted Pike, Up and Twist (Pole Vaulter)	⑧ ⑫ ⑯ ⑰ ⑱ ㉔			X	Chin-up bar
Hang Cycling	⑧ ⑪ ⑫ ⑯ ⑰ ⑱			X	Chin-up bar
Hang Giant Walk	⑧ ⑪ ⑫ ⑯ ⑰ ⑱			X	Chin-up bar

WINDSHIELD WIPER

MOVEMENTS

1. Lie supine on an exercise mat on the floor with the head on the mat.
2. Flex the hips to 90 degrees; the body will be in an L position with the legs pointing directly to the ceiling.
3. In a controlled manner, slowly lower the straight legs to one side (see consideration 2).
4. Lightly tap the floor (or don't tap at all—it's harder) and immediately raise the legs back to perpendicular.
5. Hesitate a split-second and continue to the opposite side.
6. Perform a predetermined number of repetitions.

CONSIDERATIONS

1. The difficulty of the exercise can be manipulated to a small degree. For example, if you extend the arms out onto floor perpendicular to the body, you can use leverage and a greater surface area base of support to assist with controlling leg movement. Likewise, the less involved the arms (e.g., only the elbows on the floor or the arms completely off the floor), the more difficult the exercise.
2. You can also manipulate the degree of difficulty by limiting range of motion in the rotation movement. That is, do not lower the legs completely to the floor until sufficient strength allows for such intensity.

SPECIFIC BENEFITS

NOTE

Try these Windshield Wiper variations:

- Both legs drop to the side, one leg up then next leg up, repeat opposite (see next exercise)
- One leg drops to the side, other leg drops to side, one leg up then next leg up, repeat opposite
- One leg drops to the side, other leg drops to the side, both legs simultaneously up, repeat opposite
- Flutter kick throughout the exercise
- Scissor kick throughout exercise
- Both legs drop to the side, one leg up then next leg up, flutter or scissor kick from perpendicular straight forward and down to the floor, continue to flutter or scissor kick back to a straight-leg perpendicular position, repeat opposite
- Both legs drop to the side, while in this position flex the knees and extend back to straight, return the legs back to perpendicular via any of above-mentioned actions, repeat opposite
- Spread the legs throughout the exercise: down left, up, down right, up
- In the up position, lift the upper body off the floor and catch and return pass a tossed medicine ball from a training partner: down left; up; down right; up; lift, catch, and pass; repeat

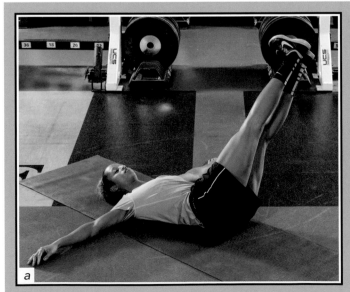

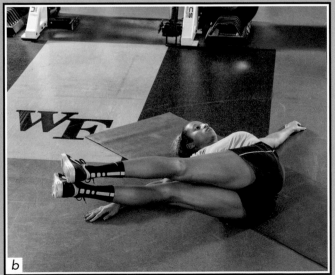

▪ WINDSHIELD WIPER VARIATION ▪

Modifications

1. Assume the Windshield Wiper start position.
2. In a controlled manner, slowly lower the straight legs to the left side.
3. Lightly tap the floor (or don't tap at all—it's harder).

4. Separate and raise only the right leg back to perpendicular. Continue by raising the left leg back to perpendicular (start position).
5. Hesitate for a split-second and continue to the opposite side.

Specific Benefits

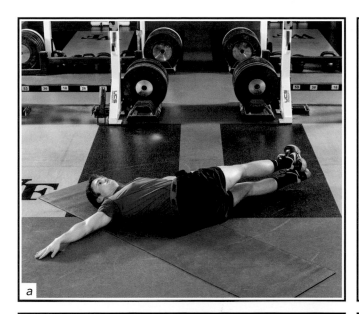

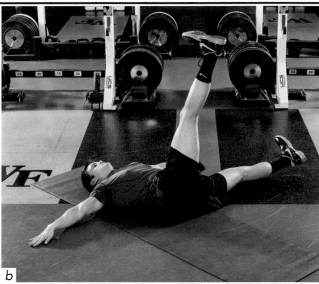

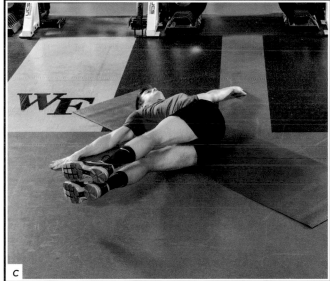

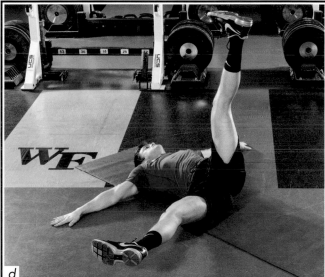

▪ WINDSHIELD WIPER ▪
WITH FLUTTER KICK

Modifications

1. The start position and action are the same as described for the Windshield Wiper with the addition of a flutter kick throughout the exercise. A flutter kick is a straight-leg, short-arc action in which the legs move rapidly up and down in opposition within the sagittal plane. For example, flutter kick drop both legs left; flutter kick both legs back to neutral; flutter kick drop both legs right; flutter kick both legs back to neutral.

Specific Benefits ❺ ⓬

Note This exercise can also be done using a scissor kick, which is a straight-leg, rapid, side-to-side action in opposition, primarily within the frontal plane.

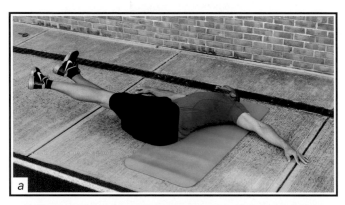

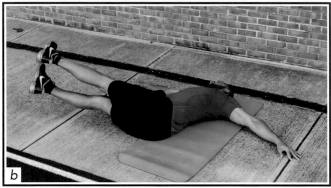

STRAIGHT-ARM PLANK

COMPLEX 1: OVERHEAD PULL

MOVEMENTS

1. Set the resistance cable or band about shoulder high when in a plank position (i.e., about a perpendicular arm's length from the floor).

2. Assume a straight-arm plank position with the head positioned *toward* the cable machine (or band attachment). The left hand is on the floor with the arm perpendicular to the floor; the right hand grips the handle. Lift the body so only the balls of the feet, toes, and left hand are on the floor. Throughout the exercise, maintain a completely straight line in the body.

3. The complex action is as follows:

   a. In a three-point plank position, the right arm is straight with the palm down (facing the floor). The right arm should be a straight-line extension of the planked body.

   b. Flex the elbow and pull the right hand to a position near the right armpit. The right hand will rotate from a palm-down position at the start of action to a palm-up position at the upper termination point (the armpit).

   c. In a controlled manner, allow the cable weight (or rubber band) to return the arm back to the start position.

4. Perform a predetermined number of repetitions; repeat on the opposite side.

CONSIDERATIONS

1. Throughout the exercise, maintain a straight line in the body (ears, shoulders, hips, knees, and ankles in alignment). Avoid sagging, hunching, or, most important, tipping opposite the cable or band hand while performing the movements.

SPECIFIC BENEFITS

 9 **12** **17**

NOTE

To add variety or increase difficulty, incorporate some of these challenges:

- Lift one leg off the floor, thereby creating only two points of contact during the exercise.
- While performing the pull action, the up leg can simultaneously perform any one or a combination of knee drives, hip extensions, abductions, mountain climber foot taps, and more.
- Position the feet on an unstable apparatus.
- Employ perturbation techniques such as gently tapping the athlete throughout the movement or positioning a resistance band around the waist, ankles, or knees.

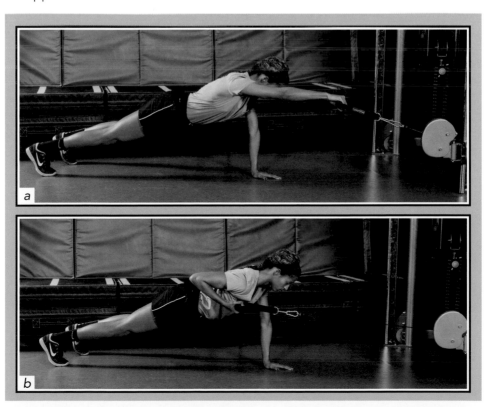

COMPLEX 2: FRONT RAISE (SAGITTAL FLEXION)

Modifications

1. Set the resistance cable or resistance band about shoulder high when in the plank position (i.e., about a perpendicular arm's length from the floor). If using a rubber band, you can incorporate two bands, one in each hand. You can then alternate the action described below.

2. Assume a straight-arm plank position with the head positioned *away* from cable machine (or band attachment). The right hand is on the floor with the arm perpendicular to the floor; the left hand grips the handle. Lift the body so only the balls of the feet, toes, and right hand are on the floor. Maintain a completely straight line in the body (ears, shoulders, hips, knees, and ankles are in alignment) throughout the exercise.

3. The complex action is as follows:
   a. While balanced in a three-point stance (both feet and right hand), front raise the straight left arm forward (sagittal plane) to a point at which the arm is in alignment with the planked body.
   b. Return the straight arm to the start position and place the left hand on the floor.

Specific Benefits ❺ ❾ ⓬ ⓱

Note The action can be a horizontal shoulder press instead of a horizontal front raise. See Straight-Arm Plank Complex 1 for ideas to increase difficulty and add variety.

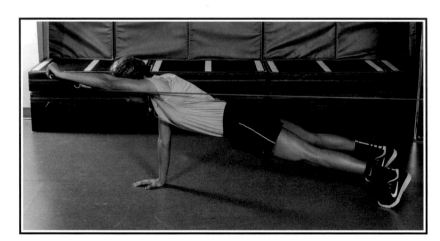

Modifications

1. Set the resistance cable or resistance band about shoulder high when in the plank position (i.e., about a perpendicular arm's length from the floor).

2. Assume a straight-arm plank position with the body perpendicular to the cable's line of pull. The left hand is on the floor with the left arm straight and perpendicular to the floor.

3. Reach through (under) the body and grab a single handle with the right hand, palm up.

4. Lift the body so only the balls of the feet, toes, and left hand are on the floor. Throughout the exercise, maintain a completely straight line in body (ears, shoulders, hips, knees, and ankles in alignment).

5. The "complex" action is as follows:

   a. In a three-point plank position, the right arm is under the body and gripping the handle.

   b. Flex the elbow and pull the right hand to the right armpit. The palm stays up throughout the exercise.

   c. In a controlled manner, return to the start position.

Specific Benefits

Note See Straight-Arm Plank Complex 1 for ideas to increase difficulty and add variety.

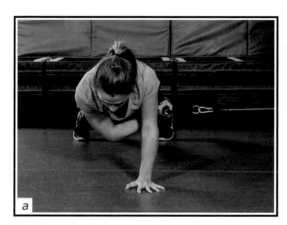

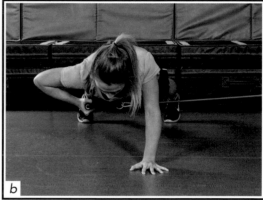

■ STRAIGHT-ARM PLANK ■
COMPLEX 4: LATERAL PULL, ELBOW EXTENSION

Modifications

1. The setup, start position, and posture are identical to Straight-Arm Plank Complex 3.
2. The complex action is as follows:
   a. In a three-point plank position, the right arm is under the body and gripping the handle.
   b. Flex the elbow and pull the right hand to the right armpit. The palm stays up until the armpit is reached.
   c. Once the hand reaches the armpit, continue the action with a lateral elbow extension to a point at which the right arm is fully extended. The palm is now down; the arm is perpendicular to the body.
   d. In a controlled manner, return to the start position.

Specific Benefits ❾ ⓬ ⓱

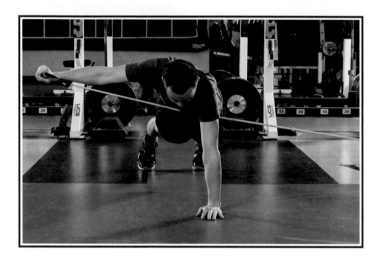

■ STRAIGHT-ARM PLANK ■
COMPLEX 5: LATERAL REAR DELTOID FLY

Modifications

1. The setup, start position, and posture are identical to Straight Arm Plank Complex 3.
2. The complex action is as follows:
   a. In a three-point plank position, the right arm is under the body and gripping the handle.
   b. Maintaining a relatively straight arm (or at least a locked elbow), pull the resistance grip under the left arm and body and continue into a rear deltoid fly to a point at which the right arm is fully extended and perpendicular to the body. At the end of the action, the palm will be facing down.
   c. Avoid twisting. Keep the right hip down when pulling with the right hand, and vice versa with the left hand.
   d. In a controlled manner, return to the start position.

Specific Benefits

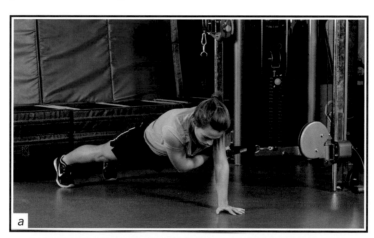

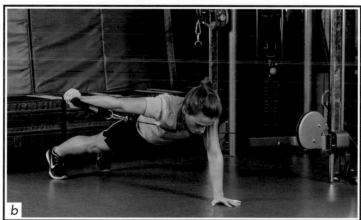

PUSH-UP COMPLEX, REAR DELTOID

MOVEMENTS

1. Assume a straight-arm plank position with the left hand on the floor and the right hand gripping a light dumbbell, also on the floor (or grip a dumbbell in each hand, as shown). Both hands are directly under the shoulders with the arms perpendicular to the floor. Lift the body so only the balls of feet, toes, and left hand are on the floor; the right hand is gripping a dumbbell, which is also on the floor. The body maintains a completely straight line (ears, shoulders, hips, knees, and ankles are aligned) throughout the exercise.

2. The complex action is as follows:

   a. Perform a push-up.

   b. While balanced in a three-point stance (both feet and left hand), front raise (flexion) the straight right arm forward (sagittal plane) to a point at which the right arm is in alignment with the planked body.

   c. Return the straight arm to the start position and place the right hand on the floor to regain balance and reposition the body prior to the next movement of the complex. (Or do not place the hand and dumbbell on the floor and instead move immediately into the next move of the complex.)

   d. Raise the straight right arm and dumbbell laterally (abduction), to a point parallel to the floor and perpendicular to the body.

   e. At this point in the complex, either continue into a core rotation or return the hand and dumbbell back to the start position prior to the core rotation. Either way, the core rotation is as follows:

      1. Rotate the entire planked body, as one unit, to a position in which the right arm is extended toward the ceiling.

      2. Both feet have remained in the same location but are fully rotated to the side of the foot.

      3. The body is in a straight-line plank (ears, shoulders, hips, knees, and ankles are in alignment)

      4. The right arm is in alignment with the left arm. You should look like a side-lying T.

      5. In a controlled manner, reverse the rotation and return to the start position.

3. Perform a predetermined number of repetitions, then repeat on the opposite side.

CONSIDERATIONS

1. Note: For safety reasons, a hex dumbbell or a dumbbell with fixed plates on the end works best. They will roll less and are more secure to the floor during the push-up phase of the complex.

2. Throughout the exercise, maintain a straight line in the body. Avoid sagging, hunching, or, most important, tipping opposite the dumbbell hand while performing the movements.

3. The exercise can also be done while holding one dumbbell in each hand as shown, which allows additional movement pattern variety. For example, you might perform one complete complex with the right arm followed by one complete complex with the left arm. Or you might alternate the complex activities, such as right arm front raise; left arm front raise; right arm rear delt raise; left arm rear delt raise; rotate right; rotate left; push-up; repeat. And much more. However, with the additional dumbbell the base of support becomes unstable, so extra caution must be taken.

4. Try adding these movements:

   • Lateral shoulder press while in the rotated position (bend the elbow, then press the dumbbell toward the ceiling).

   • Bent elbow lateral raise.

   • Rear pull (dumbbell is pulled to the chest).

   • Leave the dumbbell on the floor when rotating to the ceiling. In the up position, catch and pass a ball to a partner.

SPECIFIC BENEFITS

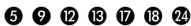

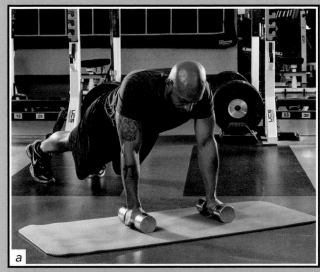

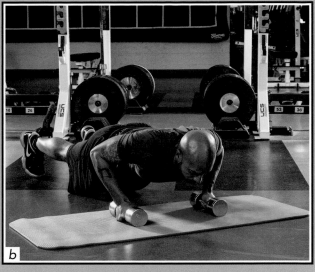

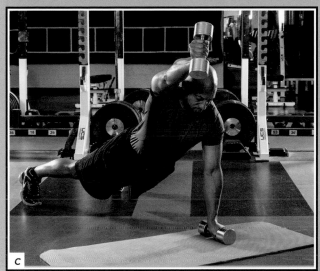

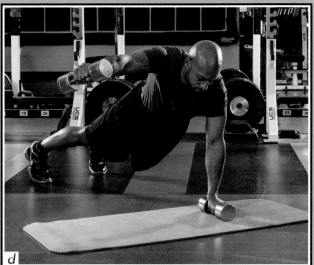

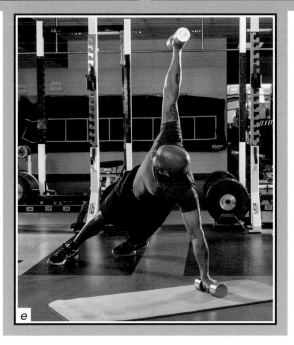

195

SLIDEBOARD HANDS

SINGLE-ARM OVERHEAD REACH

MOVEMENTS

1. Kneel on a pad (or foam mat, folded towel, etc.) positioned at one end of a slideboard. Carefully place the gloved hands on the slideboard directly under the shoulders with the arms perpendicular to the floor. Only the knees, balls of the feet, and toes are on the floor; the hands are on the slideboard.
2. Smoothly extend forward at the shoulders, hips, and knees.
3. Slide the left arm and hand forward. There should be a slight extension at the hip and a slight flexion at the right elbow, both of which facilitate the left arm movement.
4. Pull the left arm back to the start position.
5. Perform a predetermined number of repetitions; repeat on the opposite side.

CONSIDERATIONS

1. This exercise can be done with alternating arms (i.e., left arm reach and return; right arm reach and return; repeat).

SPECIFIC BENEFITS

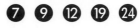

NOTE

Many movement patterns can be added. Create your own, or try the following variations:

- While in the extended position, reach and perform a circle (clockwise then counterclockwise); return to the start position.
- While circling, add a small windshield wiper action with the extended hand.
- Extend the left arm; hold the extended position; slide the right arm under the body and back; return to the start position.
- Extend the left arm; extend the right arm; return the left arm; return the right arm; repeat opposite.

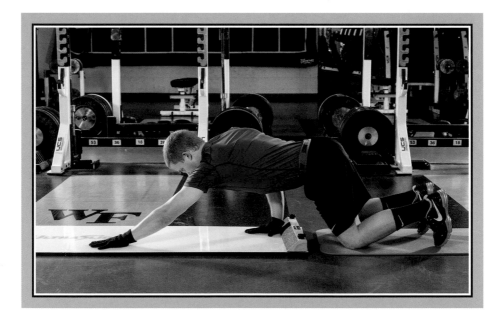

▪ SLIDEBOARD HANDS ▪
FULL-BODY EXTENSION, ALTERNATING WAX ON/WAX OFF

Modifications

1. The setup and start position are identical to Slideboard Hands Single-Arm Overhead Reach but kneel at the middle of slideboard with the body perpendicular to board.
2. Smoothly slide both arms forward and extend at the hips and knees. (Depth of the drop is dictated by the strength and comfort level of the athlete. Beginners might simply allow their arms to slide lateral while maintaining relatively straight arms.)

3. While in the extended position, perform a clockwise circle with the left hand; then stop and perform a counterclockwise circle with the right hand.
4. Maintaining full-body extension, perform a predetermined number of cycles clockwise and counterclockwise with each hand returning to the start position to end the set.

Specific Benefits **⑫ ⑲ ㉔**

▪ SLIDEBOARD HANDS ▪
FULL-BODY EXTENSION, SIMULTANEOUS WAX ON/WAX OFF

Modifications

1. The setup and start position are identical to Slideboard Hands Single-Arm Overhead Reach but kneel at the middle of slideboard with the body perpendicular to board.
2. The action is identical to Alternating Wax/Wax Off, but while in the extended position, perform a clockwise circle with the left hand and a simultaneous counterclockwise with the right hand.
3. Maintaining an upper-body extension, perform a predetermined number of cycles clockwise and counterclockwise with each hand returning to the start position to end the set.

Specific Benefits **⑫ ⑲ ㉔**

Note Try these variations:

- Pull back to start position between each hand circle.
- Circle both hands clockwise; circle both hands counterclockwise.
- Circle the left hand clockwise with simultaneous right-hand abduction and adduction; circle the left hand counterclockwise with simultaneous right-hand abduction and adduction. Repeat opposite.
- In full extension, hold position and lift the right leg lateral (fire hydrant); perform hand circle combinations; pull back to the start; repeat with the opposite leg. This can be a bit risky. Use good judgment.

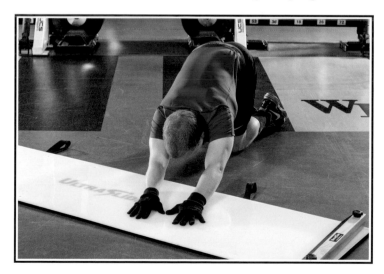

▪ SLIDEBOARD HANDS ▪
ABDUCTION AND ADDUCTION

Modifications

1. The setup and start position are identical to Slideboard Hands Single-Arm Overhead Reach but kneel at the middle of slideboard with the body perpendicular to the board.

2. From a straight-arm, perpendicular start position, slowly slide the hands lateral (abduction), allowing the body to drop toward the board.

3. Pull the arms back in (adduction); returning to the start position.

Specific Benefits   ❺ ⓬ ⓳ ㉔

Note Depth of the abduction drop depends on the strength and comfort level of the athlete. Beginners might simply allow their arms to slide lateral while maintaining relatively straight arms.

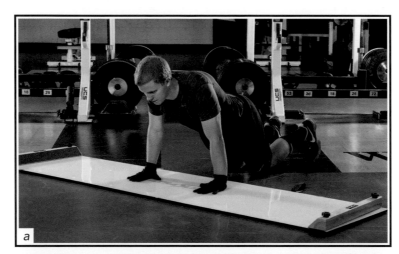

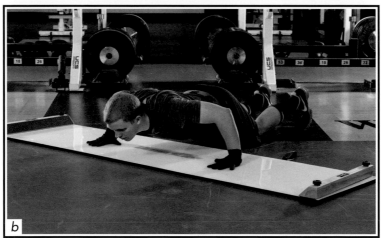

LATERAL CROSS

MOVEMENTS

1. Assume a straight-arm plank position with the arms perpendicular to the floor. The feet (in booties or socks) are on the slideboard shoulder-width apart. The hands are on the floor.
2. Carefully flex the right hip and knee and tuck slide the right leg under the straight left leg. This is the lateral cross action.
3. Return the right leg to the start position; repeat with the opposite leg.
4. Continue for a predetermined number of repetitions.

CONSIDERATIONS

1. Distance of the lateral cross depends on the strength, comfort level, and total body balance of the athlete.
2. Maintain proper posture during the exercise. Avoid tipping, hunching, or twisting at any point during the action.

SPECIFIC BENEFITS

4 **9** **12** **19** **24**

NOTE

Many movement patterns can be added. Create your own or try the following variations:

- Perform a push-up between each lateral cross action (see next exercise for something similar).
- Each hand grips a dumbbell. Perform a rear pull between each lateral cross action. Be careful. Use good judgment.

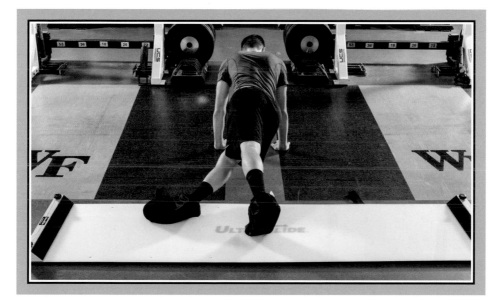

■ SLIDEBOARD FEET ■
LATERAL CROSS WITH PUSH-UP

Modifications

1. The setup and start position are identical to Slideboard Feet Lateral Cross.
2. Carefully flex the right hip and knee; tuck slide the right leg under the straight left leg. This is the lateral cross action.

3. While leg is still in the cross position (right leg crossed under the straight left leg), hold and perform a push-up.
4. Return the right leg to the start position; repeat with the opposite leg.

Specific Benefits   **4** **9** **12** **18** **19** **24**

SANDBAG PULL

MOVEMENTS

1. Assume a straight-arm plank position with the arms perpendicular to the floor. The feet (in booties or socks) are on the slideboard. A sandbag is under the right side of the body and positioned between the hands and the slideboard.
2. With the left hand, grasp the end handle (if one is available) of the sandbag and pull lateral from right to left across the midline of the body.
3. Reposition the hands. With the right hand, grasp the end handle of the sandbag and pull lateral from left to right across the midline of the body.

4. Over and back (right to left; left to right) is considered a round trip. Perform a predetermined number of round trips.

CONSIDERATIONS

1. If no end handles are available on your sandbag, use the top handles.

SPECIFIC BENEFITS

   ❺ ❾ ⑫ ⑰ ⑱ ⑲

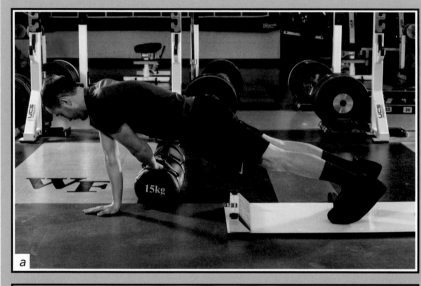

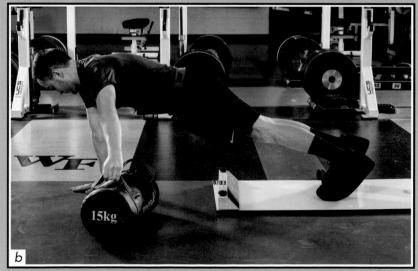

▪ SLIDEBOARD FEET ▪
SANDBAG PULL, ABDUCTION AND ADDUCTION

Modifications

1. The setup and start position are identical to Slideboard Feet Sandbag Pull except the athlete is positioned in the middle and perpendicular to the slideboard.
2. With the right hand, grasp the handle of the sandbag and pull lateral from left to right across the midline of body.
3. Reposition the hands.
4. While in neutral straight-arm plank position with the feet on the slideboard, spread the legs (abduction); bring the legs back to neutral (adduction) (a).
5. With the left hand, grasp the handle of the sandbag and pull lateral from right to left across the midline of the body (b).
6. While in neutral straight-arm plank position with the feet on the slideboard, spread the legs (abduction); bring the legs back to neutral (adduction).

Specific Benefits ❺ ❾ ⓬ ⓱ ⓲ ⓳

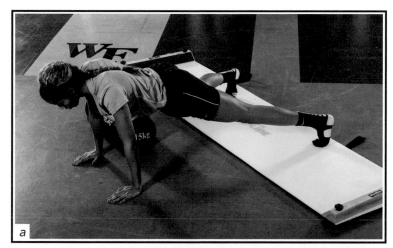

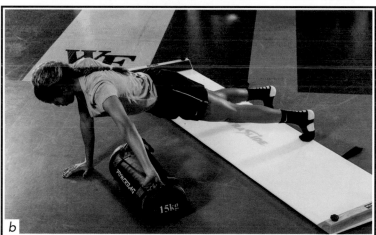

■ SLIDEBOARD FEET ■
SANDBAG PULL, MOUNTAIN CLIMBER

Modifications

1. The setup and start position are identical to Slideboard Feet Sandbag Pull, Abduction and Adduction.

2. With the right hand, grasp the handle of the sandbag and pull lateral from left to right across the midline of the body.

3. Reposition the hands.

4. While in the neutral straight-arm plank position, perform a mountain climber (drive the left knee up and under the chest; return; drive the right knee up and under the chest; return) (*a*).

5. With the left hand, grasp the handle of the sandbag and pull lateral from right to left across the midline of the body (*b*).

6. While in the neutral straight-arm plank position, perform a mountain climber (drive the right knee up and under the chest; return; drive the left knee up and under the chest; return).

Specific Benefits

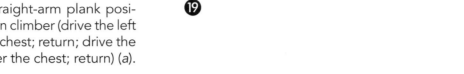

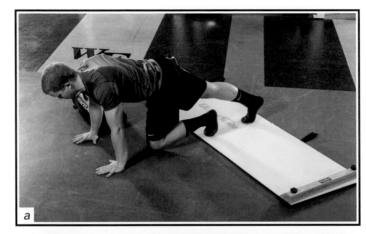

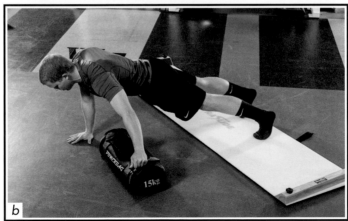

CABLE ROW

MOVEMENTS

1. Assume an elbow plank position with the body perpendicular to the cable's line of pull. The left foot is stacked on top of the right foot. Upper-body weight is on the right forearm, and the upper right arm is perpendicular to the floor.

2. The cable (or rubber band) is positioned about chest high as measured from the floor to the chest while in the lateral elbow plank position.

3. Lift the body so only the lateral side of the right foot (bottom foot) and right elbow and forearm are on the floor. The left arm is extended parallel to the floor with the left hand gripping the handle.

4. Maintain a completely straight line in the body (ears, shoulders, hips, knees, and ankles are in alignment) throughout the duration of the exercise.

5. Retract the shoulder blade of the left arm and pull (row) the handle to the armpit. Keep the left elbow close to the torso. You can either keep your palm down throughout or rotate the hand slightly so the thumb is up and the palm is semisupinated.

6. In a controlled manner, return to the start position.

7. Perform a predetermined number of repetitions; repeat on the opposite side.

CONSIDERATIONS

1. Lock the knees, tighten the glutes, and brace the abdomen throughout the duration of the exercise.

2. Maintain a straight line in the body. When performing the exercise, avoid sagging, hunching, or tipping back (away from the line-of-pull).

SPECIFIC BENEFITS

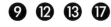 **9 12 13 17**

NOTE

To increase exercise difficulty or simply add variety, try incorporating some of the following challenges:

- Lift the top leg (abduct).
- While performing the pull action, the top leg can simultaneously do knee drives, hip extensions, abductions, front and rear foot taps, and more.
- Position the feet on an unstable apparatus.
- Employ perturbation techniques such as gently tapping the athlete throughout the movement or positioning a resistance band around the waist, ankles, or knees.

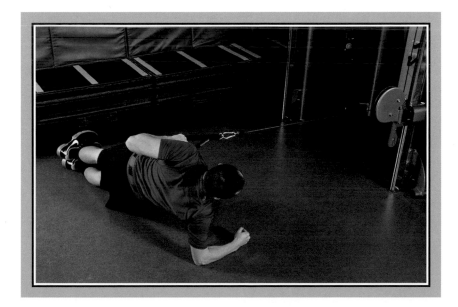

▪ LATERAL STRAIGHT-ARM PLANK ▪
CABLE ROW

Modifications

1. The left hand is on floor directly under the shoulders with the left arm perpendicular to the floor.
2. The cable (or rubber band) is positioned about chest high as measured from the floor to the chest while in the lateral straight-arm plank position.
3. Lift the body so only the lateral side of the left foot (bottom foot) and the left hand are on the floor.
4. The action and considerations are the same as for the Lateral Elbow Plank Cable Row.

Specific Benefits 9 12 13 17

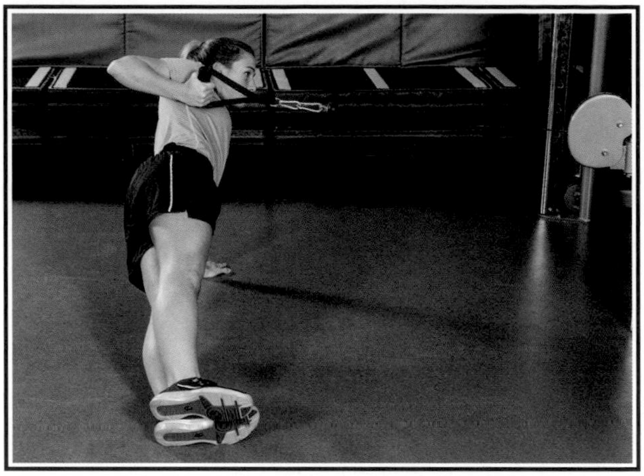

▪ LATERAL ELBOW PLANK ▪
CABLE ROW, FEET ELEVATED

Modifications

1. The start position and posture are identical to the Lateral Elbow Plank Cable Row except place the feet on a raised platform (box, bench, or stair step).
2. Lift the body so only the lateral side of the left foot (bottom foot) is on the raised platform; the left elbow and forearm are on the floor.
3. The action is identical to the Lateral Elbow Plank Cable Row.

Specific Benefits 3 9 12 13 17

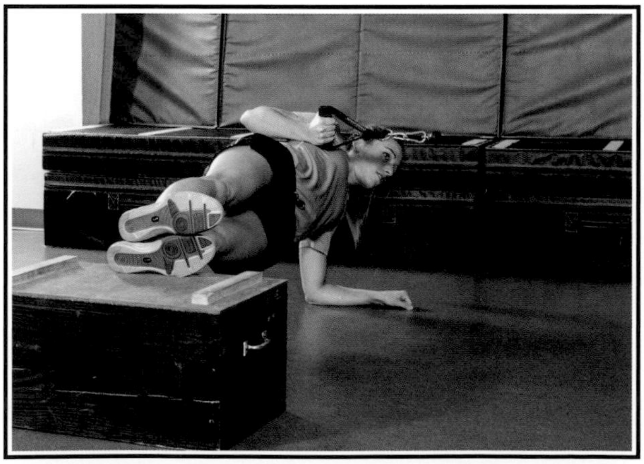

▪ LATERAL STRAIGHT-ARM PLANK ▪
CABLE ROW, FEET ELEVATED

Modifications

1. The start position and posture are identical to the Lateral Straight-Arm Plank Cable Row except place the feet on a raised platform.
2. Lift the body so only the lateral side of the left foot (bottom foot) is on the raised platform. The left hand is on the floor.
3. The action is identical to Lateral Straight-Arm Plank Cable Row.

Specific Benefits 3 9 12 13 17

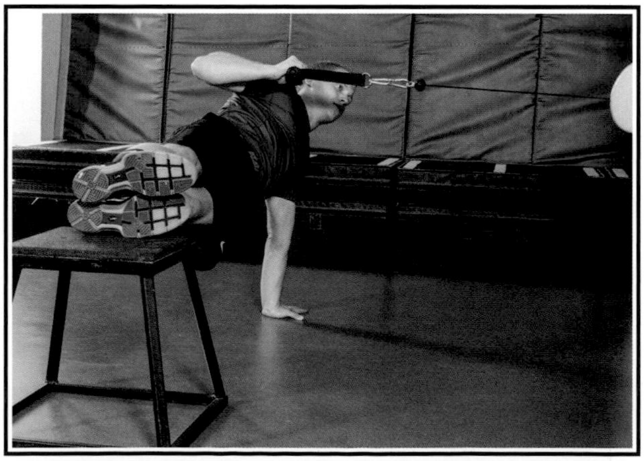

▪ LATERAL ELBOW PLANK ▪
CABLE ROW, UNSTABLE UPPER

Modifications

1. The start position and posture are identical to the Lateral Elbow Plank Cable Row except place the left elbow on a moderately unstable apparatus, such as a wobble board (or foam pad, pillow stack, etc.).

2. Lift the body so only the lateral side of the left foot (bottom foot) is on the floor. The left elbow and forearm are on the unstable apparatus.

3. The action is identical to the Lateral Elbow Plank Cable Row.

Specific Benefits

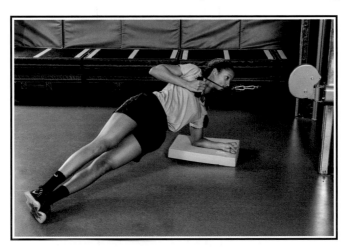

▪ LATERAL STRAIGHT-ARM PLANK ▪
CABLE ROW, UNSTABLE UPPER

Modifications

1. The start position and posture are identical to the Lateral Straight-Arm Plank Cable Row except place the hand on a moderately unstable apparatus.

2. Lift the body so only the lateral side of the left foot (bottom foot) is on the floor; the left hand is on the unstable apparatus.

3. The action is identical to the Lateral Straight-Arm Plank Cable Row.

Specific Benefits

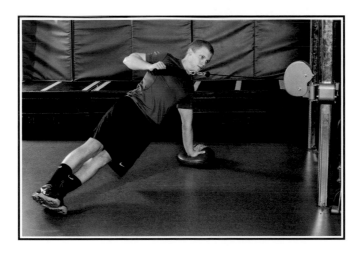

■ LATERAL ELBOW PLANK ■
CABLE ROW, UNSTABLE LOWER

Modifications

1. The start position and posture are identical to the Lateral Elbow Plank Cable Row except place the feet on a moderately unstable apparatus. For a greater challenge, elevate the feet onto a stability ball or raised platform with an unstable apparatus on top. For safety, make sure that the unstable apparatus is relatively secure.

2. Lift the body so only the lateral side of the left foot (bottom foot) is on the unstable apparatus; the left elbow and forearm are on the floor.

3. The action is identical to Lateral Elbow Plank Cable Row.

Specific Benefits   ❶ ❾ ⓬ ⓭ ⓱

If using a stability ball also ❸

Note There are many unstable apparatus options. If using a stability ball, for example, the difficulty progression might look something like this:

1. Lateral knees on the ball
2. Lateral shins (lower leg) on the ball
3. Lateral ankles on the ball

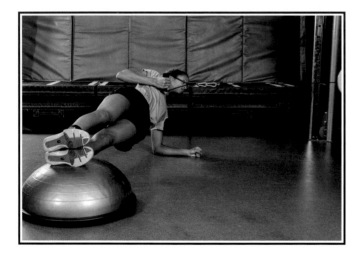

■ LATERAL STRAIGHT-ARM PLANK ■
CABLE ROW, UNSTABLE LOWER

Modifications

1. The start position and posture are identical to the Lateral Straight-Arm Plank Cable Row except place the feet on a moderately unstable apparatus. For a greater challenge, elevate the feet onto a stability ball or raised platform with an unstable apparatus on top. For safety, make sure that the unstable apparatus is relatively secure.

2. Lift the body so only the lateral side of the left foot (bottom foot) is on the unstable apparatus; the left hand is on the floor.

3. The action is identical to the Lateral Straight-Arm Plank Cable Row.

Specific Benefits   ❶ ❾ ⓬ ⓭ ⓱

If using a stability ball also ❸

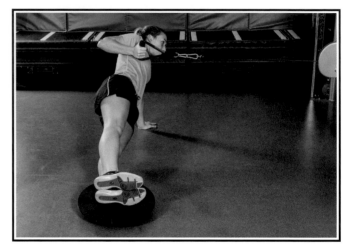

PALLOF ISOMETRIC PRESS

PROGRESSION 1: HALF-KNEELING

MOVEMENTS

1. Preset the cable's line of pull to shoulder height when in a kneeling position. Set the weight to a manageable resistance.
2. Positioned perpendicular to the cable line of pull, the knee furthest from the cable machine is flexed to 90 degrees and flat on the floor (use a mat or folded towel for knee protection). The knee closest to the cable machine is likewise bent to 90 degrees with the foot flat on the floor.
3. Grasp the handle with both hands and hold directly at the center of the chest. Brace the core; depress and retract the scapulae. Avoid leaning to the side or moving the hips.
4. Extend the arms directly in front of the body while retaining a tight grip on the handle. The arms remain parallel to the ground throughout.
5. Hold the position for a predetermined length of time; repeat to the opposite side.

CONSIDERATIONS

1. Maintain a straight torso (ears, shoulders, hips, and the ground knee are in alignment) throughout the duration of the exercise.
2. Keep the shoulders back and down at all times.
3. Maintain good posture throughout; do not break form. Never sacrifice technique for added resistance or reps.

SPECIFIC BENEFITS

12 **17** **24**

NOTE

To increase exercise difficulty or simply add variety, try incorporating some of the following challenges:

- Position the feet and knees on an unstable apparatus.
- Perform a single-arm horizontal press.
- Employ perturbation techniques such as gently tapping the athlete throughout the movement or positioning a resistance band around the waist, ankles, or knees.

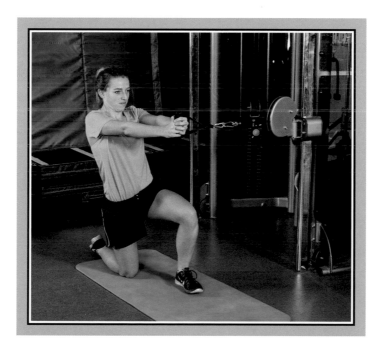

▪ PALLOF ISOMETRIC PRESS ▪
PROGRESSION 2: TALL KNEELING

Modifications

1. The setup, cable setting, action, considerations, and variations are identical to Pallof Isometric Press Progression 1: Half-Kneeling except both knees are on the floor and flexed to 90 degrees (use a mat or folded towel for knee protection).

Specific Benefits ⑫ ⑰ ㉔

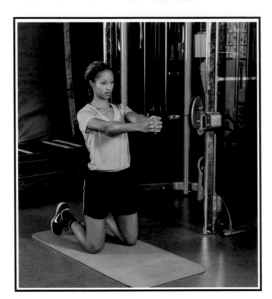

▪ PALLOF ISOMETRIC PRESS ▪
PROGRESSION 3: STANDING

Modifications

1. Preset the cable's line of pull to shoulder height when in an athletic stance.
2. The action, considerations, and variations are identical to Pallof Isometric Press Progression 1: Half-Kneeling except set up next to the cable section with both hips and knees slightly flexed. The feet are parallel and slightly wider than shoulder width. Maintain an athletic stance and brace the core throughout the exercise (ear, shoulder, and hip are in alignment).

Specific Benefits ⑫ ⑰ ㉔

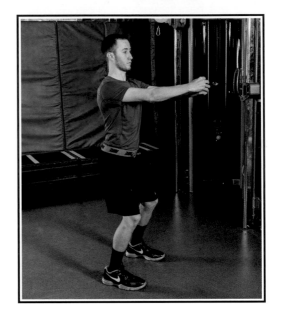

■ PALLOF ISOMETRIC PRESS ■
PROGRESSION 4: STAGGERED STANCE

Modifications

1. The setup, cable setting, action, considerations, and variations are identical to Pallof Isometric Press Progression 3: Standing except set up next to the cable section with the feet staggered one in front of the other. The foot nearest the cable machine (lead foot of the stagger) will be in front; the other foot (rear foot of the stagger) is behind.

Specific Benefits ⑫ ⑰ ⑱ ㉔

Note Moving from a highly balanced standing position into a staggered stance position creates a need to stabilize more in the frontal plane while controlling the external resistance in the transverse plane.

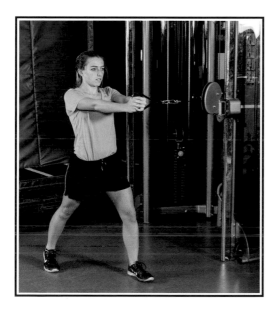

■ PALLOF ISOMETRIC PRESS ■
PROGRESSION 5: LUNGE STANCE

Modifications

1. The setup, cable setting, action, considerations, and variations are identical to Pallof Isometric Press Progression 3: Standing except set up next to the cable section with the feet staggered one in front of the other. The foot nearest the cable machine (lead foot of the stagger) will be in front; the other foot (rear foot of the stagger) is behind. Both knees are flexed to 90 degrees. You should be on the ball of the back foot (heel off the floor).

Specific Benefits ⑫ ⑰ ⑱ ㉔

Note Dropping from the staggered stance into a more dynamic lunge position creates a higher demand on the entire physiological system as the joints of the lower body are now fully loaded as well as those of the upper body.

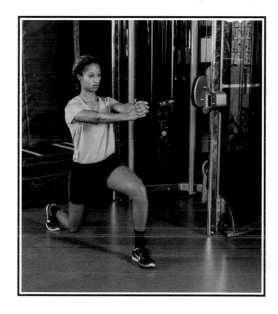

PROGRESSION 1: HALF-KNEELING

MOVEMENTS

1. Preset the cable's line of pull to shoulder height when in a kneeling position. Set the weight to a manageable resistance.
2. Positioned perpendicular to the cable line of pull, the knee furthest from the cable machine is flexed to 90 degrees and flat on the floor (use a mat or folded towel for knee protection). The knee closest to the cable machine is likewise bent to 90 degrees with the foot flat on the floor.
3. Grasp the handle with both hands and hold directly at the center of the chest.
4. Brace the core and, without leaning to the side or moving the hips, press the handle straight out in front until the elbows lock. The arms remain parallel to the ground throughout.
5. In a controlled manner, smoothly draw the handle back to the chest (start position).
6. Perform a predetermined number of repetitions; repeat on the opposite side.

CONSIDERATIONS

1. Maintain a straight torso (ears, shoulders, hips, and the ground knee are in alignment) throughout the duration of the exercise.
2. Keep the shoulders back and down at all times.
3. Maintain good posture throughout; do not break form. Never sacrifice technique for added resistance or reps.

SPECIFIC BENEFITS

12 **17** **24**

NOTE

Pressing back and forth constantly changes the lever length of the arms, increasing overall difficulty and presenting a controlled yet ever-changing challenge.

To increase exercise difficulty or simply add variety, try incorporating some of the following challenges:

- Position the feet and knees on an unstable apparatus.
- Perform a single-arm horizontal press.
- Employ perturbation techniques such as gently tapping the athlete throughout the movement or positioning a resistance band around the waist, ankles, or knees.

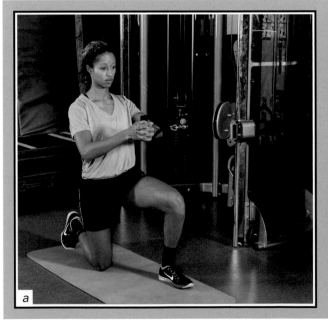

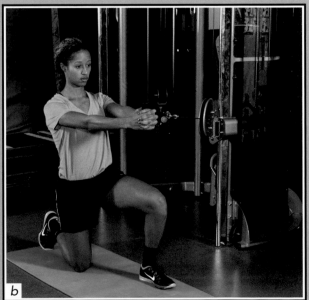

■ PALLOF HORIZONTAL PRESS ■
PROGRESSION 2: TALL KNEELING

Modifications

1. The setup, cable setting, action, considerations, and variations are identical to Pallof Horizontal Press Progression 1: Half-Kneeling except position perpendicular to the cable section with both knees flexed to 90 degrees and flat on the floor (use a mat or folded towel for knee protection).

Specific Benefits **12** **17** **24**

■ PALLOF HORIZONTAL PRESS ■
PROGRESSION 3: STANDING

Modifications

1. Preset the cable's line of pull to shoulder height when in an athletic stance.

2. The action, considerations, and variations are identical to Pallof Horizontal Press Progression 1: Half-Kneeling except set up next to the cable section with both hips and knees slightly flexed. The feet are parallel and slightly wider than shoulder width. Maintain an athletic stance and brace the core throughout the exercise (ear, shoulder and hip are in alignment).

Specific Benefits **12** **17** **24**

■ PALLOF HORIZONTAL PRESS ■
PROGRESSION 4: STAGGERED STANCE

Modifications

1. The setup, action, considerations, and variations are identical to Pallof Horizontal Press Progression 3: Standing except set up next to the cable section with the feet staggered one in front of the other. The foot nearest the cable machine (lead foot of the stagger) will be in front; the other foot (rear foot of the stagger) is behind.

Specific Benefits **12** **17** **18** **24**

Note Moving from a highly balanced standing position into a staggered stance position creates a need to stabilize more in the frontal plane while controlling the external resistance in the transverse plane.

■ PALLOF HORIZONTAL PRESS ■
PROGRESSION 5: LUNGE STANCE

Modifications

1. The setup, action, considerations, and variations are identical to Pallof Horizontal Press Progression 3: Standing except position next to the cable section with the feet staggered one in front of the other. The foot nearest the cable machine (lead foot of the stagger) will be in front; the other foot (rear foot of the stagger) is behind. Both knees are flexed to 90 degrees. You should be on the ball of the back foot (heel off the floor).

Specific Benefits **12** **17** **18** **24**

Note Dropping from the staggered stance into a more dynamic lunge position creates a higher demand on the entire physiological system as the joints of the lower body are now fully loaded as well as those of the upper body.

CABLE CHOP

PROGRESSION 1: HALF-KNEELING

MOVEMENTS

1. Adjust the cable to the highest setting and attach a long lever bar or rope. Set the weight to a manageable resistance.

2. Positioned perpendicular to the cable line of pull, the knee furthest from the cable machine is flexed to 90 degrees and flat on the floor (use a mat or folded towel for knee protection). The knee closest to the cable machine is likewise bent to 90 degrees with the foot flat on the floor.

3. Take as wide a grip as possible (see considerations). Brace the core, depress and retract the scapulae. Avoid leaning to the side or moving the hips.

4. Pull the bar (or rope) straight toward the floor with emphasis on the low hand. The sensation should be a chopping action in which the bottom hand chops down and back. Do not move or rotate the torso. Push the bar or rope down toward the side so that the arms cross the body.

5. In a controlled manner, smoothly draw the bar (or rope) across the body and back to the start position.

6. Perform a predetermined number of repetitions; repeat on the opposite side.

CONSIDERATIONS

1. If using a bar, use a wide grip with both hands in a palms-down position. If using a rope (typically a triceps push down rope), pull the rope through the ring attachment until the entire rope is on one side of the ring. Again use a wide hand position in a palms-down grip. Keep the rope taut throughout the action.

2. Keep the shoulders back and down for the entirety of the drill.

3. Maintain good posture throughout; do not break form. Never sacrifice technique for added resistance or reps.

4. The action will look similar to rowing a kayak.

SPECIFIC BENEFITS

 12 **17** **24**

NOTE

To increase exercise difficulty or simply add variety, try incorporating some of the following challenges:

- Position the feet and knees on an unstable apparatus.
- Close the eyes.
- Employ perturbation techniques such as gently tapping the athlete throughout the movement or positioning a resistance band around the waist, ankles, or knees.

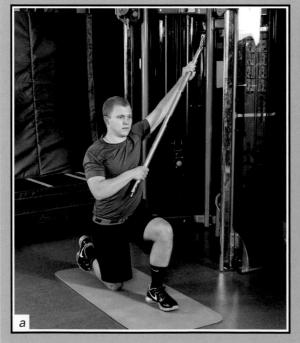

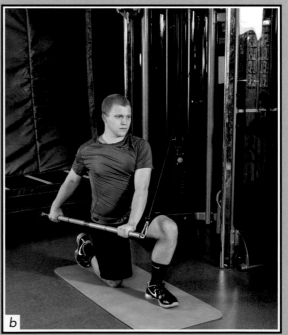

▪ CABLE CHOP ▪
PROGRESSION 2: TALL KNEELING

Modifications

1. The setup, cable setting, action, considerations, and variations are identical to Cable Chop Progression 1: Half-Kneeling except position perpendicular to the cable section with both knees flexed to 90 degrees and flat on the floor (use a mat or folded towel for knee protection).

Specific Benefits ⓲ ⓱ ㉔

▪ CABLE CHOP ▪
PROGRESSION 3: STANDING

Modifications

1. The setup, cable setting, action, considerations, and variations are identical to Cable Chop Progression 1: Half-Kneeling except position next to the cable section with both hips and knees slightly flexed. The feet are parallel and slightly wider than shoulder width. Maintain an athletic stance and braced core throughout (ear, shoulder and hip are in alignment).

Specific Benefits ⓲ ⓱ ㉔

▪ CABLE CHOP ▪
PROGRESSION 4: STAGGERED STANCE

Modifications

1. The setup, cable setting, action, considerations, and variations are identical to Cable Chop Progression 3: Standing except position next to the cable section with the feet staggered one in front of the other. The foot nearest to the cable machine (lead foot of the stagger) will be in front; the other foot (rear foot of the stagger) is behind.

Specific Benefits ⓲ ⓱ ⓳ ㉔

Note Moving from a highly balanced standing position into a staggered stance position creates a need to stabilize more in the frontal plane while controlling the external resistance in the transverse plane.

▪ CABLE CHOP ▪
PROGRESSION 5: LUNGE STANCE

Modifications

1. The setup, cable setting, action, considerations, and variations are identical to Cable Chop Progression 3: Standing except position next to the cable section with the feet staggered one in front of the other. The foot nearest to the cable machine (lead foot of the stagger) will be in front; the other foot (rear foot of the stagger) is behind. Both knees are flexed to 90 degrees. You should be on the ball of the back foot (heel off the floor).

Specific Benefits ⓲ ⓱ ⓳ ㉔

Note Dropping from the staggered stance into a more dynamic lunge position creates a higher demand on the entire physiological system as the joints of the lower body are now fully loaded as well as those of the upper body.

CABLE LIFT

PROGRESSION 1: HALF-KNEELING

MOVEMENTS

1. Adjust the cable to the lowest setting and attach a long lever bar or rope. Set the weight to a manageable resistance.
2. Positioned perpendicular to the cable line of pull, the knee closest to the cable machine is flexed to 90 degrees and flat on the floor (use a mat or folded towel for knee protection). The knee furthest from the cable machine is also bent to 90 degrees with the foot flat on the floor.
3. Take as wide a grip as possible (see considerations).
4. Brace the core; depress and retract the scapulae. Avoid leaning to the side or moving the hips.
5. Pull the bar (or rope) upward with the top hand; then push the bar out with the low hand. Do not move or rotate the torso.
6. In a controlled manner, smoothly draw the bar (or rope) across the body and back to the start position.
7. Perform a predetermined number of repetitions; repeat on the opposite side.

CONSIDERATIONS

1. If using a bar, use a wide grip with both hands in a palms-down position throughout. If using a rope (typically a triceps push down rope), simply pull the rope through the ring attachment until the entire rope is on one side of the ring. Again use a wide hand position in a palms-down grip. Keep the rope taut throughout the action.
2. Keep the shoulders back and down for the entirety of the drill.
3. Maintain good posture throughout; do not break form. Never sacrifice technique for added resistance or reps.

SPECIFIC BENEFITS

 ⑫ ⑰ ㉔

NOTE

To increase exercise difficulty or simply add variety, try incorporating some of the following challenges:

- Position the feet and knees on an unstable apparatus.
- Close the eyes.
- Employ perturbation techniques such as gently tapping the athlete throughout the movement or positioning a resistance band around the waist, ankles, or knees.

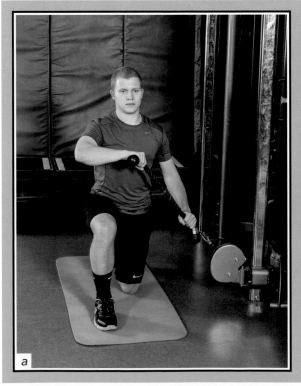

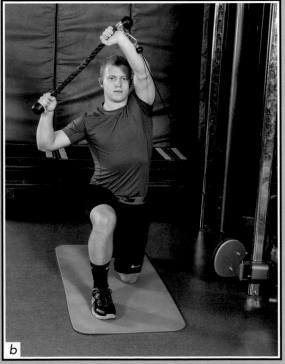

■ CABLE LIFT ■
PROGRESSION 2: TALL KNEELING

Modifications

1. The setup, cable setting, action, considerations, and variations are identical to Cable Lift Progression 1: Half-Kneeling except position perpendicular to the cable line of pull with both knees flexed to 90 degrees and flat on the floor (use a mat or folded towel for knee protection).

Specific Benefits ⑫ ⑰ ㉔

■ CABLE LIFT ■
PROGRESSION 3: STANDING

Modifications

1. The setup, cable setting, action, considerations, and variations are identical to Cable Lift Progression 1: Half-Kneeling except position next to the cable section with both hips and knees slightly flexed. The feet are parallel and slightly wider than shoulder width. Maintain an athletic stance and braced core throughout the exercise (ear, shoulder and hip are in alignment).

Specific Benefits ⑫ ⑰ ㉔

■ CABLE LIFT ■
PROGRESSION 4: STAGGERED STANCE

Modifications

1. The setup, cable setting, action, considerations, and variations are identical to Cable Lift Progression 3: Standing except position next to the cable section with the feet staggered one in front of the other. The foot nearest to the cable machine (rear foot of the stagger) will be behind; the other foot (lead foot of the stagger) is in front.

Specific Benefits ⑫ ⑰ ⑱ ㉔

Note Moving from a highly balanced standing position into a staggered stance position creates a need to stabilize more in the frontal plane while controlling the external resistance in the transverse plane.

■ CABLE LIFT ■
PROGRESSION 5: LUNGE STANCE

Modifications

1. The setup, cable setting, action, considerations, and variations are identical to Cable Lift Progression 3: Standing except position next to the cable section with the feet staggered one in front of the other. The foot nearest the cable section (rear foot of the stagger) will be behind; the other foot (lead foot of the stagger) is in front. Both knees are flexed to 90 degrees. You should be on the ball of the back foot (heel off the floor).

Specific Benefits ⑫ ⑰ ⑱ ㉔

Note Dropping from the staggered stance into a more dynamic lunge position creates a higher demand on the entire physiological system as the joints of the lower body are now fully loaded as well as those of the upper body.

MOVEMENTS

1. Preset the cable's line of pull to shoulder height when in a kneeling position and attach a long lever bar or rope. Set the weight to a manageable resistance.

2. Positioned with the cable section behind and slightly to the side, one knee is flexed to 90 degrees and flat on the floor (use a mat or folded towel for knee protection). The other knee is also bent 90 degrees with the foot flat on the floor.

3. Take as wide a grip as possible (see considerations).

4. Brace the core; depress and retract the scapulae. Avoid leaning to the side or moving the hips.

5. Pull the bar (or rope) away from the cable column; then push the bar out and around in front of the chest. Do not move or rotate the torso.

6. In a controlled manner, smoothly draw the bar (or rope) across the body and back to the start position.

7. Perform a predetermined number of repetitions; repeat on the opposite side.

CONSIDERATIONS

1. If using a bar, use a wide grip with both hands in a palms-down position throughout. If using a rope (typically a triceps push down rope), simply pull the rope through the ring attachment until the entire rope is on one side of the ring. Again use a wide hand position in a palms-down grip. Keep the rope taut throughout the action.

2. Keep the shoulders back and down for the entirety of the drill.

3. Maintain good posture throughout; do not break form. Never sacrifice technique for added resistance or reps.

SPECIFIC BENEFITS

 12 17 24

NOTE

To increase exercise difficulty or simply add variety, try incorporating some of the following challenges:

- Position the feet and knees on an unstable apparatus.
- Close the eyes.
- Employ perturbation techniques such as gently tapping the athlete throughout the movement or positioning a resistance band around the waist, ankles, or knees.

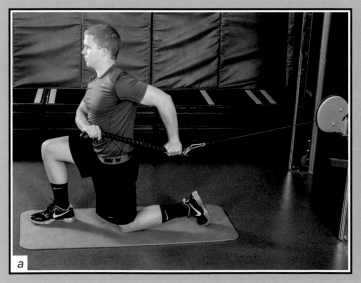

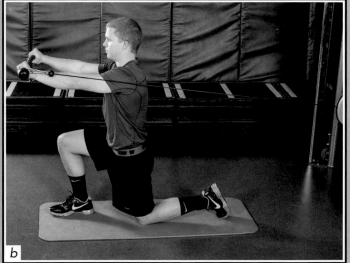

■ ANTI-ROTATION PRESS ■
PROGRESSION 2: TALL KNEELING

Modifications

1. The setup, cable setting, action, considerations, and variations are identical to Anti-Rotation Press Progression 1: Half-Kneeling except both knees are flexed to 90 degrees and flat on the floor (use a mat or folded towel for knee protection).

Specific Benefits **12** **17** **24**

■ ANTI-ROTATION PRESS ■
PROGRESSION 3: STANDING

Modifications

1. Preset cable's line of pull to shoulder height when in an athletic stance.
2. The setup, action, considerations, and variations are identical to Anti-Rotation Press Progression 1: Half-Kneeling except position in front of the cable section with both hips and knees slightly flexed. The feet are parallel and slightly wider than shoulder width. Maintain an athletic stance and braced core throughout (ear, shoulder and hip are in alignment).

Specific Benefits **12** **17** **24**

■ ANTI-ROTATION PRESS ■
PROGRESSION 4: STAGGERED STANCE

Modifications

1. The setup, cable setting, action, considerations, and variations are identical to Anti-Rotation Press Progression 3: Standing except position in front of the cable section with the feet staggered one in front of the other.

Specific Benefits **12** **17** **18** **24**

Note Moving from a highly balanced standing position into a staggered stance position creates a need to stabilize more in the frontal plane while controlling the external resistance in the transverse plane.

■ ANTI-ROTATION PRESS ■
PROGRESSION 5: LUNGE STANCE

Modifications

1. The setup, cable setting, action, considerations, and variations are identical to Anti-Rotation Press Progression 3: Standing except position in front of the cable section with the feet staggered one in front of the other. Both knees are flexed to 90 degrees. You should be on ball of back foot (heel off floor).

Specific Benefits **12** **17** **18** **24**

Note Dropping from the staggered stance into a more dynamic lunge position creates a higher demand on the entire physiological system as the joints of the lower body are now fully loaded as well as those of the upper body.

MOVEMENTS

1. If you have two cable machines facing each other, preset the line of pull of two bands or two cables at shoulder height when in a kneeling position. Set the weight to a manageable level. Grasp both handles (see considerations).

2. Facing one band or cable attachment, the left knee and hip are flexed at 90 degrees with the left foot flat on the floor. The right knee is also flexed to 90 degrees and positioned on the floor (use a mat or folded towel for knee protection).

3. Maintain a completely straight line in the body (ears, shoulders, hips, and ground knee are in alignment) throughout the exercise.

4. Firmly grasp the front band or cable handle with the right hand. The right arm is fully extended with the palm facing down.

5. Firmly grasp the back band or cable handle with the left hand. The left arm is flexed to a position at which the elbow is pointing to the floor; the left palm is facing up and is located at the armpit (to start).

6. Brace the core; depress and retract the scapulae. Avoid leaning to the side or moving the hips.

7. Press the left arm straight forward (parallel to the ground) while simultaneously pulling the right arm back toward body. During the press, the left hand will rotate from a palm-up start position to a palm-down termination (full arm extension). Conversely, the right hand will rotate from a palm-down start position to a palm-up termination (at armpit).

8. In a controlled manner, smoothly return to the start position.

9. Perform a predetermined number of repetitions; repeat on the opposite side.

CONSIDERATIONS

1. Experiment when selecting the appropriate load. For example, there is a natural imbalance between pull and press strength, so weight pulled will likely be greater than weight pressed.

2. Maintain good posture throughout; do not break form. Avoid excessive rotation. The upper torso remains fixed throughout the exercise. Never sacrifice technique for added resistance or reps.

3. Keep the shoulders back and down for the entire exercise.

4. During the pull action, the hand may pull to the armpit, hip, or any point between.

SPECIFIC BENEFITS

9 **12** **17** **24**

NOTE

To increase exercise difficulty or simply add variety, try incorporating some of the following challenges:

- Switch pull and press arms and legs. That is, instead of the left leg forward and a right hand pull as shown, try the left leg forward and a left arm pull.

- Perform a single-arm Pallof Press combined with a pull (cables must obviously be set accordingly: 90-degree line of pull).

- Position the feet and knees on an unstable apparatus.

- Close the eyes.

- Employ perturbation techniques such as gently tapping the athlete throughout the movement or positioning a resistance band around the waist, ankles, or knees.

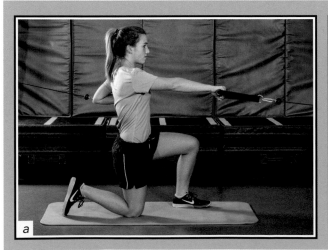
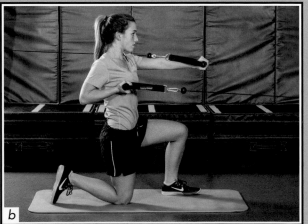

▪ PULL AND PRESS ▪
PROGRESSION 2: TALL KNEELING

Modifications

1. The setup, cable setting, action, considerations, and variations are identical to Pull and Press Progression 1: Half-Kneeling except both knees are flexed to 90 degrees and flat on the floor (use a mat or folded towel for knee protection).

Specific Benefits **9 12 17 24**

Note Drills like this increase the muscular and neural challenge to maintain a neutral posture.

▪ PULL AND PRESS ▪
PROGRESSION 3: STANDING

Modifications

1. Preset the cable's line of pull to shoulder height when in an athletic stance.
2. The setup, action, considerations, and variations are identical to Pull and Press Progression 1: Half-Kneeling except stand facing one machine or band with both hips and knees slightly flexed. The feet are parallel and slightly wider than shoulder width. Maintain an athletic stance and braced core throughout (ear, shoulder and hip are in alignment).

Specific Benefits **9 12 17 24**

▪ PULL AND PRESS ▪
PROGRESSION 4: STAGGERED STANCE

Modifications

1. The setup, cable setting, action, considerations, and variations are identical to Pull and Press Progression 3: Standing except the feet are staggered one in front of the other. Facing one band or cable attachment, the left leg is forward. With the knees slightly flexed and the body's center of mass directly between the base of support (right and left foot), you should be in an athletic (although split) stance.

Specific Benefits **9 12 17 18 24**

Note Moving from a highly balanced standing position into a staggered stance position creates a need to stabilize more in the frontal plane while controlling the external resistance in the transverse plane.

▪ PULL AND PRESS ▪
PROGRESSION 5: LUNGE STANCE

Modifications

1. The setup, cable setting, action, considerations, and variations are identical to Pull and Press Progression 3: Standing except the feet staggered one in front of the other in a lunge stance. Facing the band or cable attachment, the left leg is forward. The left knee is flexed to 90 degrees with the left foot flat on the floor. The right leg is back with the knee flexed 90 degrees. You should be on the ball of the back foot (heel off the floor).

Specific Benefits **9 12 17 18 24**

Note Dropping from the staggered stance into a more dynamic lunge position creates a higher demand on the entire physiological system as the joints of the lower body are now fully loaded as well as those of the upper body.

LANDMINE ROTATION

MOVEMENTS

1. Place one end of an Olympic bar in the center hole of a 45-pound plate (~20 kg) or larger (see considerations).
2. Grip the opposite end of bar firmly with both hands at about eye level. Assume an athletic stance with the feet wider than shoulder width; knees are flexed.
3. Brace the core and maintain a tall posture of the torso. Depress and retract the scapulae, chest out.
4. Rotate the bar in an arcing pattern to one side. The termination point is somewhat subjective. You should stop the movement when body rotation is unavoidable.
5. Controlling the downward movement, immediately reverse the action in the opposite direction.
6. Continue right to left to right rotation for a predetermined number of repetitions.

CONSIDERATIONS

1. Any plate 45 pounds (~20 kg) or larger will suffice. Other alternatives would include a solid corner (90-degree angle).
2. Use good judgment when integrating this exercise. The athlete might find it more comfortable to have a slight pivot action with the feet during the action. For example, when rotating far to the left the athlete could pivot the right (back) foot, similar to the foot action during a golf swing.

SPECIFIC BENEFITS

12 **17** **24**

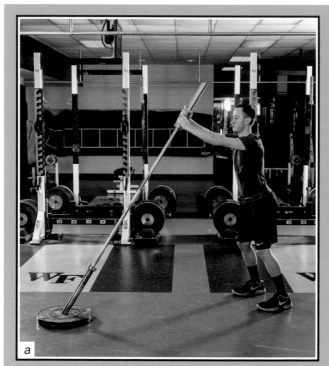

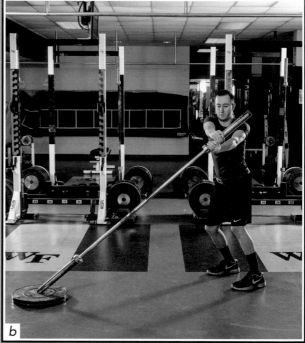

▪ LANDMINE ROTATION ▪
WITH HANDLE

Modifications

1. The setup, action, and considerations are identical to the Landmine with the exception of incorporating a landmine handle (specifically designed for landmine exercises).

Specific Benefits **12** **17** **24**

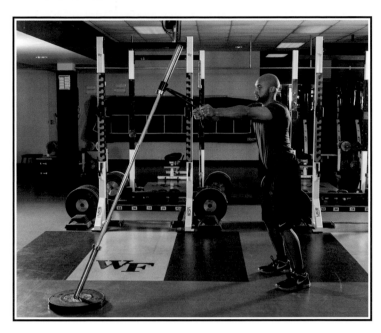

▪ LANDMINE ROTATION ▪
WITH HANDLE AND LOAD

Modifications

1. The setup, action and considerations are identical to the Landmine With Handle with the exception of adding a manageable amount of weight. (Note: You must always be in control of the bar. Never sacrifice technique for additional resistance or reps).

Specific Benefits **12** **17** **24**

CABLE ROTATION WITH STABILITY BALL, STANDING

MOVEMENTS

1. Preset the line of pull of two bands (or two cables of a functional trainer or cable-X machine) at chest height regardless of stance position (e.g., kneeling, low squat, split stance, etc.). If using a cable machine, set both weight stacks to a manageable resistance level.

2. Position the body in between both cables.

3. Maintaining a stability ball (or similar; see considerations) at chest height, wrap the arms around the ball and grasp the handles. Note that the right hand grips the left handle and the left hand the grips right handle. Wrap the arms tightly around the stability ball. Stand with the knees slightly flexed in a balanced athletic stance.

4. Brace the core; depress and retract the scapulae. Maintain an upright torso throughout the exercise.

5. Contract the rotators (primarily the obliques) and, *as a single unit,* rotate the torso clockwise (left to right). Avoid arm and shoulder action (see consideration 2).

6. In a controlled manner, allow the resistance to return to the start position. Again, control this action. This is the true purpose of the exercise.

7. Perform a predetermined number of repetitions; repeat on the opposite side.

CONSIDERATIONS

1. Cable rotations can use stability balls, weighted balls, or other similar devices.

2. The hands, arms, and shoulders are basically extensions of the cables. That is, all rotational action, be it concentric (positive) or eccentric (negative), is from the core and not the arms.

3. The sensation of action should be as though pivoting in precisely the transverse plane around a rod that runs from the floor through the spine and out the top of the head.

SPECIFIC BENEFITS

12 **17**

NOTE

To increase exercise difficulty or simply add variety, try incorporating some of the following challenges:

- Adjust stance position (e.g., half-kneeling, tall kneeling, staggered stance, lunge stance, etc.).
- Stand or kneel on an unstable apparatus.
- Close the eyes.
- Employ perturbation techniques such as gently tapping the athlete throughout the movement or positioning a resistance band around the waist, ankles, or knees.

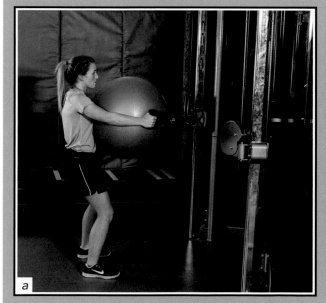

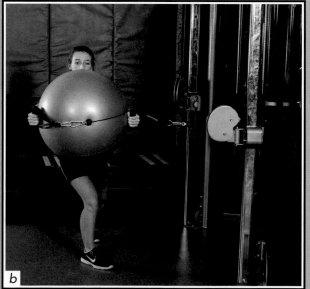

CONDITIONING TO THE CORE

The following hanging exercises are a small sample of the many hanging exercises and complexes that incorporate a suspended action. While most of the exercises are shown on a chin-up bar, there are many other options for suspension, including slings, ropes, dangling handles, overhand grip bar, underhand grip bar, and more.

Grip choice greatly influences the exercise's effectiveness and difficulty. For example, because of greater muscle involvement and lever advantage, an underhand grip might be to one athlete's advantage, but that same athlete might find it difficult to take an overhand wide grip, which might be the strength of another athlete. Our advice is to incorporate a variety of grips and apparatus to promote total musculature and mechanical development.

The following grip and elbow positions are listed in order of physical difficulty from most to least difficult:

- Neutral grip (palms facing each other), elbows flexed to 90 degrees or less
- Underhand grip, elbows flexed to less than 90 degrees
- Underhand grip, elbows flexed to 90 degrees or more
- Underhand grip, arms fully extended
- Overhand grip, elbows flexed to 90 degrees or less
- Overhand grip, arms fully extended

Note that a narrow grip tends to be easier for most athletes than a wider grip.

If choosing the straight-arm (fully extended) position, avoid subluxation of the shoulder. Maintain a depressed and retracted scapulae.

MOVEMENTS

1. Grasp a sturdy chin-up bar with an underhand grip; lift the body into a position in which the elbows are flexed to 90 degrees or less (see consideration 2).
2. Maintain a neutral pelvic tilt throughout. Controlling anterior and posterior pelvic tilt helps to eliminate swinging, which interferes with the exercise's effectiveness and compromises the structural integrity of the lower lumbar region.
3. Flex the hips and knees to about 90 degrees. This posture is the bent-knee start position (also called knee-tuck position) shown in the photo.
4. Extend the hips and knees; allow the legs to hang straight down.
5. Flex the hips and knees to 90 degrees returning to the bent-knee start position
6. Perform a predetermined number of repetitions.

CONSIDERATIONS

1. It is important to avoid an extreme kyphotic lumbar curve during this and all exercises.
2. Grip choices vary from wide to narrow, underhand to over hand, and elbow flexed to elbow straight. However, one constant is retraction and thus stabilization of the scapula.

SPECIFIC BENEFITS

NOTE

To increase exercise difficulty or simply add variety, try incorporating some of the following challenges:

- Extend legs with a slight twist—left, neutral, right, repeat.
- Hold a medicine ball or similar weighted apparatus between the knees or ankles.
- Place a resistance band around the ankles.
- Employ perturbation techniques such as gently tapping the athlete throughout the movement or positioning a resistance band around the waist, ankles, or knees.

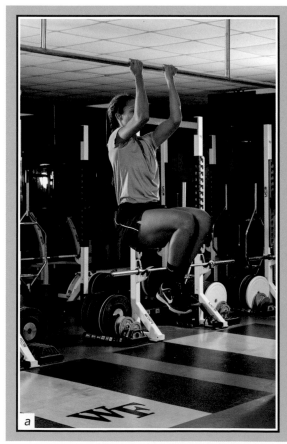

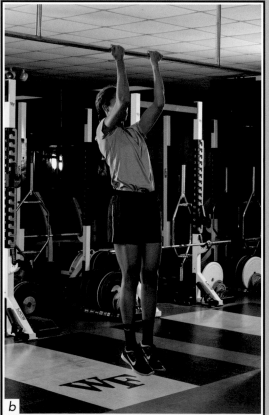

▪ HANGING KNEE TUCK ▪
EXTENDED L

Modifications

1. The setup, posture, and considerations are identical to the Hanging Knee Tuck.
2. Extend the knees with the legs moving straight out parallel to the ground to form an L position. The hips remain flexed to about 90 degrees.
3. Flex the knees and return to the start position.

Specific Benefits

Note To increase exercise difficulty or simply add variety, try incorporating some of the following challenges:

- Hold the L position for a set time period (isometric).
- Extend the legs at different angles (e.g., above parallel, parallel, below parallel, parallel, etc.).
- Hold a medicine ball or similar weighted apparatus between the knees or ankles.
- Place a resistance band around the ankles.
- Employ perturbation techniques such as gently tapping the athlete throughout the movement or positioning a resistance band around the waist, ankles, or knees.

▪ HANGING KNEE TUCK ▪
EXTENDED L TWIST

Modifications

1. The setup, posture, and considerations are identical to the Hanging Knee Tuck.
2. During the knee extension action, add a twist—literally. From the start position, extend the knees with the legs moving straight out parallel to the ground and return to the start position.
3. Next, extend the knees and twist to the left. Return to the start position.
4. Next, extend the knees forward parallel to the ground again. Return to the start position.
5. Next extend the knees and twist to the right. Return to the start position.
6. Steps 2 through 5 equal one repetition.

Specific Benefits

▪ HANGING KNEE TUCK ▪
UP AND TWIST

Modifications

1. The setup, posture, and considerations are identical to the Hanging Knee Tuck.
2. From the start position, lift the legs up and simultaneously twist, attempting to bring the left knee to the right elbow. Effectiveness of the exercise is not determined by actually touching the knee to the elbow. It is simply a directive goal.
3. In a controlled manner, slowly lower back to the start position; immediately repeat in the other direction: right knee toward the left elbow.
4. Steps 2 and 3 equal one repetition.

Specific Benefits

HANGING KNEE TUCK
BENT-KNEE WINDSHIELD WIPER

Modifications

1. The setup, posture, and considerations are identical to the Hanging Knee Tuck.
2. Rock back, lifting the knees up and back toward the chest. While in this up-and-back position, contract the rotators (primarily the obliques) and twist the legs to the right; then immediately twist to the left.
3. Return to the neutral up-and-back position.
4. In a controlled manner, slowly lower back to the knee tuck start position.
5. Repeat steps 2 through 4 but in opposition: twist left, then immediately twist right.

Specific Benefits [12] [16] [17] [18] [24]

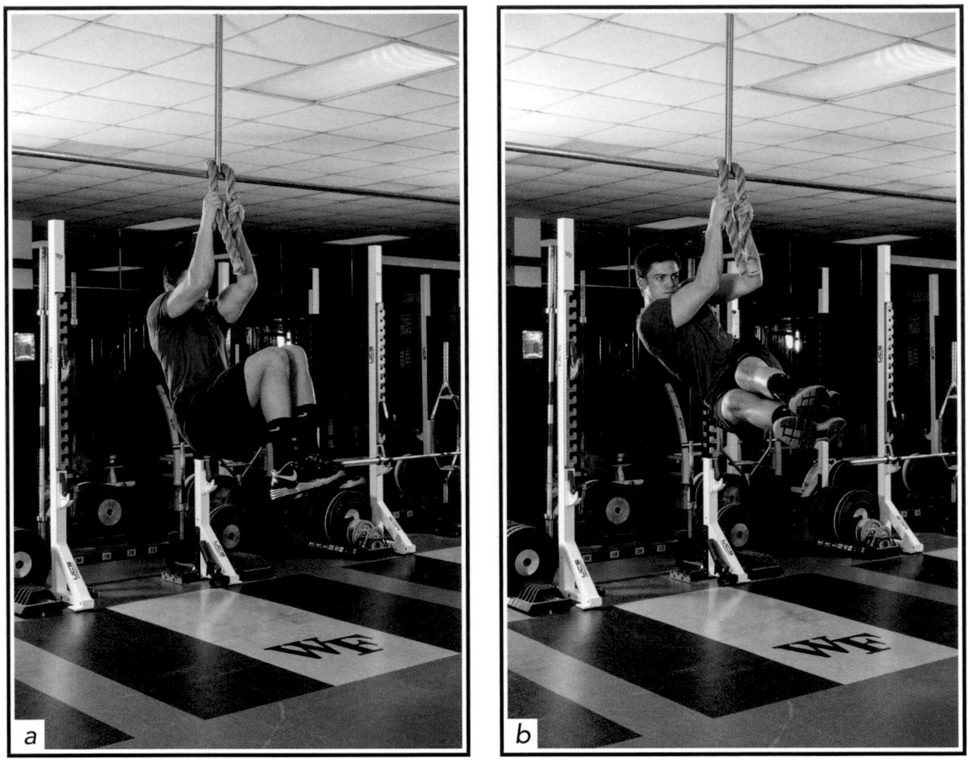

HANGING KNEE TUCK
BENT-KNEE WINDSHIELD WIPER FOR SPEED

Modifications

1. The setup, posture, and considerations are identical to the Hanging Knee Tuck, Bent-Knee Windshield Wiper.
2. The action is also the same, except once in the up-and-back position, perform the wiper movement in a controlled but accelerated motion. In other words, go as fast as possible without sacrificing technique or risking injury.
3. Do not return to the start position; maintain the up-and-back posture throughout the exercise. The action is simply left, right, left, right, and so on.

Specific Benefits [12] [16] [17] [18] [22] [23] [24]

HANGING INVERTED PIKE

DOUBLE-LEG WINDSHIELD WIPER

MOVEMENTS

1. Grasp a sturdy chin-up bar with an underhand grip. Lift to a position in which the elbows are flexed to 90 degrees or less (see consideration 2). Maintain a neutral pelvic tilt throughout the exercise. Controlling anterior and posterior pelvic tilt helps eliminate swinging, which interferes with the effectiveness of the exercise and compromises the structural integrity of the lower lumbar.

2. Lift the legs from a straight hang to an inverted position. The knees are locked and the feet and straight legs point toward the ceiling. The shins (lower leg) are very near the bar (this is elbow flexion dependent).

3. In a controlled manner, lower (drop) the legs to one side. Stop the downward movement no lower than parallel to the ground (see consideration 5).

4. Reverse the action and lift the legs back to the start position. Either stop at the inverted pike start position to regain control or simply continue directly into lowering the legs to the opposite side.

5. Steps 3 and 4 equal one repetition.

6. Perform a predetermined number of repetitions.

CONSIDERATIONS

1. Avoid the chicken head. Do not extend the head and neck in opposition to scapular retraction. Yes, this is a hard exercise. But lifting your chin toward the bar does nothing to assist with the intended movement and could cause a cervical spine impingement.

2. For this exercise—and any exercise in this book, for that matter—your strength and comfort level should determine range of motion of movement. With this specific exercise, the wiper action might simply be a few inches (or centimeters) left and right of vertical. As strength and confidence improve, greater distances can be attempted. Always use a spotter to help with control and mechanics. Never try to progress to a more difficult exercise until you have mastered the antecedent exercises.

SPECIFIC BENEFITS

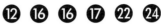 **12** **16** **16** **17** **22** **24**

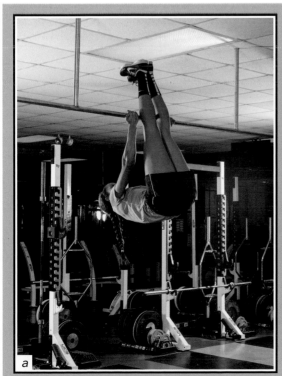

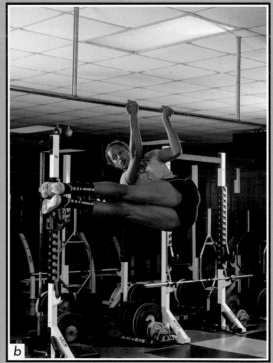

■ HANGING INVERTED PIKE ■
WINDSHIELD WIPER ABDUCTION AND ADDUCTION

Modifications

1. The setup, posture, and considerations are identical to the Hanging Inverted Pike, Double-Leg Windshield Wiper.
2. From the inverted pike start position, lower the right leg to the right. Stop the downward movement of the right leg no lower than parallel to the ground (see consideration 5 of the primary exercise).
3. Lower the left leg to the right leg.
4. Return both legs to the start position.
5. Repeat the action to the opposite (left) side.
6. Steps 2 through 5 equal one repetition.

Specific Benefits

Note Try these abduction and adduction variations:

- Both legs to right side; left leg up; right leg up; both legs to left side; right leg up; left leg up. Continue.
- Legs are spread (abducted). Drop legs to left; return to neutral; spread and drop both abducted legs to right.
- Abduct and drop right leg to right; drop left leg to right; return left leg to neutral; return right leg to neutral (inverted pike start position).
- Flutter-kick both legs to right; abduct and return left leg up; adduct and return right leg up; both legs are now back in inverted pike start position. Repeat to the opposite side.

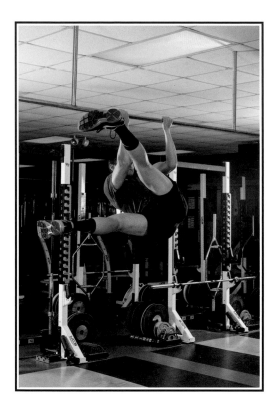

■ HANGING INVERTED PIKE ■
UP AND TWIST (POLE VAULTER)

Modifications

1. The setup, posture, and considerations are identical to the Hanging Inverted Pike, Double-Leg Windshield Wiper.

2. From the start position, contract the flexors and lift the hips along with the straight legs toward the ceiling (make sure you have ceiling height clearance). Simultaneously contract the rotators (oblique musculature) and twist to the left. For those of you who have ever pole vaulted, the action is similar to "shooting" prior to piking over the bar.

3. In a controlled manner, slowly lower back to the start position; repeat on the opposite side.

4. Steps 2 and 3 equal one repetition.

Specific Benefits ⑧ ⑫ ⑯ ⑰ ⑱ ㉔

Note A good precursor to this exercise is to eliminate the twist action and perform the movement by simply lifting the straight legs up toward the ceiling from the inverted pike start position. Remember that all grip positions and elbow flexion options apply for this and all other hanging drills.

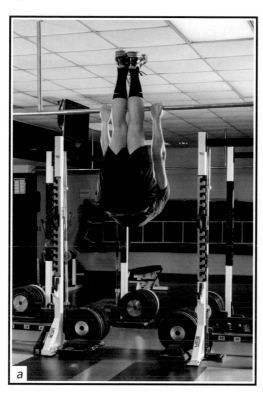 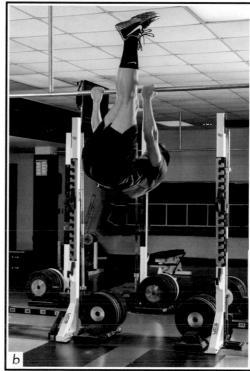

MOVEMENTS

1. Grasp a sturdy chin-up bar with an underhand grip (or place your arms in the slings as shown). Lift into a position in which slings elbows are flexed 90 degrees or less (see consideration 2). Both legs will hang straight toward floor with the feet dorsiflexed.

2. Maintain a neutral pelvic tilt throughout the exercise. Controlling anterior and posterior pelvic tilt helps eliminate swinging, which interferes with the effectiveness of the exercise and compromises the structural integrity of the lower lumbar.

3. Lift the right knee toward the chest (at least as high as the upper thigh), parallel to the floor. Extend the right foot out and around slightly—not a full foreleg reach but just enough to resemble a slight leg cycle action.

4. As the right leg starts its downward motion, simultaneously lift the left knee toward the chest.

5. The right leg and foot will move past the neutral hanging start position to a point slightly behind the body's vertical line. That is, the right hip will extend slightly. Again, mimic the leg cycle of a running stride.

6. Continue this alternating leg cycle action for a predetermined number of repetitions or length of time.

CONSIDERATIONS

1. To increase difficulty or simply add variety, try the exercise in an inverted position: leg cycling with legs pointed toward the ceiling.

SPECIFIC BENEFITS

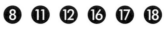

8 11 12 16 17 18

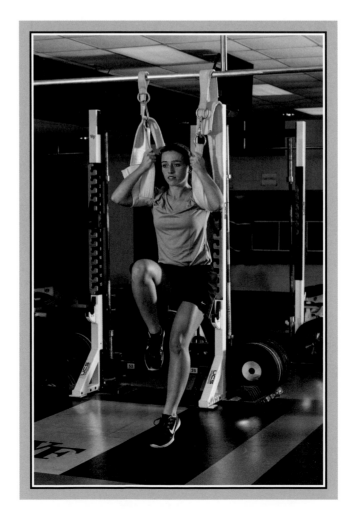

MOVEMENTS

1. Grasp a sturdy chin-up bar with an underhand grip. Lift into a position in which the elbows are flexed to 90 degrees or less. Maintain a neutral pelvic tilt throughout the exercise. Controlling anterior and posterior pelvic tilt helps to eliminate swinging, which interferes with the effectiveness of the exercise and compromises structural integrity of the lower lumbar.

2. Lift the legs from a straight hang to an inverted position. The knees are locked and the feet and straight legs point toward the ceiling.

3. In a controlled manner drop the right leg parallel to the ground. The left leg remains pointing straight up.

4. Simultaneously drop the left leg perpendicular to the floor while the right leg returns to the start position.

5. Steps 3 and 4 equal one repetition.

6. Perform for a predetermined number of repetitions or length of time.

CONSIDERATIONS

1. To decrease difficulty or simply add variety, start the exercise with the legs hanging straight down and alternate bringing each leg up to parallel.

SPECIFIC BENEFITS

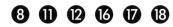

❽ ⓫ ⓬ ⓰ ⓱ ⓲

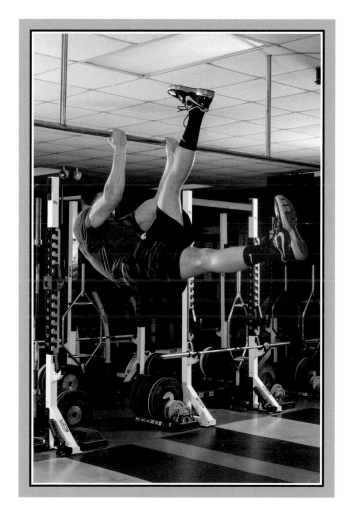

Scapulothoracic Exercises

A stable scapulothoracic joint is the foundation for all effective upper-body movement. But improving the stability of an area without improving its strength is completing only part of the puzzle. As we have stressed, a joint or joint system must be stable to function properly and reduce injury risk. But if this system is not prepared to deal with forces—be they external forces from impact or internal forces from transference of ground reaction—bad things can happen.

Basketball, water polo, tennis, football, badminton, and volleyball are a just a few of the sports that have a high degree of overhead kinesis. The junction formed by the ribcage and scapula is called the scapulothoracic joint and is one of the two primary joints critical to the athlete involved in sports with overhead movements. The other critical joint is the glenohumeral joint, which is formed by the scapula and the humerus; together these two joints make up the shoulder complex.

Stabilization not-withstanding, shoulder injuries in athletes are often the result of a lack of strength of the scapulothoracic joint. The primary reason for this deficiency is a strength imbalance between the various muscles that attach to the scapula. A significant strength discrepancy between the typically strong upper trapezius and the weaker middle and lower trapezius and the serratus anterior is often the principal culprit. If the upper trapezius persistently contracts too soon and with greater force than the middle and lower trapezius and the serratus, the result is an aberrant scapular motion. It is this disturbed symmetry that further adversely stresses the rest of the shoulder complex and specifically the rotator cuff musculature of the glenohumeral joint.

Athletes whose sports routinely involve overhead movements typically overemphasize these same movements in their training. Standing, seated, and supine incline activities tend to elicit the big muscles of the shoulders. Upright exercises, which greatly encourage upper trapezius activation and consequently place little emphasis on the middle and lower portion of the same muscle complex, will contribute to scapular muscle imbalances and scapulothoracic dysfunction. The resultant heightened instability will decrease functionality, which in turn will adversely affect performance or in the worst-case scenario lead to the onset of serial distortion patterns.

To develop scapulothoracic strength and reinstate a purposeful kinetic chain, strengthening exercises must be implemented that will target the lower and middle trapezius and serratus anterior with minimal emphasis on the upper trapezius and deltoid complex. Scapula retraction strength exercises that are movement focused as opposed to muscle focused should, for the most part, be performed while in a prone or side-lying posture. Therefore, exercises that target scapula retraction strength while in the aforementioned postures will address the underlying biomechanical factors that strengthen the scapulothoracic structure.

The rotator cuff, which provides stability to the glenohumeral joint, is only effective when operating from a strong and stable foundation. That base of support is a firmly established scapulothoracic structure. Overhead presses and similar strengthening exercises from an erect posture should not be eliminated entirely; instead, take an integrated approach that includes drills that provide the foundation for further strength development in the extremities.

The exercises in this chapter have been selected to increase strength levels in the scapulothoracic area, improve posture, streamline force summation, and keep the entire area sound during contact with the floor (e.g., goalie diving for a save) or with another athlete (e.g., clean rugby tackle). Like all core exercises, there is a primary focus (anti-extension, anti-rotation, etc.), but because the body is an all-inclusive physiological unit, for some exercises the scapulothoracic region is a major player in the ability to execute a multifaceted task (e.g., Band Pull Apart as compared to Hanging 90-90 Complex).

The following exercise finder lists the benefits, difficulty level, and equipment needed for every exercise that appears in this chapter. Primary exercises are highlighted in blue, with their progressions in red. The primary exercises are also noted in the text with a red title bar.

Scapulothoracic Strength Exercise Finder

Exercise Name	Specific Benefits (see chapter 5)	Difficulty Level			Equipment
		Easy	Medium	Hard	
Band Pull Apart	⑤ ⑫ ⑰	X			Band
Prone Loaded Scaption (Y), Incline Bench	② ⑤ ⑫ ⑰		X		Two dumbbells or weight plates, incline bench
Prone Loaded Scaption (Y), Stability Ball	① ② ⑤ ⑫ ⑰		X		Two dumbbells or weight plates, stability ball
Prone Loaded Shoulder Abduction (T), Incline Bench	⑤ ⑫ ⑰		X		Two dumbbells or weight plates, incline bench
Prone Loaded Shoulder Abduction (T), Stability Ball	① ② ⑤ ⑫ ⑰		X		Two dumbbells or weight plates, stability ball
Prone Loaded Scapular Retraction and Depression (A), Incline Bench	⑤ ⑫ ⑰		X		Two dumbbells or weight plates, incline bench
Prone Loaded Scapular Retraction and Depression (A), Stability Ball	① ② ⑤ ⑫ ⑰		X		Two dumbbells or weight plates, stability ball
Prone Loaded Scapulothoracic Combination (YTA), Incline Bench	② ⑤ ⑫ ⑰ ⑱ ㉔			X	Two dumbbells or weight plates, incline bench
Prone Loaded Scapulothoracic Combination (YTA), Stability Ball	① ② ⑤ ⑫ ⑰ ⑱ ㉔			X	Two dumbbells or weight plates, stability ball
Suspended Prone Retract and Protract	② ⑥ ⑫		X		Suspension trainer
Suspended Supine Rear Pull	② ⑥ ⑫ ⑯		X		Suspension trainer
Suspended Supine Rear Pull, Single Leg	② ⑥ ⑫ ⑯		X		Suspension trainer
Suspended Supine Alternating Knee Drive	② ⑥ ⑧ ⑪ ⑫ ⑯ ⑱		X		Suspension trainer
Suspended Supine Up and Twist	② ⑥ ⑫ ⑯ ⑱ ㉔		X		Suspension trainer
Hanging Rock-Back Pull-Up	⑫ ⑯ ⑰ ⑱			X	Chin-up bar
Hanging 90-90 Complex With Medicine Ball	⑥ ⑫ ⑯ ⑰ ⑱ ㉔			X	Chin-up bar, sandbag or medicine ball

MOVEMENTS

1. Assume an athletic stance with the feet positioned slightly wider than shoulder width, parallel, and pointing forward. The knees are slightly flexed, and the pelvis is in a neutral position.
2. With a rigid elbow, the arms are relatively straight and parallel to the floor (shoulder flexion within the sagittal plane). Grasp the band in a palms-down position (can also be done with the palms facing one another).
3. Brace the core; depress and retract the scapula.
4. Simultaneously pull the ends of the band "apart" to a position in which the arms are fully outstretched to the sides (frontal plane).
5. In a controlled manner, return the arms and hands to the start position.
6. Perform a predetermined number of repetitions.

CONSIDERATIONS

1. The elbows are locked, shoulders are relaxed, and shoulder blades remain depressed and retracted throughout the exercise.
2. Keep the chin pushed straight back, and don't let head fall forward. The cervical vertebrae should remain straight with the head tilted neither forward nor back.
3. Avoid the chicken head. Do not lift and then extend the head and neck in opposition to the band pull.

SPECIFIC BENEFITS

❺ ⓬ ⑰

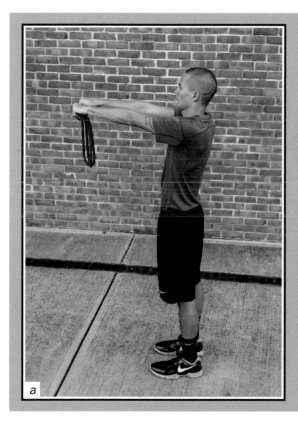

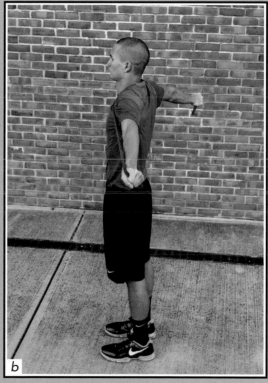

MOVEMENTS

1. Lie prone (face down) on an incline bench with the legs straight and feet securely on the floor.
2. Hold a dumbbell or weight plate in each hand; the weight should be challenging but not so great that it affects technique.
3. Outstretch the arms to form a Y position (relative to body orientation). The hands are in a neutral thumbs-up position. This is critically important.
4. Keep the chin pushed back (think double chin) and avoid dropping the head (cervical vertebrae are straight, with the head tilted neither forward or back). The chest remains on the incline bench throughout the exercise.
5. Consciously depress and retract the scapulae.
6. Raise the arms up, maintaining a thumbs-up position throughout.
7. Lower the arms to the start position.
8. Perform a predetermined number of repetitions.

CONSIDERATIONS

1. The shoulder blades remain depressed and retracted throughout the exercise.
2. Avoid the chicken head. Do not lift and then extend the head and neck in opposition to the arm raise.
3. Raise the arms as high as comfortably possible without additional body compensation (the sensation is one of extending the arms outward simultaneous to the lift action).

SPECIFIC BENEFITS

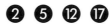

NOTE

Possible variations include the following:

- Alternate arms, lifting only one at a time.
- Attach bands to the bench and hold the opposite ends, using the stretching elastic as resistance.
- Hold a light medicine ball in each hand to work on grip strength at the same time as scapular thoracic strength.

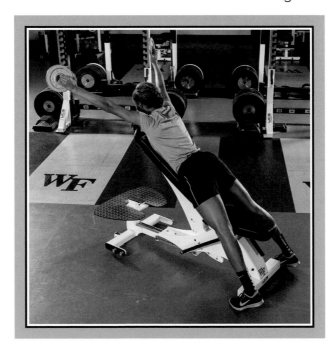

▪ PRONE LOADED SCAPTION (Y) ▪
STABILITY BALL

Modifications

1. Lie prone (face down) on a stability ball with the legs straight and feet securely on the floor.
2. Follow the steps for the Prone Loaded Scaption (Y), Incline Bench.

Specific Benefits

PRONE LOADED SHOULDER ABDUCTION (T)
INCLINE BENCH

MOVEMENTS

1. Lie prone (face down) on an incline bench with the legs straight and feet securely on the floor.
2. Hold a dumbbell or weight plate in each hand; the weight should be challenging but not so great that it affects technique.
3. Outstretch the arms to form a T position (90 degrees relative to the torso). The palms are down. This is critically important.
4. Keep the chin pushed back (think double chin) and avoid dropping the head (cervical vertebrae are straight, with the head tilted neither forward or back). The chest remains on the incline bench throughout the exercise.
5. Consciously depress and retract the scapulae.
6. Raise the arms, keeping them in the T position.
7. Lower the arms to the start position.
8. Perform a predetermined number of repetitions.

CONSIDERATIONS

1. The shoulder blades remain depressed and retracted throughout the exercise.
2. With the arms raised and outstretched, consciously draw these limbs back inward (squeeze the shoulder blades together).
3. Raise the arms as high as comfortably possible without additional body compensation.

SPECIFIC BENEFITS

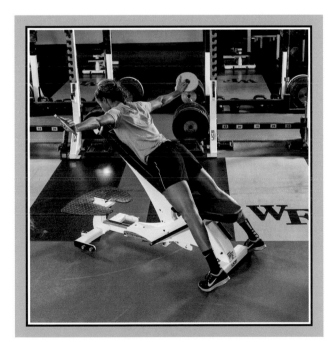

▪ PRONE LOADED SHOULDER ABDUCTION (T) ▪
STABILITY BALL

Modifications

1. Lie prone (face down) on a stability ball with the legs straight and feet securely on the floor.

2. Follow the steps for the Prone Loaded Shoulder Abduction (T), Incline Bench.

Specific Benefits

PRONE LOADED SCAPULAR RETRACTION AND DEPRESSION (A)

INCLINE BENCH

MOVEMENTS

1. Lie prone (face down) on an incline bench with the legs straight and feet securely on the floor.
2. Hold a dumbbell or weight plate in each hand; the weight should be challenging but not so great that it affects technique.
3. Outstretch the arms to the sides of the body to form an A position (relative to the torso). The palms are down at the start of the exercise.
4. Keep the chin pushed back (think double chin) and avoid dropping the head (cervical vertebrae are straight, with the head tilted neither forward or back); the chest remains on the incline bench throughout the exercise. The chest remains on the incline bench throughout the exercise.

5. Consciously depress and retract the scapulae.
6. Raise the arms, keeping them in the "A" position.
7. Lower the arms to the start position.
8. Perform a predetermined number of repetitions.

CONSIDERATIONS

1. The shoulder blades remain depressed and retracted throughout the exercise.
2. Raise arms as high as comfortably possible without additional body compensation.

SPECIFIC BENEFITS

5 **12** **17**

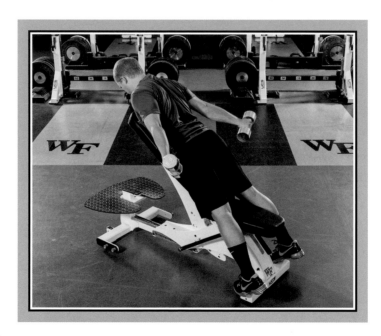

PRONE LOADED SCAPULAR RETRACTION AND DEPRESSION (A)

STABILITY BALL

Modifications

1. Lie prone (face down) on a stability ball with the legs straight and feet securely on the floor.

2. Follow the steps for Prone Loaded Scapular Retraction and Depression (A), Incline Bench.

Specific Benefits **1** **2** **5** **12** **17**

PRONE LOADED SCAPULOTHORACIC COMBINATION (YTA)

INCLINE BENCH

MOVEMENTS

1. Lie prone (face down) on an incline bench with the legs straight and feet securely on the floor.
2. Hold a dumbbell or weight plate in each hand; the weight should be challenging but not so great that it affects technique.
3. Outstretch the arms to form a "Y" position (relative to body orientation). The hands are in a neutral thumbs-up position. This is critically important.
4. Keep the chin pushed back (think double chin) and avoid dropping the head (cervical vertebrae are straight, with the head tilted neither forward or back); the chest remains on the incline bench throughout the exercise. The chest remains on the incline bench throughout the exercise.
5. Consciously depress and retract the scapulae.
6. To start this three-part move, first raise the arms up in the "Y" position.
7. Lower to the start position; immediately reposition the arms to a "T" position. The palms are down (still important!). Consciously depress and retract the scapulae and raise the arms. The arms are outstretched forming a "T" position (90 degrees relative to the torso).
8. Lower the arms; immediately reposition the arms to the "A" position. Consciously depress and retract the scapulae and raise the arms. The arms are outstretched forming an "A" position (relative to the torso). The palms are down (again, important!). During the lift, externally rotate the straight arm from the shoulder so the thumbs point up and out. As you lift, reach outward as if extending the arms during the movement.
9. Lower the arms and reposition to the original "Y."
10. The entirety of the combination is equal to one repetition. Perform a predetermined number of repetitions.

CONSIDERATIONS

1. The shoulder blades remain depressed and retracted throughout the exercise.
2. Raise the arms as high as comfortably possible without additional body compensation.

SPECIFIC BENEFITS

2 **5** **12** **17** **18** **24**

◾ PRONE LOADED SCAPULOTHORACIC COMBINATION (YTA) ◾

STABILITY BALL

Modifications

1. Lie prone (face down) on a stability ball with the legs straight and feet securely on the floor.

2. Follow the steps for the Prone Loaded Scapulothoracic Combination (YTA), Incline Bench.

Specific Benefits   **1** **2** **5** **12** **17** **18** **24**

SUSPENDED PRONE RETRACT AND PROTRACT

MOVEMENTS

1. Kneel on the floor and place the hands in the grip or straps.
2. Brace the core and lift the body into a suspended plank position (shoulders, hips, knees, and ankles are in alignment). The feet are dorsiflexed with only the toes and balls of the feet in contact with the floor (or bench, box, etc.).
3. Depress and retract the scapulae and drive the chest toward the floor. The body remains in alignment and the arms are straight throughout.
4. Protract the shoulder blades, but do not sacrifice body alignment (do not sag). A coaching cue is "chest out, chest in" (i.e., retract, protract).
5. Keep the chin pushed back (think double chin) and avoid dropping the head (cervical vertebrae are straight, with the head tilted neither forward or back).
6. Maintain a completely straight line in the body throughout a predetermined number of repetitions.

CONSIDERATIONS

1. Avoid subluxation of the shoulder.
2. Avoid the chicken head. Do not lift and then extend the head and neck in opposition to retraction.

SPECIFIC BENEFITS

 ❷ ❻ ⓬

NOTE

Specific benefits will vary depending on the body angle (i.e., feet elevated or upper body elevated and degree of either).

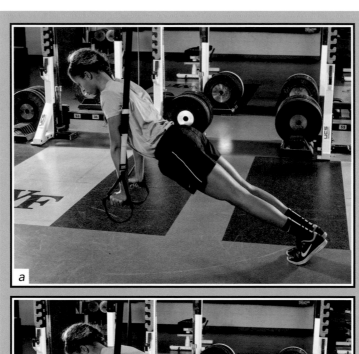

a

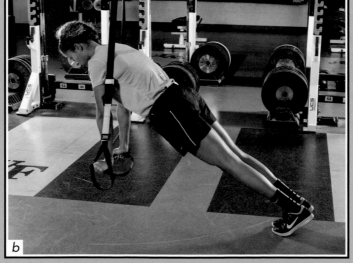

b

SUSPENDED SUPINE REAR PULL

MOVEMENTS

1. To begin, sit on the floor and place the hands in the grips (or straps). This drill can be performed with any combination of three hand positions:
   a. Neutral grip: palms face one another throughout the drill
   b. Pronated grip: palms face the feet throughout the drill
   c. Combination: palms start pronated and turn to neutral during the repetition

2. Brace the core and lift the body into a suspended plank position (shoulders, hips, knees, and ankles are aligned). The feet are dorsiflexed with only the heels are in contact with the floor (or bench, box, etc.).

3. Consciously depress and retract the scapulae; maintain this position throughout the exercise.

4. Keep the chin pushed back (think double chin) and avoid dropping the head (cervical vertebrae are straight, with the head tilted neither forward or back).

5. Engage the back (focus on the middle and lower back) and biceps musculature and pull the upper body to a position in which the hands are close to the armpits.

6. Return to the start position in a controlled manner.

7. Maintain a completely straight line in the body throughout the entirety of the set.

CONSIDERATIONS

1. Avoid subluxation of the shoulder.

2. Lift the body as high as comfortably possible without additional body compensation.

3. Avoid the chicken head. Do not lift and then extend the head and neck in opposition to the pull.

SPECIFIC BENEFITS

2 **6** **12** **16**

NOTE

Benefits will vary depending on body angle (i.e., feet elevated or upper body elevated and the degree of either).

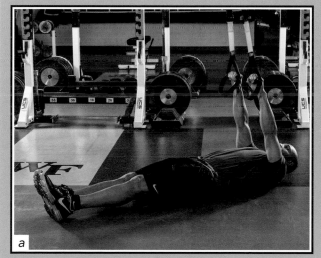
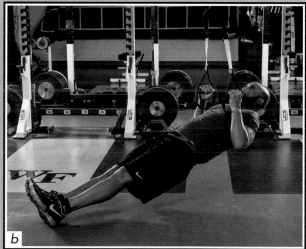

■ SUSPENDED SUPINE REAR PULL ■
SINGLE LEG

Modifications

1. Action is the same as for the Suspended Supine Rear Pull, except one foot remains on the floor while the opposite foot and leg are raised up and remain so throughout the exercise. The hip should be flexed and the leg straight throughout. Maintain a completely straight line in the body throughout the entirety of the set.

Specific Benefits **2** **6** **12** **16**

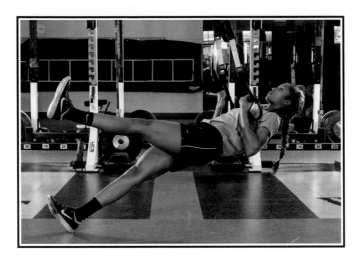

■ SUSPENDED SUPINE ALTERNATING KNEE DRIVE ■

Modifications

1. Assume the plank position and body alignment as previously described for Suspended Supine Rear Pull; heels are on the floor.

2. Pull the upper body into a position in which the elbows are at 90 degrees. Maintain this locked-arm position throughout the drill.

3. With a strongly braced core, lift (drive) one knee toward the chest; hold for a second and return to the start position.

4. Continue to maintain a straight body plank.

5. "Lift" (drive) the opposite knee toward the chest and repeat.

Specific Benefits **2** **6** **8** **11** **12** **16** **18**

■ SUSPENDED SUPINE UP AND TWIST ■

Modifications

1. This exercise requires a single handle. Depending on the apparatus used, you can simply hold one handle, hold both handles as one handle, or cross-twist one handle into the other to prevent slippage. Regardless of the method you choose, a spotter is recommended.

2. Assume the plank position and body alignment as previously described for Suspended Supine Rear Pull; the heels are on the floor.

3. Simultaneously pull and twist the body. Pull the body as far as comfortably possible.

4. During the pull action, the feet will drop (turn) toward the direction of the twist. This decreases joint torque stress.

5. Continue for a predetermined number of repetitions. Repeat on the opposite side.

Specific Benefits ❷ ❻ ⓬ ⓰ ⓲ ㉔

Note Maintain a plank position throughout the exercise. Initially, the angle of the body might be fairly close to vertical to make the effort less challenging. As strength and comfort levels improve, the angle should become more extreme, requiring greater strength to perform the movement.

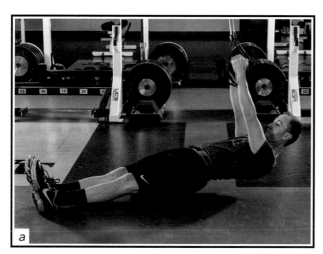

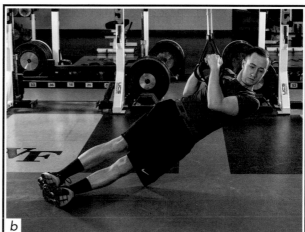

MOVEMENTS

1. Step on a box and grasp a chin-up bar with an underhand grip (photographs demonstrate utilizing a rope, and in this case a typical overhand grip should be used) The arms can be straight or flexed depending on strength and control levels. If the arms are straight, do not allow subluxation of the shoulders at the bottom of the hang.

2. Depress and retract the scapulae.

3. Brace the core; flex the hips and knees to 90 degrees. The upper legs (thighs) are parallel to the floor at the start position. Dorsiflex the feet. Assume a slight anterior pelvic tilt.

4. In a controlled manner, engage the core musculature and posteriorly tilt the pelvis.

5. Hold this position and do a pull-up (chin to the bar).

6. Return to the start position and slowly lower the pelvic tilt back to the anterior position.

7. Repeat steps 2 through 6 in a continuous movement for a predetermined number of repetitions.

CONSIDERATIONS

1. The pelvic action is limited. It should be a sensation of rolling the pelvis back and then rolling the pelvis forward. Rarely is this rolling movement much more than 6 to 12 inches (15-30 cm) total.

2. Never jerk or throw the lower body up into position.

3. A spotter might be necessary. If so, the spotter kneels on floor and places the hands out at the appropriate height to provide a contact point for the athlete's feet. This accomplishes two things: First, it provides the athlete with a visual and tactile stopping point between repetitions; second, it allows the spotter to provide assistance at the beginning of the movement, when needed most to overcome inertia. If a spotter is unavailable, use a box or a bench. If the tilt portion of the exercise is not too difficult, then the spotter can assist the athlete by standing behind him and placing the hands at the upper or middle back and help to push the athlete toward the chin-up bar.

4. The upper legs never drop below parallel to the floor.

SPECIFIC BENEFITS

12 **16** **17** **18**

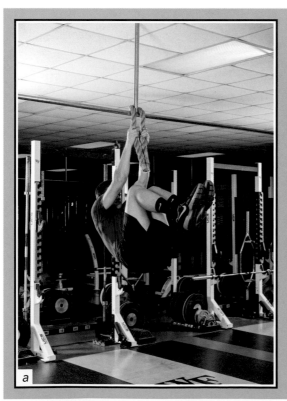
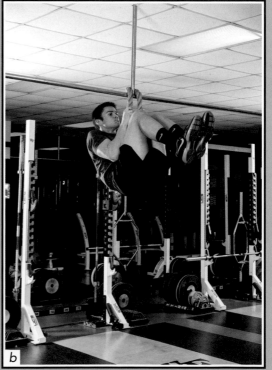

▪ HANGING 90-90 COMPLEX WITH MEDICINE BALL ▪

Muscle synergies and the central nervous system's control of the efficiency of kinetic chain functionality is the goal of an integrated and balanced global training regimen. Our goal, whenever possible, is to avoid training isolated muscles. Thus the following is a multipart exercise (a complex) in which many combinations of static and dynamic movements can be executed. The idea is to train comprehensively using an assortment of planes, tempo, and movement patterns. With safety at the forefront of the conceptual program design, we encourage you to develop your own unique and progressively challenging complexes.

Modifications

1. Place a medicine ball between the knees (or use a sandbag on the knees across the thighs or a weight belt around the legs above the knees, or even a band resistance held from behind).

2. Assume the start position described in steps 1 through 3 of Hanging Rock-Back Pull-Up. In our demonstration, we use the chin-up bar instead of the rope (a).

3. The complex action is as follow:

   a. In a controlled manner, engage the core musculature and posteriorly tilt the pelvis. Hold this position and do a pull-up (chin to the bar).

   b. In the up position, perform a corn-on-the-cob move (i.e., shift the entire body weight from left to right and back—b-c).

   c. Lower the body to a point at which the elbows are flexed at 90 degrees. In this position, with the elbows locked, cocontract the oblique musculature and "twist lift" to the left (d) and then under control "twist lift" to the right (e).

   d. Lower to the start position and do a predetermined number of repetitions.

Specific Benefits ⓫ ⓰ ⓱ ⓲ ㉔

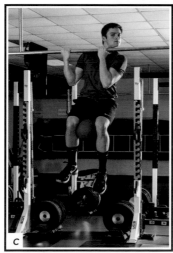
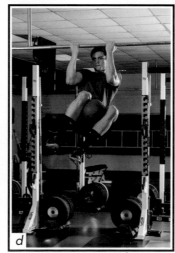
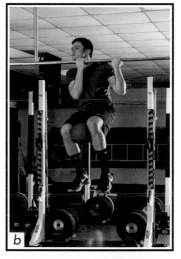
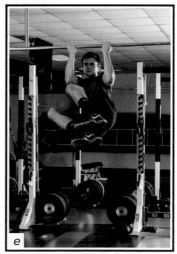
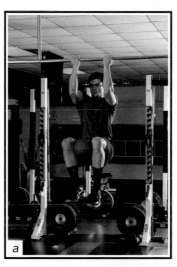

13

Lumbo-Pelvic Hip Exercises

The core is made up of an intricate spider web of musculature that interweaves its way throughout the torso collaboratively linking the shoulders, spine, and pelvis to establish a solid foundation from which all mobilization can occur. In the absence of a deep stabilizer equilibrium, the strong, flexible, and free-moving actions of the core musculature, specifically the outer mobilizers, would be quite ineffective. During athletic movements, the lumbo-pelvic hip complex (LPHC) functions primarily to conserve dynamic postural control by maintaining precise positioning of the body's center of mass above its base of support. Without this critical function, performance limitations would unquestionably exist, along with a heightened risk of injury.

The LPHC plays an incredibly important role in establishing and executing strength. It serves as the conduit for force and power transfer throughout the body. The LPHC should not be taken lightly. The complex influences every movement the body makes—from providing a dynamic foundation from which to transfer power when throwing a discus to osteoarticular stabilization when using a squidger to flip a tiddlywink into the pot. All things equal, the stronger athlete will usually win. Strengthening the lumbo-pelvic hip complex pays big performance dividends.

The following exercise finder lists the benefits, difficulty level, and equipment needed for every exercise that appears in this chapter. Primary exercises are highlighted in blue, with their progressions in red. The primary exercises are also noted in the text with a red title bar.

Lumbo-Pelvic Hip Strength Exercise Finder

Exercise Name	Specific Benefits (see chapter 5)	Difficulty Level			Equipment
		Easy	Medium	Hard	
Hip Lift, Shoulders Elevated	12 17	X			Raised platform*
Hip Lift With Resistance Band, Shoulders Elevated	5 12 17	X			Raised platform, mini-band
Loaded Hip Lift With Resistance Band, Shoulders Elevated	5 12 17		X		One weight, raised platform, mini-band
Loaded Hip Lift, Shoulders Elevated	12 17		X		One weight, raised platform
Hip Lift, Shoulders Elevated, Single Leg	4 12 17		X		Raised platform
Loaded Hip Lift, Shoulders Elevated, Single Leg	4 12 17		X		One weight, raised platform
Overhead Squat Series Progression 1: Prisoner Squat With Resistance Band	5 12 17		X		Mini-band
Overhead Squat Series Progression 2: Overhead Squat With Resistance Band	5 12 17		X		Broomstick or PVC pipe, mini-band
Overhead Squat Series Progression 3: Weighted Overhead Squat	12 17			X	Barbell
Overhead Squat Series Progression 4: Weighted Overhead Squat With Resistance Band	5 12 17			X	Barbell, mini-band
Overhead Squat Series Progression 5: Single-Arm Weighted Overhead Squat	11 12 17 18			X	Dumbbell or kettlebell
Overhead Squat Series Progression 6: Single-Arm Weighted Overhead Squat With Resistance Band	5 11 12 17 18			X	Dumbbell or kettlebell, mini-band
Sumo Squat Series Progression 1: Sumo Squat	12 17		X		Dumbbell or kettlebell
Sumo Squat Series Progression 2: Lateral Slide	8 12 17 18		X		Dumbbell or kettlebell
Sumo Squat Series Progression 3: Lateral Leg Lift	8 9 12 17 18 22 23		X		Dumbbell or kettlebell
Sumo Squat Series Progression 4: Lateral Slide and Lateral Leg Lift	8 9 12 17 18 22 23		X		Dumbbell or kettlebell
Lateral Band Slide	5 8 9 12 17	X			One or two resistance bands
Lateral Band Slide, Straight Legs	5 8 9 12 17	X			Resistance band
Lateral Band Slide, Skating	5 8 9 12 17 24	X			Resistance band
X-Band Walk	5 8 9 12 17		X		Elastic tubing

* Many options are available for the raised platform, including a box, bench, stair, or step.

SHOULDERS ELEVATED

MOVEMENTS

1. Positioned perpendicular to a utility bench, lie supine (face up) with the shoulders and neck (back of the head) completely supported by the pad. The knees are bent with the feet flat on the floor.
2. With the core braced, allow the hips to drop toward the floor. Note that depending on your height and/or the height of the bench, your butt may or may not touch the floor. However, a short box or some folded mats placed under you might help with the "butt tap" on the floor.
3. From the down position, under control, engage the core and lift the hips smoothly toward the ceiling (i.e., lift hips to parallel).
4. Slowly return to the down position and perform a predetermined number of repetitions.

CONSIDERATIONS

1. Contract the glutes and brace the core throughout the exercise.
2. Lift the hips to a position in which the ear, shoulder, hip, and knee are in a straight line. Avoid lumbar hyperextension.
3. If at any point you feel the upper hamstrings or lower back tightening, return to the start position and begin again.
4. Never sacrifice technique for added reps or sets. Maintain precision with mechanics.

SPECIFIC BENEFITS

12 **17**

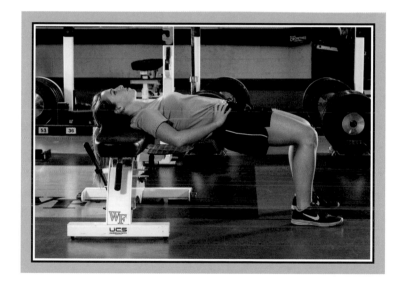

■ HIP LIFT ■
WITH RESISTANCE BAND, SHOULDERS ELEVATED

Modifications

1. The setup, start position, action, and considerations are the same as for the Hip Lift, Shoulders Elevated except that a rubber power band is positioned above and around both knees.

Specific Benefits ⑤ ⑫ ⑰

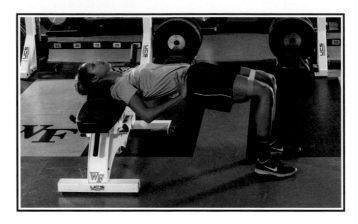

■ LOADED HIP LIFT ■
WITH RESISTANCE BAND, SHOULDERS ELEVATED

Modifications

1. The setup, start position, action, and considerations are the same as for the Hip Lift With Resistance Band, Shoulders Elevated except that in addition to the power band above and around both knees, place a weight or barbell across the front of the hips.

Specific Benefits ⑤ ⑫ ⑰

■ LOADED HIP LIFT ■
SHOULDERS ELEVATED

Movements

1. The setup, start position, action, and considerations are the same as for the Hip Lift, Shoulders Elevated except place an Olympic plate (or similar load such as a barbell, sandbag, or medicine ball) across the front of the hips. It is typically necessary to hold the weight in place with the hands.

Specific Benefits ⑫ ⑰

▪ HIP LIFT ▪
SHOULDERS ELEVATED, SINGLE LEG

Modifications

1. The setup, start position, action, and considerations are the same as the Hip Lift, Shoulders Elevated except keep one knee bent and that foot on the floor while the opposite leg is fully extended.

Specific Benefits ❹ ⓬ ⓱

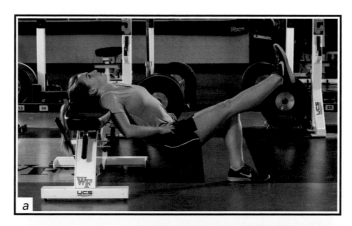

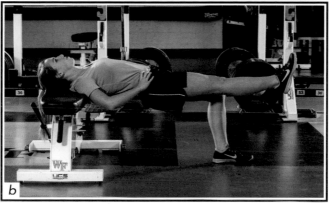

▪ LOADED HIP LIFT ▪
SHOULDERS ELEVATED, SINGLE LEG

Modifications

1. The setup, start position, action, and considerations are the same as the Hip Lift, Shoulders Elevated, Single Leg except place an Olympic plate (or similar load such as a barbell, sandbag, or medicine ball) across the front of the hips. It is typically necessary to hold the weight in place with the hands.

Specific Benefits ❹ ⓬ ⓱

Raising the arms overhead during a squatting movement as shown in the following drills places a higher demand on your body as your upper half is now in complete extension while your lower half is experiencing complete flexion. Through many force couple relationships working up and across the body, you are now in one of the most challenging primitive movement patterns and your LPHC must work at its most optimum to deal with this extreme bodyweight challenge. Only attempt such challenging and high-risk exercises after mastering the exercises and preliminary skills that prepare for them, and always use a spotter.

OVERHEAD SQUAT SERIES

PROGRESSION 1: PRISONER SQUAT WITH RESISTANCE BAND

MOVEMENTS

1. Place a resistance band around the legs directly above the knees. Stand erect with the scapulae depressed and retracted. The feet are parallel and slightly wider than shoulder width. Some individuals might find it more comfortable with a slight hip external rotation—toes pointed out.
2. Clasp the hands gently behind the head. Pull the elbows back and "lift" the chest slightly.
3. Brace the core, sit down and back. The first sensation is the butt moving back.
4. When in the low-squat position, the lower legs should be perpendicular to the floor. The knees should be directly over the front third of the foot.
5. Maintain a constant lateral pressure against the resistance band (hip abduction). Do not allow the resistance band to pull the knees in.
6. While maintaining a braced core, return to the stand-tall position.
7. Repeat for a predetermined number of repetitions.

CONSIDERATIONS

1. A spotter is suggested for all overhead squat drills. Use caution.
2. Do not pull forward on the head or neck with the hands.
3. When the thighs are parallel to floor, or slightly below parallel, the knees should not extend beyond the feet. Glance down to check!
4. Weight distribution should be toward the back half of the feet. A quick test of weight distribution is to simply lift the big toe inside the shoe. If the weight is too far forward, lifting the big toe will be difficult.
5. Ensure that the knees do not collapse inward into a knock-kneed position (valgus). This tendency might be eliminated via the slight foot flare noted above in addition to the tactile sense to maintain hip abduction caused by the resistance band around the knees.

SPECIFIC BENEFITS

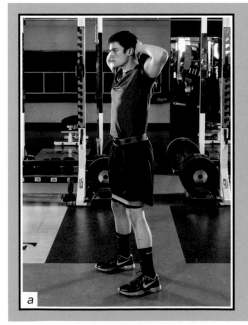

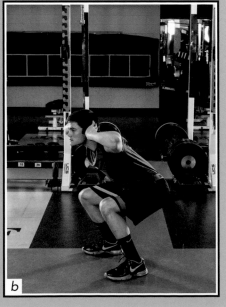

■ OVERHEAD SQUAT SERIES ■
PROGRESSION 2: OVERHEAD SQUAT WITH RESISTANCE BAND

Modifications

1. Grasp a lightweight bar such as a broomstick or a PVC pipe. The hands should be wider than shoulder width. Raise the bar directly overhead to a position resembling a Y. Be careful not to press the bar too far behind your head at the risk of subluxing the shoulder.

2. The posture, action, and considerations are identical to Overhead Squat Series Progression 1.

Specific Benefits

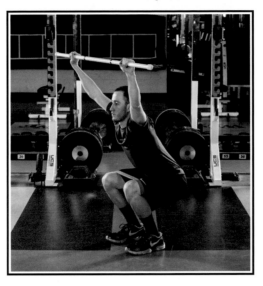

■ OVERHEAD SQUAT SERIES ■
PROGRESSION 3: WEIGHTED OVERHEAD SQUAT

Modifications

1. The setup, start position, posture, action, and considerations are identical to Overhead Squat Series Progression 2 except remove the resistance band around the legs and use a weighted bar overhead.

Specific Benefits ⑫ ⑰

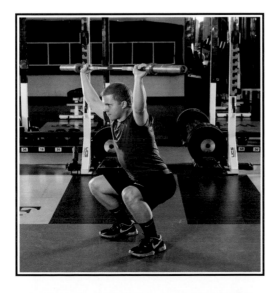

■ OVERHEAD SQUAT SERIES ■
PROGRESSION 4: WEIGHTED OVERHEAD SQUAT WITH RESISTANCE BAND

Modifications

1. The setup, start position, posture, action, and considerations are identical to Overhead Squat Series Progression 3 except a resistance band is placed around the legs directly above the knees.

2. Ensure that the resistance band does not collapse the knees inward.

Specific Benefits ❺ ⑫ ⑰

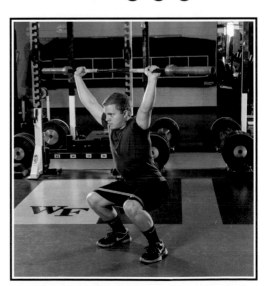

▪ OVERHEAD SQUAT SERIES ▪
PROGRESSION 5: SINGLE-ARM WEIGHTED OVERHEAD SQUAT

Modifications

1. The setup, start position, posture, action, and considerations are identical to Overhead Squat Series Progression 3 except a single weight is used as resistance instead of a bar.

2. Grasp a dumbbell (or a kettlebell, sandbag, medicine ball with a grip). Carefully lift the resistance directly overhead. Select a weight that is manageable and does not interfere with the proper mechanics of the exercise.

Specific Benefits ⑪ ⑫ ⑰ ⑱

Note Asymmetric loading provides a new challenge to the body as not only does the required amount of force have to be produced to move the weight, but stabilization becomes critical to maintain the balance of the weight. Neuromuscular control and efficiency have to be maintained without the body compensating at any of the major joints.

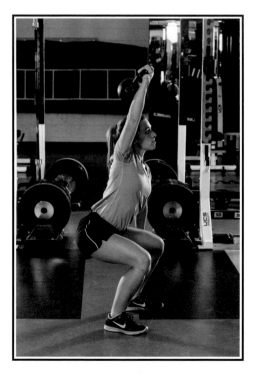

▪ OVERHEAD SQUAT SERIES ▪
PROGRESSION 6: SINGLE-ARM WEIGHTED OVERHEAD SQUAT WITH RESISTANCE BAND

Modifications

1. The setup, start position, posture, action, and considerations are identical to the Overhead Squat Series Progression 5 except a resistance band is placed around the legs directly above the knees.

2. Ensure that the resistance band does not collapse the knees inward into a knock-kneed position (valgus).

Specific Benefits ⑤ ⑪ ⑫ ⑰ ⑱

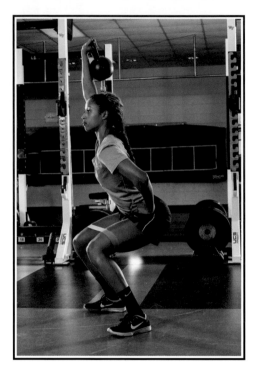

SUMO SQUAT SERIES

PROGRESSION 1: SUMO SQUAT

MOVEMENTS

1. Assume a wide "defensive stance" position with the feet parallel and slightly flared.
2. Grip a dumbbell or similar weight (e.g., medicine ball, kettlebell, Olympic plate).
3. Maintain a wide stance, pick the weight up off the floor, and stand tall. The pelvis is in a neutral position. The arms hang straight down. Do not allow the weight to pull on the shoulders; maintain a retracted scapulae throughout.
4. Brace the core and sit down and back. The first sensation is the butt moving back. The Shoulders are retracted; chest is out.
5. When in the low-squat position, the lower legs should be relatively perpendicular to the floor. The knees should be directly over the front third of the foot.
6. While maintaining a braced core, return to the stand-tall position.
7. Repeat for a predetermined number of repetitions.

CONSIDERATIONS

1. Avoid the chicken head. Keep the chin pushed back (think double chin) and avoid dropping the head (cervical vertebrae are straight, with the head tilted neither forward or back).
2. Ensure that the knees do not collapse inward into a knock-kneed position (valgus) especially when pressing back up to the start position. This tendency should be eliminated via the slight foot flare.

SPECIFIC BENEFITS

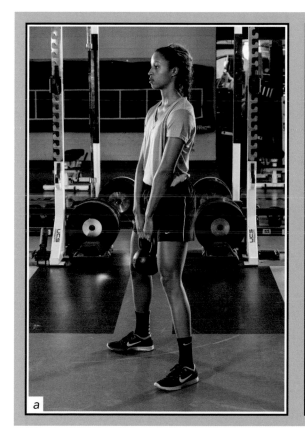
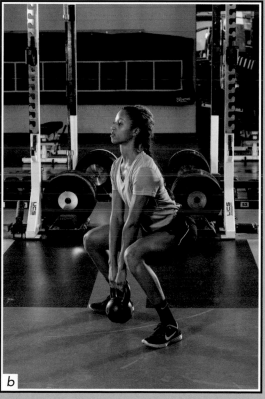

▪ SUMO SQUAT SERIES ▪
PROGRESSION 2: LATERAL SLIDE

Modifications

1. The setup, posture, and initial action are identical to Sumo Squat Series Progression 1.

2. In the low-squat position, take two to four slide steps to the right. Slide steps are performed as follows:

   a. Lift the right leg up and drive (push) off the left leg laterally to the right.

   b. The right foot comes down to the floor and the trailing left leg slides to a position in which the feet are the same distance apart as when Sumo Squat stance was first established.

   c. Repeat the lateral step, ending again in a wide Sumo Squat stance.

   d. Following two to four steps to the right, press up to the tall position.

   e. Immediately reverse the action: brace the core and sit down and back. The first sensation is the butt moving back.

   f. Lift the left leg and drive (push) off of the right leg lateral to the left.

3. Down and back equals one round trip. Perform a predetermined number of round trips.

Specific Benefits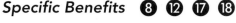

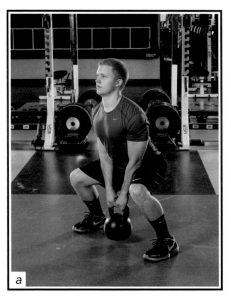 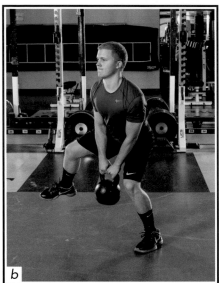

▪ SUMO SQUAT SERIES ▪
PROGRESSION 3: LATERAL LEG LIFT

Modifications

1. The setup, posture, and initial action are identical to Sumo Squat Series Progression 1.

2. In the low-squat position, explosively drive up and lateral onto the right leg.

3. In continuation of the movement, the left leg and foot leave the floor and all of the body weight shifts onto the right leg. In the up position, the right ankle, right knee, and right hip should be in a straight line with the right leg perpendicular to the floor. The upper body might lean slightly to the right for a balanced weight distribution.

4. Now here is the whole point of the exercise. It's not the drive into the tall position that is the focus (although this is important) but rather the following action that creates the adaptive qualities we strive for: Allow the body weight and dumbbell to *fall* back to the left. *Catch* the drop in a comfortably low-squat position. The *catch* should be soft with the bent ankle, hip, and knee acting as shock absorbers. Do not land on a stiff left leg.

5. Immediately reverse the action by driving up onto the left leg while lifting the right leg in preparation for the return action.

6. Over and back equals one round trip. Perform a predetermined number of round trips.

Specific Benefits

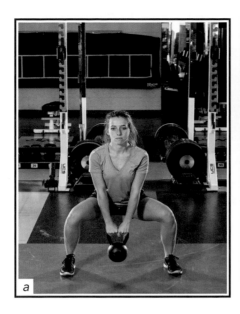
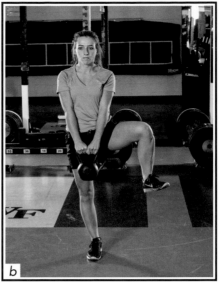

■ SUMO SQUAT SERIES ■
PROGRESSION 4: LATERAL SLIDE AND LATERAL LEG LIFT

Modifications

1. The setup, posture, and initial lateral slide action are identical to Sumo Squat Series Progression 2 except that at the end of the lateral slide, execute a lateral leg lift as just described in Sumo Squat Series Progression 3.

2. Down and back equals one round trip. Perform a predetermined number of round trips.

Specific Benefits ❽ ❾ ⑫ ⑰ ⑱ ㉒ ㉓

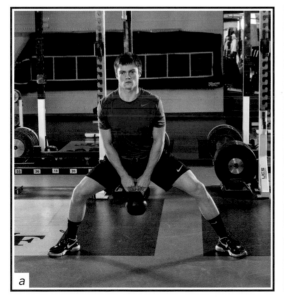
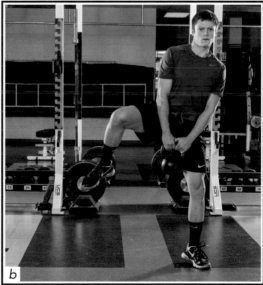

There are hundreds of resistance band movement patterns to choose from. Included here are several exercises that we hope will stimulate your creativity. If not performed correctly, resistance bands can elicit poor mechanics, so be mindful of proper technique to reap the full benefits.

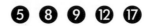

LATERAL BAND SLIDE

MOVEMENTS

1. Stand tall with a resistance band positioned around both legs directly above knees or directly above the ankles (or both, for maximum challenge, as shown). The feet are slightly wider than shoulder-width apart and parallel.
2. Depress and retract the scapulae. Brace the core and place the hands on the hips.
3. Flex the hips and knees slightly; drop into an athletic position.
4. Lift the left foot and leg a few inches off the ground and simultaneously drive (push) off the right leg laterally to the left.
5. Side step to the left and place the left foot back on the floor.
6. Lift and move (slide) the right foot to the left toward (but not to) the left foot. Maintain tension in the resistance band (do not let the band go slack). You are now back in the start position (posture and stance).
7. Continue the action—lift, drive, step, and slide—for a predetermined number of repetitions or distance. Repeat in the opposite direction.

CONSIDERATIONS

1. Maintain proper posture throughout the exercise. There should be no seesaw motion with the hips or upper body.
2. The simultaneous lift and drive is critical to the purpose of the exercise. When done correctly, there is no need to tip to the right to leverage a move to the left in steps 4 and 5).
3. The body's center of mass remains directly between the feet, which are the base of support. So again, no tipping outside the base.

SPECIFIC BENEFITS

[5] [8] [9] [12] [17]

NOTE

Variations might include but are certainly not limited to the following:

- Band positioned around the ankles.
- Band positioned around the calves.
- Band positioned directly below the knees.
- Slide pattern option 1: two steps down, one step back, and repeat.
- Slide pattern option 2: four steps down, two steps back, and repeat.
- Right knee in; right knee out; left knee in; left knee out; lateral slide step; repeat.
- Wide-stance lateral quick jumps (feet simultaneously leave and land on the ground).
- Wide-stance jump lateral, narrow jump, wide-stance jump lateral.
- Wide-stance jump lateral with lower body rotation; the upper body remains perpendicular to the direction of travel.
- Maintain wide stance; forward jump; backward jump; lateral jump right; forward jump; backward jump; lateral jump right. Continue.
- Maintain wide stance; forward jump; backward jump; lateral (step slide or wide stance jump) down two; back one; forward jump; backward jump; lateral down two; back one and repeat.
- Wide-stance step slide; react to coach's command.
- With all of these lateral band slides and variations noted here (and any that you develop), you can add a visual tracking and reaction component by incorporating a ball toss.

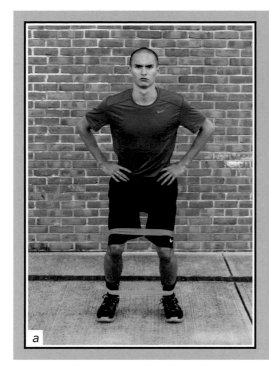
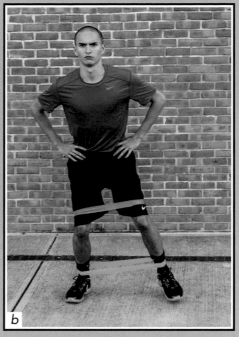

a

b

▪ LATERAL BAND SLIDE ▪
STRAIGHT LEGS

Modifications

1. The start position, posture, considerations, and variations are identical to the Lateral Band Slide except the resistance band is positioned above the ankles and both legs remain straight throughout the exercise. Toe in the right foot slightly; the left foot remains perpendicular to the line of travel.

2. Brace the core, depress and retract the scapulae, place the hands on the hips, and maintain straight legs throughout.

3. Lift the right foot a few inches off the floor while simultaneously driving (pushing) to the right with the left leg. Do not push with a flexed knee; the work should be felt in the glutes and surrounding musculature of the hip.

4. Lead with the heel (the right leg is slightly rotated inward so that the ball of the right foot contacts the ground first, however, the right heel is ahead of the toes at the point of contact).

5. Lift and move (slide) the left foot to the right toward (but not to) the right foot. Maintain tension in the resistance band (do not let the band go slack). You are now back in the start position (posture and stance).

6. Continue the action—lift, drive, step, and slide—for a predetermined number of repetitions or distance. Repeat in the opposite direction.

Specific Benefits   ⑰

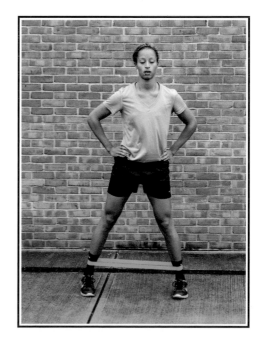

▪ LATERAL BAND SLIDE ▪
SKATING

Modifications

1. The start position, considerations, and variations are identical to the Lateral Band Slide. This exercise can also be done with the resistance band positioned around the calves, directly below the knees, or directly above the knees. The feet are slightly wider than shoulder-width apart and parallel.

2. Brace the core, depress and retract the scapulae, and place the hands on the hips.

3. Lift the left foot and leg a few inches off the ground and step both forward and at a 45-degree angle while simultaneously driving (pushing) with the right leg against the band's resistance.

4. Place the left foot on the ground; hold a split stance for a second or so.

5. Bring the right foot forward and tap the left ankle before pushing the right foot into the next step, both forward and at a 45-degree angle. Place the right foot on the floor; hold the split stance for a second or so.

6. Continue skating for a predetermined number of repetitions or distance.

Specific Benefits   ❺ ❽ ❾ ⑫ ⑰ ㉔

Note   This drill can also be performed backward.

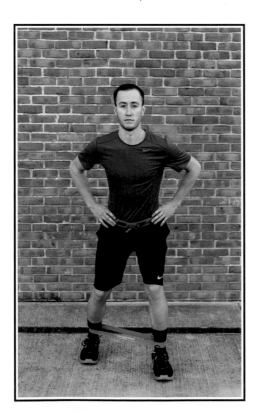

▪ X-BAND WALK ▪

Modifications

1. Step into a large band. Crisscross the band in front and grasp it between the hips and chest (depending on the tension required). Stand straight with the shoulders retracted and feet pointing forward.

2. Step laterally with a slight bend in the knees.

3. Ensure the hips stay level throughout and there does not appear to be a rocking motion back and forth.

Specific Benefits   ❺ ❽ ❾ ⑫ ⑰

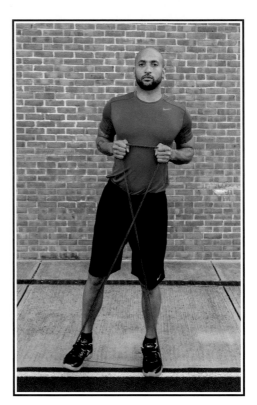

Total Core Exercises

To this point, we've built strong argument with regard to training the body from a global, or total body, perspective and limiting (or eliminating) a muscle isolation focus. Having said that, muscle isolation training does have its place in a total athletic development program design, primarily from the standpoint of rehabilitation and preventative methodologies.

However, to claim that poor performance or injury potentiation can be traced to a single nonfiring muscle, such as the gluteus medius, is absurd. This does not lessen the importance of an effective glute muscle from the standpoint of total body functionality, but it does suggest that, in an attempt to find an excuse and place blame on poor performance, a specific anatomical anomaly is often identified as being the culprit when in actuality, the athlete simply lacked the necessary total body development to get the job done.

Total core exercises are the final bridge to integrating regional core training into full athletic movement patterns. Many exercises can fall into the total core category, including such classics as squats and deadlifts as well as the many variations of the Olympic lifts. These types of exercises are often complex and multitask related, requiring higher levels of focus, conditioning, and experience. Because of this and the mix of possible equipment used, these exercises can also be a lot of fun.

Assuming that the athlete is healthy and assessment results suggest that there are no serious structural integrity compromises, then the modality of choice should be one of training the entire body as it was designed to function. To take this concept of global training one step further we have included a number of total core exercises. These are designed to place a larger amount of stress on a greater physiological area, thereby allowing you to get more bang for the core training buck in an intensified and efficient manner.

All that said, exercises that fall into this category should be picked with purpose and not just thrown into a regimen because they look cool or seem different. The incorporation of these exercises into your program should be through purposeful systematic training. Although global in design, they are of course not all encompassing, and although extremely useful in many ways, an individual drill may miss one or two important areas in the total athletic development perspective. When organizing your individual program, our advice is to incorporate a variety of exercises so that the combination of drills will achieve a global objective. This program will thus be implemented into the same cyclical plan as all other exercises in accordance with the results of your individualized testing and ultimately performance goals. Any time a new drill is introduced into a training regimen, use good judgment when determining load. The weight of the resistance can greatly affect the mechanics of the drill. Start with a resistance that is manageable and progress from there. Again, it can't be stated enough, never sacrifice technique for additional reps, sets, or load.

The following exercise finder lists the benefits, difficulty level, and equipment needed for every exercise that appears in this chapter. Primary exercises are highlighted in blue, with their progressions in red. The primary exercises are also noted in the text with a red title bar.

Total Core Strength Exercise Finder

Exercise Name	Specific Benefits (see chapter 5)	Difficulty Level			Equipment
		Easy	Medium	Hard	
Bilateral Farmer's Walk	❽ ⑫ ⑰		X		Two kettlebells or dumbbells
Unilateral Farmer's Walk	❽ ❾ ⑩ ⑪ ⑫ ⑰		X		One kettlebell or dumbbell
Bilateral Waiter's Walk	❽ ⑩ ⑪ ⑫ ⑰		X		Two kettlebells or dumbbells
Unilateral Waiter's Walk	❽ ❾ ⑩ ⑪ ⑫ ⑰		X		Kettlebell or dumbbell
Cross Walk	❽ ❾ ⑩ ⑪ ⑫ ⑰		X		Two kettlebells or dumbbells
Turkish Get-Up	❽ ❾ ⑪ ⑫ ⑰ ⑱ ㉔			X	One kettlebell, dumbbell, medicine ball, or plate
Split-Stance Cable Pull Complex 1: Dumbbell Squat	❾ ⑪ ⑫ ⑰ ⑱		X		Cable section with handle, kettlebell or dumbbell
Split-Stance Cable Pull Complex 2: Squat With Dumbbell Overhead Press	❾ ⑪ ⑫ ⑰ ⑱		X		Cable section with handle, kettlebell or dumbbell
Sandbag Complex 1: Burpee, Overhead Press	❽ ⑩ ⑪ ⑫ ⑰ ⑱ ⑳ ㉑ ㉒ ㉓			X	Sandbag
Sandbag Complex 2: Cross-Body Lawnmower	❾ ⑪ ⑫ ⑰ ⑱ ⑳ ㉑ ㉒ ㉓ ㉔			X	Sandbag
Sandbag Complex 3: How-De-Do Shoulder Squat	❾ ⑫ ⑰ ⑱ ⑳ ㉑ ㉒ ㉓			X	Sandbag
Sandbag Complex 4: Lunge, Press, Round-the-World	❽ ❾ ⑩ ⑪ ⑫ ⑰ ⑱ ⑳ ㉑ ㉒ ㉓ ㉔			X	Sandbag
Sandbag Complex 5: Suspended Push-Up, Flamingo Rear Pull, Overhead Press	❸ ❹ ❻ ❼ ❽ ❾ ⑩ ⑪ ⑫ ⑰ ⑱ ⑳ ㉑ ㉒			X	Sandbag, suspension trainer

MOVEMENTS

1. Stand between two identical weights (e.g., kettlebells, dumbbells).
2. Brace the core and sit down and back. The first action is the hips moving backward.
3. Depress and retract the scapulae. A good coaching cue it to "keep the chest up."
4. Grasp one weight in each hand. Maintaining a braced core, return to the stand-tall position.
5. Keep a tight grip on the weights and take slow and controlled steps forward.
6. Walk for a predetermined number of repetitions or distance.

CONSIDERATIONS

1. Maintain a braced core throughout the exercise.
2. Maintain an upright, lifted torso with the shoulder blades depressed and retracted throughout the exercise.

SPECIFIC BENEFITS

8 12 17

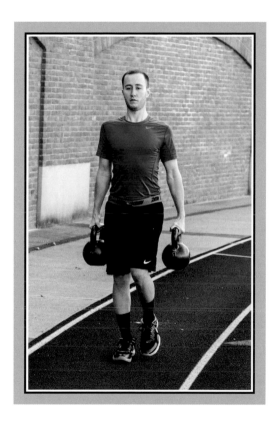

▪ UNILATERAL FARMER'S WALK ▪

Modifications

1. The start position, posture, and initial action are identical to the Bilateral Farmer's Walk, but for this exercise use a single weight.
2. Squat down and grasp the single weight in one hand. Maintaining a braced core, return to the stand-tall position.
3. Keep a tight grip on the weight and take slow and controlled steps forward.

Specific Benefits

▪ BILATERAL WAITER'S WALK

Modifications

1. The start position and initial action are identical to the Bilateral Farmer's Walk. Grasp a weight in each hand and return to a stand-tall position
2. Extend both arms carefully overhead. Keep the shoulder blades back and down throughout; do not shrug upward.
3. Keep a tight grip on the weights and take slow and controlled steps forward.

Specific Benefits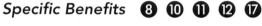

Note Raising weights over your head requires a strong core engagement to maintain control and balance of the load as well as to ensure the lumbar spine does not slip into extension.

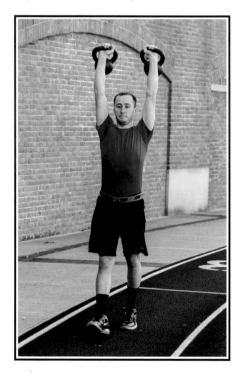

▪ UNILATERAL WAITER'S WALK ▪

Modifications

1. The start position and initial action are the identical to the Unilateral Farmer's Walk. Grasp a weight in one hand and return to a stand-tall position.
2. Extend one arm carefully up overhead.
3. Keep a tight grip on the weight and take slow and controlled steps forward.

Specific Benefits ❽ ❾ ❿ ⓫ ⓬ ⓱

Note Asymmetric loading of the body provides a new challenge to the body. Not only does the required amount of force have to be produced to move the weight, but stabilization also becomes critical to maintain the balance of the weight. Neuromuscular control and efficiency have to be maintained without the body compensating at any of the major joints.

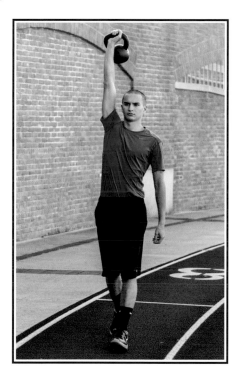

▪ CROSS WALK ▪

Modifications

1. The start position, posture and initial action are identical to the Bilateral Farmer's Walk. Grasp one weight in each hand and return to the stand-tall position while maintaining a braced core. Note that the weight you intend to lift overhead should be lighter than the weight that will remain by the side.
2. Extend one arm straight up over head and keep the other arm at the side.
3. Keep a tight grip on the weights and take slow and controlled steps forward.

Specific Benefits ❽ ❾ ❿ ⓫ ⓬ ⓱

Note This exercise utilizes not only asymmetric positioning but also asymmetric loading (the overhead load will always be lighter). This challenges the core to maintain control and balance of the load to ensure the lumbar spine does not slip into extension and the torso does not lean to the side of the heavier down weight. Neuromuscular control and efficiency have to be maintained without the body compensating at any of the major joints.

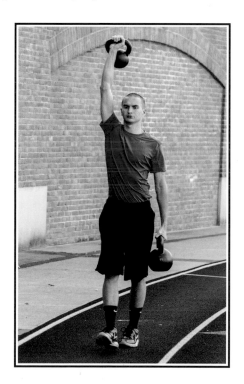

MOVEMENTS

1. Lie flat on the floor in a supine position (face up) with the legs straight and a medicine ball or other weight (e.g., kettlebell, dumbbell, or weight plate) placed near the biceps of one arm. Bend the knees and draw the feet inward. Roll to the side and grasp the weight with one hand; roll back flat again. (This protects against any shoulder issues that could come from picking the weight up in an awkward position.)

2. The leg on the side of the weight should remain bent with the foot flat on the floor; the opposite leg should be extended straight out.

3. Extend the arm holding the weight straight up over chest; the opposite arm remains flat on the floor, palm down and slightly out from the hip.

4. Keep the foot flat and the weight pointing to the ceiling. Sit up straight, pushing lightly with the down arm for support.

5. Pushing through the flat foot, fully extend the hips up off the floor. With the weight pointed to the ceiling and the entire body supported by one hand and one foot, swing the other leg through into a lunge position.

6. Push up through the legs until standing straight up with your feet side by side.

7. Moving into a reverse action, step back; bend the knees to return to the lunge position.

8. With the weight still pointed to the ceiling, in a controlled manner, lean down, and again support the upper body with the opposite hand.

9. With the hips extended, swing the back leg through to the original front position. Gently lower the torso back to the floor.

10. Slowly lower the arm holding the weight back to the start position.

11. Perform a predetermined number of repetitions; repeat on the opposite side.

CONSIDERATIONS

1. Brace the core throughout the exercise.

2. Keep the shoulders back and down throughout; do not shrug.

SPECIFIC BENEFITS

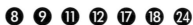 ❽ ❾ ⑪ ⑫ ⑰ ⑱ ㉔

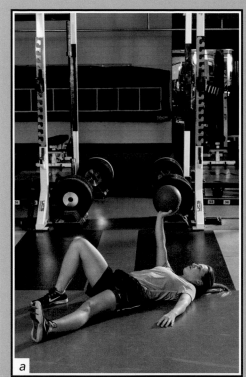

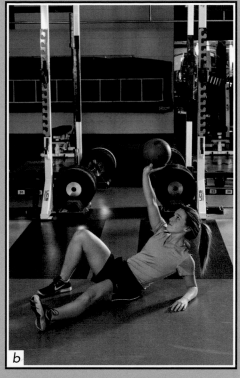

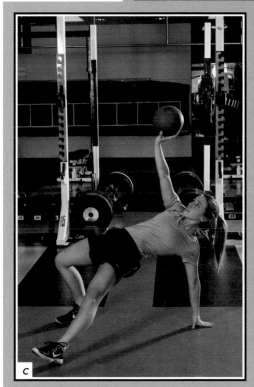

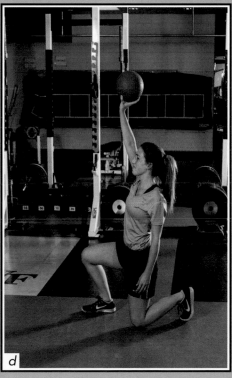

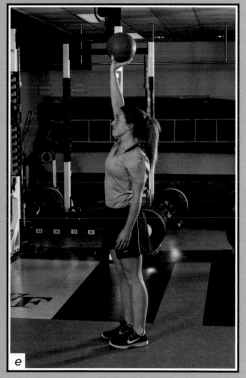

MOVEMENTS

1. While standing, position the cable handle at about chest height (or slightly lower).

2. Assume a split stance with the left foot in front of the right foot. Both feet point straight ahead and are directly in line with the cable's line of pull.

3. With an overhand grip (palm facing down to start), grasp the cable handle with the left hand.

4. Hold a kettlebell or similar weight (e.g., dumbbell, medicine ball with a grip) in the opposite (right) hand. The right arm is straight with the weight hanging down directly in front of the rear right leg.

5. Maintain a neutral scapular posture: chest out. The upper body should be directly between the base of support (feet) and perpendicular to the floor. The ear, shoulder, and hip are in alignment.

6. The double complex action is as follows:

   a. Simultaneously pull the cable to the armpit with the left hand and drop into a low-split squat position. When pulling the handle, the arm follows a natural external rotation (palm down at the start of the pull; palm up at the end of the pull). In the low-squat position, the back knee is bent and *almost* touches the floor; the front *lower* leg is perpendicular to the floor.

   b. Press back to the split-stance start position while allowing the cable resistance to pull the left arm back to the horizontally extended (sagittally flexed), palm-down position; make sure to control this action (do not let the weight jerk the arm back to the start position).

   c. Perform a predetermined number of repetitions; repeat on the opposite side.

CONSIDERATIONS

1. Do not allow the kettlebell (or the cable weight stack) to pull the shoulder into an excessive protracted position (subluxation).

2. Avoid rotating the upper body and torso during all facets of the action.

3. Never sacrifice technique for additional resistance, reps, or sets.

SPECIFIC BENEFITS

9 **11** **12** **17** **18**

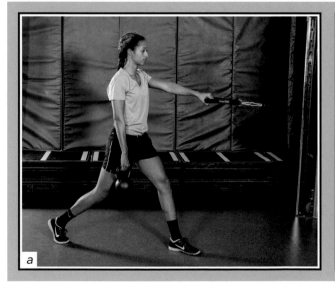

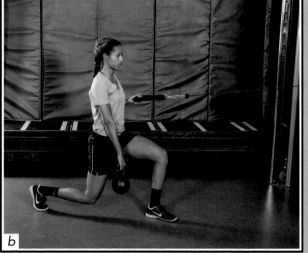

To add variety and possibly make the exercise more challenging, try these alternatives:

- Position the cable handle *high* (above the head) so the line of pull is from high to low.
- Position the cable handle *low* (about ankle height) so the line of pull is from low to high.
- Stand perpendicular to the line of cable pull and pull lateral to the chest.
- Overhand to underhand pull (shown).
- Underhand to overhand pull.
- Neutral (hammer grip) pull.
- Position the handle at knee height and perform a biceps curl instead of a rear pull.

- Position the handle at knee height; stand perpendicular to the line of pull; underhand grip the handle with the opposite hand (e.g., if the left shoulder is closest to the cable, grip the handle with the right hand); pull the handle across the body and up into a lateral deltoid raise.
- Incorporate perturbation techniques: A partner pulls on a rubber band positioned around the ankle, knee, or waist.
- Place the front foot, rear foot, or both feet on an unstable surface (use extreme caution).
- Start in a stand-tall position and lunge forward into a split stance. Follow steps 2 through 6 and then stand tall again.

■ SPLIT-STANCE CABLE PULL COMPLEX 2 ■
SQUAT WITH DUMBBELL OVERHEAD PRESS

Modifications

1. While standing, position the cable handle at about chest height.
2. Assume a split stance with the right foot in front of the left foot. Both feet point straight ahead and are directly in line with the cable's line of pull.
3. With an overhand grip (palm facing down to start), grasp the cable handle with the left hand. Note: In contrast to the previous exercise, grasp the handle with the opposite hand of the front leg.
4. In the right hand, hold a dumbbell (or similar weight) at shoulder height. The palm is in (facing the body) with the right elbow pointing toward the floor.
5. Maintain a neutral scapular posture: chest out. The upper body should be directly between the base of support (feet) and perpendicular to the floor. The ear, shoulder, and hip are in alignment.
6. The triple complex action is as follows:
   a. Simultaneously pull the cable handle to the armpit with the left hand, drop into a low-split squat position, and press the dumbbell overhead. In the up position the dumbbell will be slightly behind the head. When pulling the handle, the arm follows a natural external rotation (palm down at the start of the pull; palm up at the end of the pull). In the low-squat position, the back knee is bent; the front *lower* leg is perpendicular to floor.
   b. Press back to the split-stance start position while allowing the cable resistance to pull the left arm back to the horizontally extended (sagittally flexed), palm-down position; make sure to control this action (do not let the weight jerk the arm back to the start position). The dumbbell in the overhead press is lowered, under control, back to the neutral start position.

Specific Benefits ❾ ⓫ ⓬ ⓱ ⓲

Note The considerations and variations noted for the Split-Stance Cable Pull Complex 1 apply, but take extra caution any time a weight is over the head. Don't perform this complex on an unstable surface.

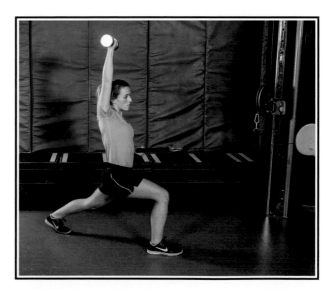

MOVEMENTS

1. Stand tall in an athletic stance with the feet shoulder-width apart. Grip the sandbag's handles and cradle it to the chest. Brace the core throughout the exercise.

2. The complex action is as follows:

   a. In a controlled manner, allow the sandbag to roll forward while simultaneously flexing the ankles, knees, and hips. The sandbag continues to the floor with the handles on the top of the bag and the body behind the bag in a squat position. There should be a slight anterior tilt of the pelvis. The core remains braced and the head is up with the eyes focused forward. The hands remain on the top of the sandbag.

   b. Perform a burpee: Jump the lower body backward, landing in a bent arm push-up position with the ears, shoulders, hips, knees, and ankles in alignment.

   c. Jump forward, returning to the above mentioned posture where the ankles, knees, and hips are flexed with the hands gripping the handles of the sandbag.

   d. With the hands still gripping the sandbag, forcefully stand erect while simultaneously flipping the sandbag to the chest.

   e. Without hesitation, immediately press the sandbag overhead (Note: This is a continuation of the movement from the floor). Focus on maintaining control of the load. The weight should be directly over the base of support (feet on the ground, and shoulder-width apart).

   f. Return the sandbag to the start position.

3. One complete complex action equals one repetition. Perform a predetermined number of repetitions.

CONSIDERATIONS

1. You can either maintain your grip on the sandbag handles and perform the Burpee from a knuckle position (fists down), or you may want to release the tight grip on the handles and instead place the hands (palms down) on the sandbag. Either way, be careful of the wrists.

SPECIFIC BENEFITS

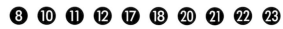

NOTE

To add variety and possibly make the exercise more challenging, try these alternatives:

- Jump press (jerk) the bag overhead.

- Use a parallel stance or split stance during the overhead press.

- Some sandbags have no handles. Others have elaborate grip options. Either way, this exercise can be adapted to fit available equipment.

- Add a push-up during the burpee down position.

- Add a push-up with a twist to the ceiling during the burpee down position.

- Add a variety of mountain climber actions to the burpee movement.

- Add a spread-leg component to the burpee: down with feet together; jump spread the legs; feet back together; continue burpee.

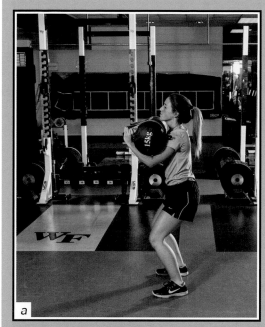

a

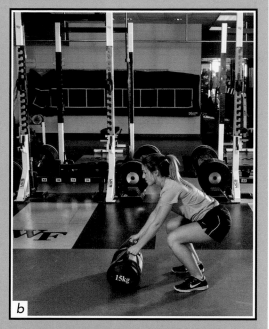

b

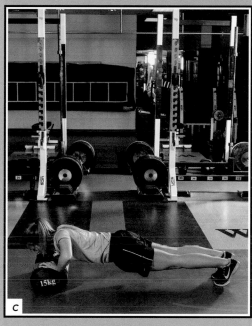

c

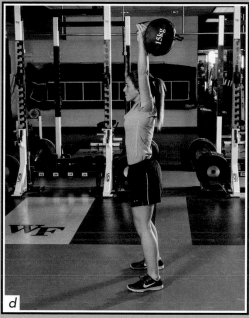

d

SANDBAG COMPLEX 2

CROSS-BODY LAWNMOWER

MOVEMENTS

1. Stand tall in an athletic stance with the feet shoulder-width apart. Grip the sandbag's handles and cradle the sandbag to the chest. Brace the core throughout the exercise.

2. The complex action is as follows:

   a. Flex the ankles, knees, and hips; rotate the torso (focus on thoracic as opposed to lumbar rotation) so that the sandbag moves across the body to a position on the outside of the left hip. In the low position, the core remains braced and the upper torso is relatively perpendicular to the floor. The knees remain directly over the feet (do not allow the knees to move forward, ahead of the feet). In other words, the lower leg is relatively perpendicular to the floor.

   b. Initiate the movement with the legs and accelerate the sandbag up and across the body. Generate as much velocity as possible.

   c. The continuation of the movement allows for control of the sandbag flip, in which the bag makes a half-turn (180-degree flip) and lands gently on the right shoulder. Allow for soft knees (slight flexion of the ankles, knees, and hips) as the sandbag lands on the shoulder. The core still remains braced

   d. Stand tall with the bag on the shoulder.

   e. Now, slightly flex the ankle, knee, and hip. With a little "pop" of the legs, lift the sandbag off the shoulder with just enough velocity to flip it back to the start position (chest cradle).

3. Perform a predetermined number of repetitions; repeat on the opposite side.

CONSIDERATIONS

1. The exercise can be performed in an alternating format (i.e., flip to right shoulder, flip to left shoulder).

SPECIFIC BENEFITS

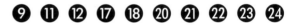

⑨ ⑪ ⑫ ⑰ ⑱ ⑳ ㉑ ㉒ ㉓ ㉔

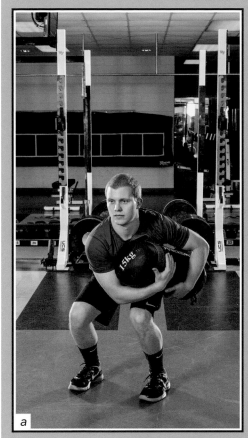

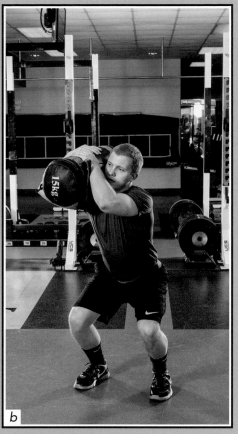

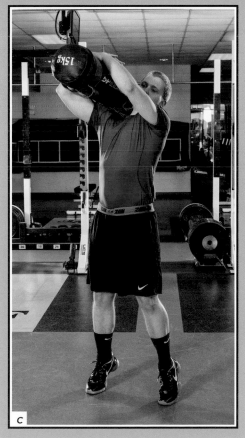

SANDBAG COMPLEX 3
HOW-DE-DO SHOULDER SQUAT

MOVEMENTS

1. Grip one handle with both hands and cradle the sandbag to the chest. Stand tall in an athletic stance with the slightly wider than shoulder-width apart. The core remains braced throughout the exercise.

2. The complex action is as follows:
   a. Slightly flex the ankles, knees, and hips; allow the sandbag to swing between the legs. Note: Extreme caution is advised. Maintain a tightly braced core throughout the exercise and generate as much velocity as possible while never losing control of the action.
   b. Through a simultaneous cocontraction, directly accelerate the sandbag. Continuation of the movement allows for a controlled flip in which the bag makes a half-turn (180-degree flip) and lands gently on the right shoulder.

   c. With the sandbag resting on the right shoulder, immediately perform a squat to a depth whereby the upper thighs are close to parallel to the floor.
   d. Explosively stand tall from the squat while simultaneously flipping the sandbag back to the start position (chest cradle).

3. Perform a predetermined number of repetitions; repeat on the opposite side.

CONSIDERATIONS

1. This exercise can be performed in an alternating format (i.e., flip to right shoulder, flip to left shoulder).

SPECIFIC BENEFITS

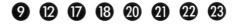

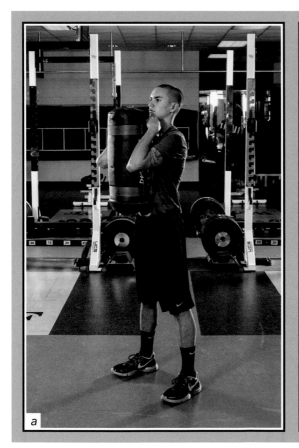

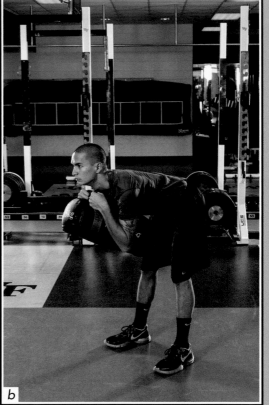

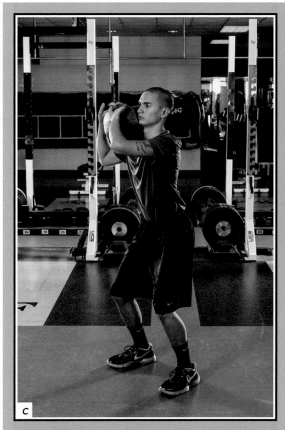

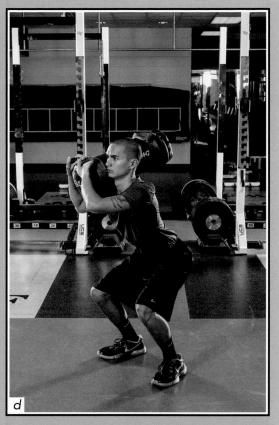

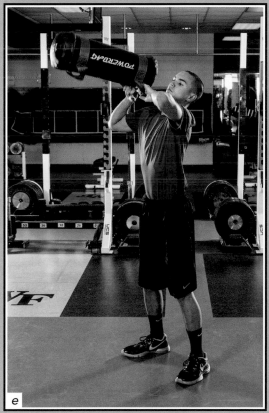

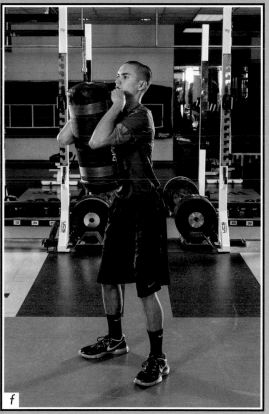

LUNGE, PRESS, ROUND-THE-WORLD

MOVEMENTS

1. Flex the ankles, knees, and hips; squat to the floor and grasp the sandbag by handles. While still in the squat position, cradle the sandbag to the chest. Brace the core throughout the exercise.

2. The complex action is as follows:

   a. Explosively stand tall and flip the sandbag to the chest. Maintain an athletic stance with the feet slightly wider than shoulder-width apart.

   b. After flipping the sandbag to the chest, immediately press the sandbag overhead. Maintain control of the load. The weight should be directly over the base of support (which is the feet on the ground, and shoulder width apart).

   c. Lower the bag and place it on the shoulders behind the head (avoid placing the sandbag high on the neck).

   d. Lunge forward with left leg; push-back with the left leg and continue past the previously mentioned start standing position whereby the feet were shoulder-width apart and the body was positioned between the base of support. Instead of stopping at this start position, immediately perform a reverse (or rear, or Bulgarian) lunge with the same left leg. Upon completion of the rear lunge, immediately push forward with the left leg, but this time stop at the neutral standing position, again maintain a slightly wider than shoulder-width stance.

   e. Maintain an athletic stance (ankles, knees, and hips are slightly flexed and the core is still braced). Lift the sandbag slightly off the shoulders and perform a round-the-world action: Brace the core and trace the sandbag around the head (the "world"). The sandbag makes a full revolution (360 degrees), starting and ending behind the head with the elbows pointing to the floor throughout. The bag remains very close but never actually touches the head. Immediately repeat one full revolution in the opposite direction. End by placing the sandbag back onto the shoulders.

   f. Perform a front and rear lunge with the opposite (right) leg (same action as d).

   g. Perform another round-the-world action, again returning the sandbag to behind the head but this time not actually resting on the shoulders.

   h. Press the bag overhead. Maintain control of the load. The weight should be directly over the base of support.

3. Lower the sandbag, first to the chest and then to the floor. Note: Do not lower the sandbag all the way from overhead to the floor. Instead lower the bag to the chest, flex the knees and hips, and then lower the bag to the floor. Maintain a braced core throughout.

4. Perform the entire complex for a predetermined number of repetitions.

CONSIDERATIONS

1. When placing the sandbag (or similar load) behind the head and resting it on the shoulders, avoid excessive anterior cervical tilt (Remember the chicken head?). Maintain a depressed and retracted scapulae with the chin tucked down slightly.

2. Any part of this drill can be performed or excluded. For example, you may not want to press the sandbag overhead, or if you have a shoulder girdle issue you might want to avoid the round-the-world action. Regardless, in its entirety or parts, this is a darn good drill.

SPECIFIC BENEFITS

8 **9** **10** **11** **12** **17** **18** **20** **21** **22** **23** **24**

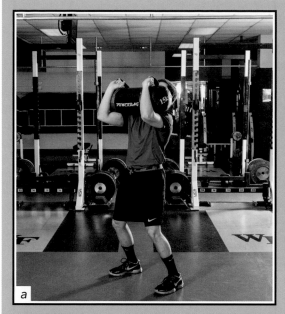

a

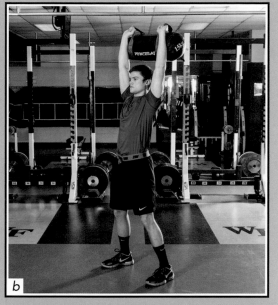

b

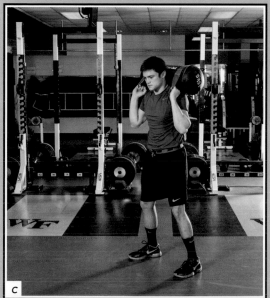

c

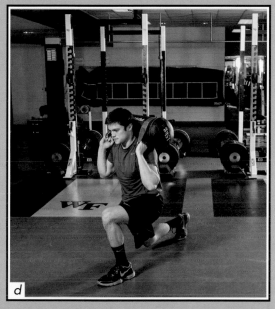

d

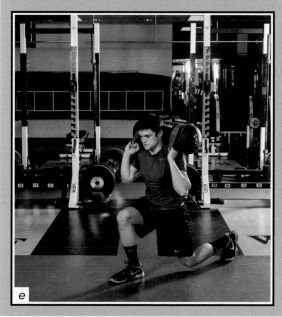

e

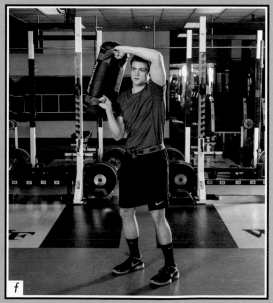

f

SANDBAG COMPLEX 5

SUSPENDED PUSH-UP, FLAMINGO REAR PULL, OVERHEAD PRESS

MOVEMENTS

1. With the assistance of a partner, place one foot in the stirrup (for descriptive purposes, let's say the left foot is in the stirrup). A sandbag is placed on the floor in front of you. Grip the sandbag handles. Brace the core throughout the exercise.

2. The complex action is as follows:

   a. Lift the right leg off the floor. Most of the body weight will shift forward and be supported by the upper body and arms. Maintain a rigid body alignment. Avoid excessive sagging or hunching of the body during the push-up/plank position phase of the exercise

   b. With the lower body suspended and the left leg up, perform a push-up. While moving into the up or straight-arm position of the push-up, smoothly move the nonsuspended (right) leg forward and place the foot on the floor directly under the chest.

   c. In one smooth action, still with a braced core, rear-pull the sandbag while simultaneously standing tall. The bag should flip and be cradled to the chest. In this position, with the left leg still suspended in the stirrup, the ear, shoulder, hip, knee, and ankle of the right leg are relatively aligned. Press the sandbag overhead.

3. Unload the action. First, lower the sandbag from overhead to the chest, then flex the ankles, knees, and hips, and lower the bag to the floor.

4. Lift the right leg off the floor again and perform a predetermined number of repetitions. Repeat on the opposite side.

CONSIDERATIONS

1. If any portion of the complex action is cause for concern, eliminate that part of the movement from the exercise. Or simply add something different. These activities are not written in stone. Be creative, with safety considerations at the forefront of that creativity.

2. If you have a history of wrist issues, extra caution should be taken. Maintain a rigid joint at the wrist while in the push-up position.

3. To add variety and possibly make the exercise more challenging, try these alternatives:
   - Add a round-the-world action.
   - Add a core rotation (twist left, then twist right, then press over head).
   - Incorporate perturbation techniques (be careful).

SPECIFIC BENEFITS

❸ ❹ ❻ ❼ ❽ ❾ ❿ ⓫ ⓬ ⓱
⓲ ⓴ ㉑ ㉒

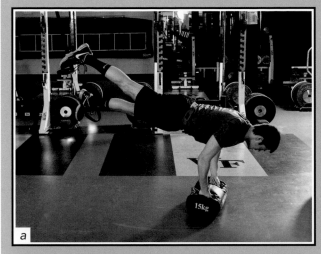

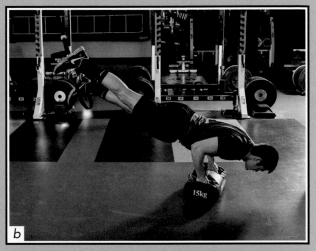

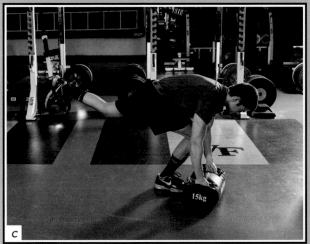

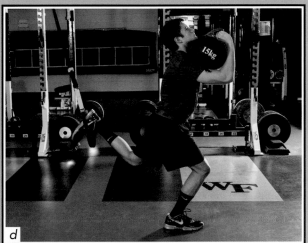

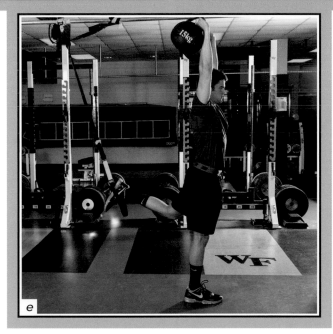

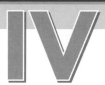

CORE POWER TRAINING

To this point, we have discussed various elements integrated to increase total body functionality. Strength, stabilization, proprioception, flexibility, and power call for a comprehensive training approach to maximize performance. Ultimately, your own goals and objectives will dictate the design of your individualized functional program, but within that design are some absolute constants. Necessary varietal inclusion, namely, multiplane activities, anti-rotational components, dynamic balance, acceleration, deceleration, and complex combination movement patterns, should all be integrated in all programming. In addition, movements that use the entire strength spectrum of eccentric (force reduction), concentric (force production), and isometric (static) muscle contractions will undoubtedly enhance your center of power–specifically, stabilization, strength, and power. Common to all sport, power is the one constantly recurring theme and is a persistent trademark of superior performance.

UNDERSTANDING POWER, FORCE, AND SPEED

Powerful, forceful, fast—these are adjectives you often hear from sports announcers describing exceptional athletic feats. Power, force, and speed are highly prized performance variables that dedicated athletes spend endless hours refining. Each of these expressive terms can be interpreted differently depending on context. In the context of core training, total body *force* is controlled by the core. The core will restructure and express force based on the needs of the individual. *Power* is a product of force and, when efficiently employed, can be devastatingly impressive. *Speed* is the link between the two—force to power. Force must be produced and synchronized at a lightning-fast rate because most sports are played at a high-intensity level. Thus power must be executed with rapid frequency. To work at its most optimal, the core section must stabilize itself (part II), thereby allowing for force application and injury reduction while withstanding a variety of loaded forces (part III), and do so when those forces come at great speed (part IV).

The discussion of using force and creating power is extremely important, but we must first understand the construct of what we are dealing with. Physics breaks force down into the following equation:

$$\text{Force} = \text{mass} \times \text{acceleration}$$

In athletics, the mass is generally our bodies, and the acceleration is the speed of movement or rate of change of velocity. Thus speed and force are directly linked.

Now, taking the performance algorithm one step further, power is mathematically broken down by this equation:

$$\text{Power} = \text{force} \times \text{velocity}$$

Once again, force plays a major role, and on the other side of the equation is velocity, which in sport is a change in position of a mass (e.g., our body) as it relates to time. Thus the most powerful athletes in sport are those most able to rapidly change position. This is possible only through superior force production. Ultimately, no matter the mathematical breakdown, how fast we move (acceleration) and the time it takes us to get there (velocity) both link us back to speed.

TRAINING THE CORE FOR POWER

Interestingly, on microscopic observance, the predominant musculature of the core is mostly comprised of type I (slow-twitch) fibers. You could thus reach the reasonable conclusion that training the core for power is a futile venture—because the ability to produce high levels of force in a quick response is typically associated with type II (fast-twitch) fibers. So some rethinking of how the core should be trained is called for here.

Thus far, we have demonstrated that the core should be fine-tuned to streamline power, not necessarily to create it. As such, it makes sense that the musculature's predominant fiber be slow twitch. This allows for the sustainability of large workloads with only moderate fatigue, which is the exact mechanical characteristic that all athletes need. For the core to fail late in the game would be unfortunate because this could certainly make the difference between a successful dynamic move to the basket or a structural breakdown that leads to injury.

The common thread to all sport participation is that the adaptive situation around the core is constantly shifting at microsecond speed. This being the case, the logical next step in core development is to perform exercises designed to maximize the speed component of power. These exercises mimic the energy system and movement mechanics specific to high-intensity, explosive athletic performance, similar to what is experienced in competition. Ordinarily, the distal extremities control the mechanics and any equipment essential to your favorite sport, but it is the proximal core—the *control hub* of all movement—that must sense instantly and respond appropriately to the imposed stimuli.

PROPRIOCEPTION AND THE CORE

To this point, we have said little about the importance of the central nervous system (CNS) and its critical involvement in everything fitness and sport related, especially the power component. As we mentioned in chapter 4, the sensory mechanisms used for proprioception include the vestibular apparatus of the inner ear, the muscle spindle, and the Golgi tendon organ (GTO). All sensory information regarding homeostasis and the structural integrity of the musculoskeletal system is relayed from these sensory mechanisms to the CNS. Thus proprioception can be broadly defined as an awareness of your body's position as it moves within its spatial surroundings. *Proprioception* and *kinesthetic sense* are frequently used interchangeably, but there are subtle differences, and these differences are often points of contention among academicians, coaches and, others. Fundamentally, kinesthesia is everything that proprioception is with the exception of managing inner ear equilibrium; for example, if an athlete had an inner ear infection, proprioception would be affected, but not kinesthesia.

In designing a comprehensive exercise regimen, it would be prudent to include a variety of training aspects that involve balance and body control, regardless of the differentiation of the senses in question. In terms of enhanced performance methodologies, activities using modalities that include unstable environs, juggling, visual tracking, eye–hand control, and eye–foot control will greatly improve total body balance and muscle memory. For example, the skill of shooting a jump shot becomes automatic for the seasoned basketball player, primarily because of the hundreds of thousands of shots taken previously. With this superior muscle memory, the player can shift focus to other aspects of the game—strategizing, processing other players on the court, rebounding, and so on.

Strategic to quality movement is the proper functioning of these sensory mechanisms. Creating a training environment rich in equilibrium challenges and whole-brain activities such as the aforementioned eye–hand control, eye–foot control, ambidexterity, and creative right-side training can enhance the functionality of proprioceptive as well as kinesthetic abilities. These proprioceptors detect changes in muscle function such as force, tension, position, stretch, and external pressures. The perception of movement and the position of the body are continuously monitored by the sensory mechanisms. This information is then relayed to the CNS, where any number of responses might occur. For our purposes, the core's ability to apply explosive or controlled force—be it production or reduction—within an ever-present athletic challenge to the equilibrium leads to a safe integration of efficient movement patterns and heightened performance.

There are two primary proprioceptors that are of concern for this discussion: the Golgi tendon organ (GTO) and the muscle spindle. The GTO is located at the insertion point where skeletal muscle fibers meld into the tendons of the muscle (figure 1). It was long thought that the GTO helped protect muscle from unexpected excessive forces. Now it is understood that the excitation, or message being transmitted to the CNS, is a form of positive feedback that can elicit greater force production via motor unit response and corresponding muscle involvement.

Another primary receptor is the muscle spindle (see figure 4.1 in chapter 4). Muscle spindles (also known as intrafusal fibers) are cone-shaped sensory mechanisms that lie in, among, and parallel to muscle fibers (extrafusal fibers). When we speak of muscles and muscle fibers, we are usually referring to extrafusal fibers. Muscle spindles are also called stretch receptors, principally because of their functioning efficacy. When the extrafusal fibers of a muscle lengthen, the intrafusal fibers are dually sensitive to the length of change and responsive to the rate of change. They then relay a message to the CNS, which in turn sends a message back to the motor units and

their corresponding muscle fibers being lengthened, directing a desired response. Conversely, when a muscle contracts, it places tension on the muscle tendon unit. Thus the GTO, which is located in the tendon muscle junction, senses the change in tension, as well as the rate of this change. The cumulative information from these muscle receptors, along with data from additional sensory sources—vestibular, sight, and tactile—allows us to determine the position of our muscles, extremities, and entire body, and the rate at which changes are occurring.

The synergy between the GTO and muscle spindles directly influences power. For example, let's look at an athlete executing a simple countermovement jump. As the player drops his center of mass, the muscles and their corresponding tendons (obviously containing GTO sensors) that span the ankles, knees, hips, and even the shoulders are placed on a rapid stretch (lengthened). The muscle spindle senses the change in length and the rate of change and sends this information to the athlete's CNS. The responding message sent back to the stretched muscle spindle unit and the surrounding muscle fibers is to contract and perform some action—in this example, that action is a vertical jump.

This stretch-shortening cycle is called the stretch reflex, or myotatic reflex. It was once thought that the speed component of power was the conduction time required for the muscle spindle to sense the muscle lengthening to the resultant response of a muscle contraction (e.g., the total nerve conduction, which was typically 40 or 50 milliseconds). Misguided coaches and trainers, ourselves included, mistakenly thought that through training protocols such as plyometrics, we could see changes in the speed of nerve conduction.

In actuality, training the stretch-shortening cycle through modalities such as plyometrics promotes the development of the muscle spindle response. If we reexamine our earlier example, during the drop phase of the countermovement jump, generally speaking, the calves, quads, glutes, and front deltoids are being lengthened (stretched). The muscle spindle senses the stretch and sends the message directly to the spine. The returning message is for the motor units and their corresponding extrafusal fibers to fire to either slow the stretch or stop it altogether. In the untrained athlete, the CNS is not quite sure how many motor units to involve to achieve the required result. Thus more and more information is sent to the CNS, and more and more motor

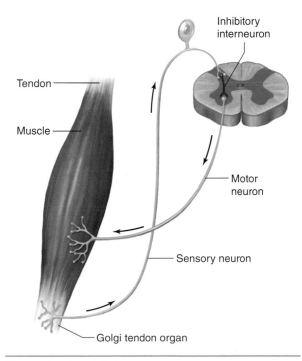

Tendon

Muscle

Inhibitory interneuron

Motor neuron

Sensory neuron

Golgi tendon organ

Figure 1 The Golgi tendon organ.

units are ultimately involved to stop the descent and reverse the action.

Conditioning the body using techniques such as plyometrics can create adaptive qualities within the muscle spindle and GTO response so that the message being sent back from the CNS is to fire everything available—in other words, to incorporate as many motor units and their corresponding fibers to stop the descent and rapidly contract with greater action potentiation. Greater force in a comparable amount of time results in speed and power, and this is trainable for all muscles of the body, including the core.

The GTO works in tandem with the muscle spindle in monitoring the structural integrity of the tendon unit and the closely associated joints, building an additional argument in support of incorporating balance training into a regimen for the enrichment of proprioception. When the lumbo-pelvic hip complex is unstable, the message from the CNS will be to either suppress the prime movers in an attempt to minimize structural risks and hinder kinetic chain functionality or to incorporate the prime movers to work as structural stabilizers. This in turn creates synergistic imbalances, opening up an overabundance of functional stabilization issues, not to mention performance hindrances.

Thus with proprioception and kinesthesis in mind, our training protocols will challenge the magnitude of muscle length, the rate of change of muscle length, stabilization, balance, and body control to ensure further muscular strength and power development. Sensitivity of the stretch-shortening cycle and muscle spindle response maximizes the use of these variables and thus positively influences athletic performance. If you maximize the core, you maximize performance. If you limit the core, you limit performance.

It must be understood that a continuum of training is vital. An exercise that looks challenging and exciting might not be functionally effective. Stability must be improved before strength—only after strength can we integrate speed into the power equation. An ill-prepared core attempting to perform the power exercises in the upcoming chapters could easily lead to setbacks, including injury. Such training is analogous to a person who has just begun jogging for the first time in years to suddenly attempt an all-out 40-yard dash. Something bad is likely to happen.

All science aside, when effectively integrated, the ensuing exercises have been at the heart of our training championship teams and are key to developing some of the best athletes in the world.

Anti-Extension Exercises

Speed is one of the most highly coveted attributes in sport. However, of equal if not greater importance to acceleration is the ability to regulate speed. In fact, one could argue that deceleration is even more crucial to sport performance than acceleration. To decelerate quickly and under control is a vastly underappreciated yet critically essential quality for optimal athletic performance.

Traditionally, the highest significance has been placed on an athlete's ability to accelerate. Draft picks, starting positions, scholarships, and many other talent-based decisions are made simply on an athlete's ability to run fast, only to discover that the athlete is ineffectual on the field. The speediest athlete is not always the most effective athlete. The much slower gazelle often eludes the fastest animal on earth—the cheetah—not by outrunning him but by outmaneuvering him. How does this happen?

Let's look at football as an example. If acceleration were the determining factor for superior athletic performance in football, why aren't world-class sprinters dominating the sport? I realize that this is an over-simplification and that there are far more variables to consider when isolating the rationale for unimpressive performance. Sticking with the football analogy, let's consider the 40-yard dash. Among the many tests that potential draft picks must perform at the pro football combine is a simple 40-yard sprint, which is used primarily to determine absolute speed but also serves as a means for player comparison. You might assume that the fastest athlete in the test would be the most effective

player on the field because he can simply run away from his opponents. Scouts, coaches, and general managers make this same assumption, which is why millions of dollars are sometimes spent to sign a player with no consideration of his dynamic functionality. Yes, he has superior speed, but can he *control* his speed? To understand the importance of controlling speed, let's return to the 40-yard dash:

- Wide receiver 1 (WR1) runs the 40-yard dash in 4.2 seconds.

- Wide receiver 2 (WR2) runs the 40-yard dash in 4.8 seconds.

At first glance, many would assume that WR1 is a superior athlete who would dominate WR2 on the playing field. But what if WR1 can control only 50 percent of his maximum speed, whereas WR2 can control 90 percent? In other words, in the open field, if a play calls for WR1 to run a simple down-and-out pattern, he would have to slow his speed by half before making a sharp 90-degree cut. WR2 will have to slow his speed by only 10 percent to make the same cut. WR2 thus controls a far greater percentage of his absolute speed even though his speed is considerably less than that of his rival. Many records in the books are not by those with superior speed but rather those who have greater control over what speed they have. WR2 is just such an athlete. The athlete who controls a greater percentage of his or her athleticism will typically dominate. Now just imagine if WR1 could control 90% of his speed—there rests our goal.

The ability to control a greater percentage of speed directly correlates to a superior ability to decelerate. The drills in this chapter, although emphasizing great explosiveness and acceleration, also require a strong focus on controlling the decelerative (or anti-acceleration) portion of the action. This control allows for superior athletic performance. This is why the most well fed cheetahs on the Serengeti are not only fast but can also cut and dodge with the best gazelles on the plains.

The following exercise finder lists the benefits, difficulty level, and equipment needed for every exercise that appears in this chapter. Primary exercises are highlighted in beige with their progressions in green. The primary exercises are also noted in the text with a green title bar.

Anti-Extension Power Exercise Finder

Exercise Name	Specific Benefits (see chapter 5)	Difficulty Level			Equipment
		Easy	Medium	Hard	
Box Drop and Jump, Upper Body	❷ ⑫ ㉒ ㉓			X	Two raised platforms*
Straight-Arm Plank Walk-Out Jump	❼ ❽ ⑪ ⑫ ㉒ ㉓			X	Medicine ball
Kneeling Overhead Wall Toss	⑫ ⑭ ⑮ ⑰ ⑳ ㉑ ㉒ ㉓		X		
Supine Overhead Wall Toss Complex	⑫ ⑭ ⑮ ⑰ ⑳ ㉑ ㉒ ㉓		X		Medicine ball
Overhead Medicine Ball Slam Progression 1: Tall Kneeling	⑫ ⑭ ⑮ ⑰ ⑳ ㉑ ㉒ ㉓		X		Medicine ball
Overhead Medicine Ball Slam Progression 2: Standing	⑫ ⑭ ⑮ ⑰ ⑳ ㉑ ㉒ ㉓		X		Medicine ball
Overhead Medicine Ball Slam Progression 3: Tall Kneeling With Wind-Up	⑫ ⑭ ⑮ ⑰ ⑳ ㉑ ㉒ ㉓		X		Medicine ball
Overhead Medicine Ball Slam Progression 4: Standing With Wind-Up	⑫ ⑭ ⑮ ⑰ ⑳ ㉑ ㉒ ㉓		X		Medicine ball

* Many options are available for the raised platform, including a box, bench, stair, or step.

MOVEMENTS

1. Place two mats or boxes of the same height on the floor; they should be 3 to 12 inches (7.6-30 cm) high and slightly wider than shoulder-width apart.
2. Place one hand on each mat close to edges, with the body positioned between the two mats.
3. Lock the knees, tighten the glutes, and brace the abdomen.
4. Lift the body so that only the balls of the feet and toes are on the floor. Maintain a completely straight body line (ears, shoulders, hips, knees, and ankles are in alignment).
5. Remove both hands simultaneously from the boxes, allowing the body to drop toward the floor between the two boxes. The hands should contact the floor between the boxes and directly under the shoulders.
6. Immediately "touch and go," "jumping" explosively back to the start position.
7. Perform a predetermined number of repetitions.

CONSIDERATIONS

1. When on the box in the start position, the arms should be slightly angled to perpendicular to the floor.
2. Upon landing on the floor, there should be a natural give (think shock absorption) at the wrist and elbow. *Do not land with locked elbows.*
3. Emphasize a quick "jump" off the floor.
4. The decelerative elements mentioned in the introduction are best demonstrated in this drill. Upon contacting the floor with the hands, the athlete attempts to limit the amount of time spent on the ground (amortization phase) prior to jumping back onto the boxes.
5. This drill has the potential for joint discomfort or injury. A sensible progression from a short drop to more challenging heights should absolutely be implemented. Never perform a drill without first determining the risk/reward benefits. Use good judgment.

SPECIFIC BENEFITS

❷ ⓬ ㉒ ㉓

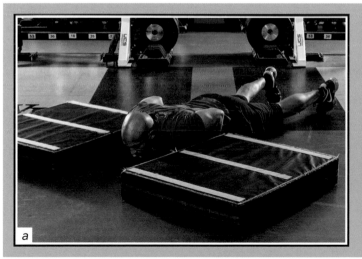

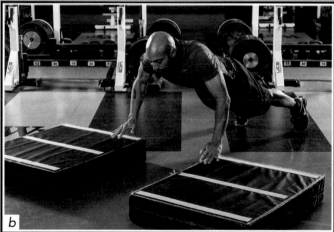

Modifications

1. Position the hands on the floor directly under the shoulders with the arms perpendicular to the floor.
2. Lift the body up so that only the balls of the feet and toes are in contact with the floor.
3. Brace the core and keep entire the body straight.
4. Drop the body's center of mass and jump explosively into the air (hands and feet leave the ground).

Specific Benefits   ⑫ ㉓

Note To add variety and possibly make the exercise more challenging, try these alternatives:

- Jump and move forward.
- Jump and move lateral.
- Left hand, right hand, jump; left leg, right leg, jump.
- Add push-ups between jumps.

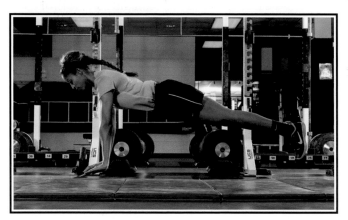

KNEELING OVERHEAD WALL TOSS

MOVEMENTS

1. Kneel about three feet (.9 m) from a solid wall (see consideration 1).
2. Hold an appropriately weighted medicine ball overhead. The elbows are flexed not quite to 90 degrees.
3. Brace the core and maintain a completely straight line in the body (ears, shoulders, hips, knees are in alignment).
4. Extend the elbows and throw the ball against the wall. The ball should be thrown from behind the head. That is, try to release the ball before the hands cross over the top of the head. This might take some practice but, once successful, will ultimately further challenge the core.
5. The ball should be thrown high enough such that the rebound will facilitate a subsequent catch of the ball overhead. Make the catch, flex the elbows, and immediately repeat for a predetermined number or repetitions.

CONSIDERATIONS

1. Distance from the wall is determined by the athlete's current level of strength and the resiliency (bounciness) of the medicine ball.
2. The height of the pass is determined by the athlete's current level of strength and the resiliency (bounciness) of the medicine ball. If strength level is low then a lighter medicine ball should be used. The toss must be high enough to facilitate subsequent fluid catches and tosses.
3. The wall should be solid (concrete, cinderblock, brick, solid wood, etc.).
4. To add variety and possibly make the exercise more challenging, try these alternatives:
   - Kneel on an unstable apparatus.
   - Increase and decrease the weight of the medicine ball.
   - Increase the speed (velocity) of the reps—be careful.

- Add movements such as thoracic (spinal) rotations, wood choppers, or lateral tosses to a partner (on return catch, use an overhead toss). The inclusion of these types of movements will make the drill a complex action. Be careful and never sacrifice technique.
- Avoid excessive core involvement (flexion and extension). Maintain a stable spine throughout.

- Benefit 23, gravity load, is a bit of a misnomer for this particular drill and the following one. In actuality, the rubber medicine ball and its resiliency and therefore responsive energy stored in the rubber and subsequent horizontal energy released upon contact with the wall act in much the same fashion as vertical gravity load.

SPECIFIC BENEFITS _____

⑫ ⑭ ⑮ ⑰ ⑳ ㉑ ㉒ ㉓

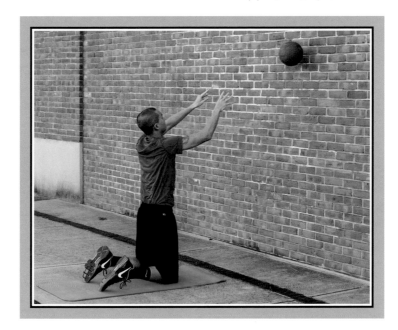

■ SUPINE OVERHEAD WALL TOSS COMPLEX ■

Modifications

1. Sit about three feet (.9 m) from a solid wall with the knees slightly flexed and with upright posture.
2. Start in the up position, holding the ball over and behind the head.
3. Drop and tap the shoulder blades to the floor, immediately followed by tapping the medicine ball to the floor (the ball will tap over and behind the head).
4. Contract the core and forcefully raise back up, releasing the ball toward the wall. Do not throw the ball. The momentum generated through a forceful core flexion is enough to accelerate the ball toward the wall with enough force that the ball returns to the hands, which remain above the head.

Specific Benefits ⑫ ⑭ ⑮ ⑰ ⑳ ㉑ ㉒ ㉓

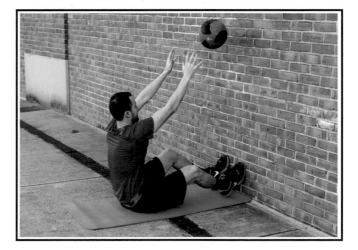

OVERHEAD MEDICINE BALL SLAM

PROGRESSION 1: TALL KNEELING

MOVEMENTS

1. Kneel on both knees with an upright torso.
2. Extend the arms and raise the ball overhead.
3. Tighten the glutes and brace the abdomen. Maintain a completely straight line in the body (ears, shoulders, hips, and knees are in alignment).
4. Accelerate the arms and slam the ball as hard as possible to the ground directly in front of the body.
5. Maintain good posture throughout; flex the hips slightly if necessary.
6. Perform a predetermined number of repetitions.

CONSIDERATIONS

1. Select a medicine ball light enough to be thrown with great velocity but heavy enough to provide resistance.
2. Maintain good posture. Depress and retract the scapulae.
3. Control the speed of the recoil and allow momentum to assist in raising the ball back overhead
4. Benefit 23, gravity load, is a bit of a misnomer for this particular drill and the following progressions. In actuality, the rubber medicine ball and its resiliency and therefore responsive energy stored in the rubber and subsequent horizontal energy released upon contact with the wall act in much the same fashion as vertical gravity load.

SPECIFIC BENEFITS

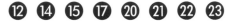 12 14 15 17 20 21 22 23

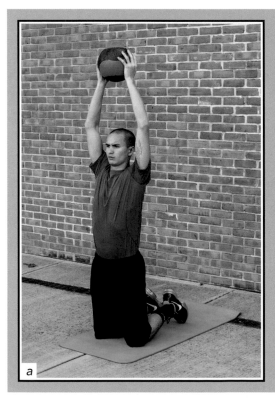
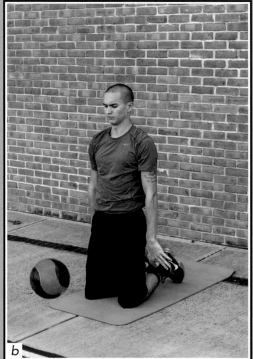

▪ OVERHEAD MEDICINE BALL SLAM ▪
PROGRESSION 2: STANDING

Modifications

1. Stand with the feet parallel and hip-width apart. Flex the knees and hips to an athletic stance.
2. Extend the arms and raise the ball overhead.
3. The action is identical to Overhead Medicine Ball Slam Progression 1.

Specific Benefits ⑫ ⑭ ⑮ ⑰ ⑳ ㉑ ㉒ ㉓

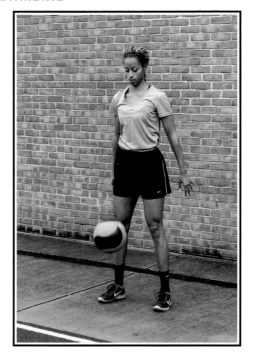

▪ OVERHEAD MEDICINE BALL SLAM ▪
PROGRESSION 3: TALL KNEELING WITH WIND-UP

Modifications

1. To begin, kneel on both knees with an upright torso.

2. Grip the medicine ball with both hands and hold at the midsection of the body.

3. Tighten the glutes and brace the abdomen. Maintain a completely straight line in the body (ears, shoulders, hips, and knees are in alignment).

4. Sweep the ball out and around to one side of the body and then up over the head in a sledgehammer fashion.

5. Accelerate the arms and slam the ball as hard as possible to the ground directly in front of the body. Maintain good posture throughout; flex the hips slightly if necessary.

6. Immediately repeat the sweep action on the opposite side of the body.

Specific Benefits ⑫ ⑭ ⑮ ⑰ ⑳ ㉑ ㉒ ㉓

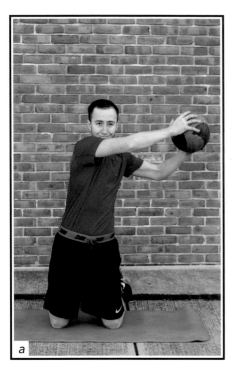 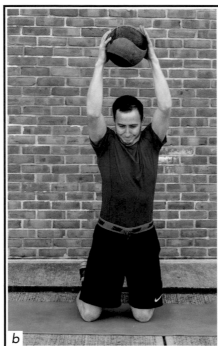 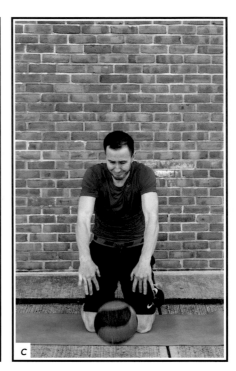

▪ OVERHEAD MEDICINE BALL SLAM ▪
PROGRESSION 4: STANDING WITH WIND-UP

Modifications

1. Stand with the feet parallel and hip-width apart. Flex the knees and hips to an athletic stance.

2. Grip the medicine ball with both hands and hold at the midsection of the body.

3. The action is identical to Overhead Medicine Ball Slam Progression 3.

4. Immediately repeat the sweep action on the opposite side of the body.

Specific Benefits ⑫ ⑭ ⑮ ⑰ ⑳ ㉑ ㉒ ㉓

Anti-Rotation Exercises

Rotational power is an often overlooked athletic trait. On close examination of most action in all sports, one sees a surprisingly disproportionate number of rotational movement patterns. If we were to itemize a "whole" gross movement pattern, in observing the "parts" of that pattern we would see persistent rotational activity. For example, in tennis, the fingers, wrist, elbow, shoulder, hip, knee, ankle, and toes all exhibit a rotational component during a simple forehand stroke. However, a significant limiting factor in the further production of concentric acceleration is the subconscious fear of being unable to control (decelerate) the rotational action. Consequently, while the athletes might be fully capable of expanded acceleration while executing a rotational action, they might not fully apply this acceleration in fear of being unable to safely decelerate the momentum, thus opening themselves to the possibility of injury. This rotation can be either localized at a specific joint or through the entire body (multijoint). Regardless, the body has mechanisms in place to sense and control the risk–reward potential of increased velocity.

Consistent with the precept of *specificity of training*, to fully realize the appropriate adaptive response, it is imperative that the appropriate training stimulus be implemented that is conditional to the desired results. For example, the core stabilizers are primarily type I slow-twitch muscle fibers. Therefore, if stabilization is the focus of a training session, or even of a specific exercise, then adaptation will best respond to exercises lasting between 6 and 20 seconds. In general, type II fibers are more closely associated with fast and powerful muscular contractions. Regardless of the intended adaptive focus, in generality type I or type II, each repetition duration within a set is referred to as time under tension (explosive action, 6 seconds, 20 seconds, etc.). Anti-rotational, power-oriented exercises like those presented here help athletes better understand their limitations and further develop the ability to control explosive rotational movement.

The following exercise finder lists the benefits, difficulty level, and equipment needed for every exercise that appears in this chapter. Primary exercises are highlighted in beige with their progressions in green. The primary exercises are also noted in the text with a green title bar.

Anti-Rotation Power Exercise Finder

Exercise Name	Specific Benefits (see chapter 5)	Difficulty Level			Equipment
		Easy	Medium	Hard	
Around the World	⑫ ⑰		X		Weight plate, sandbag, or medicine ball
Around the Universe	⑫ ⑰		X		Weight plate, sandbag, or medicine ball
Kneeling Angle Toss	⑨ ⑫ ⑭ ⑮ ⑰ ⑳ ㉑ ㉒ ㉓ ㉔		X		Medicine ball, wall
Seated Angle Toss	⑨ ⑫ ⑭ ⑮ ⑰ ⑳ ㉑ ㉒ ㉓ ㉔		X		Medicine ball, wall
Kneeling Reverse Half-Rotation	⑨ ⑫ ⑭ ⑮ ⑰ ⑳ ㉑ ㉒ ㉓		X		Medicine ball, wall
Standing Reverse Half-Rotation	⑨ ⑫ ⑭ ⑮ ⑰ ⑳ ㉑ ㉒ ㉓		X		Medicine ball, wall
Kneeling Reverse Full Rotation	⑨ ⑫ ⑭ ⑮ ⑰ ⑳ ㉑ ㉒ ㉓		X		Medicine ball, wall
Standing Reverse Full Rotation	⑨ ⑫ ⑭ ⑮ ⑰ ⑳ ㉑ ㉒ ㉓		X		Medicine ball, wall
Kneeling Scoop Pass	⑨ ⑪ ⑫ ⑭ ⑮ ⑰ ㉑ ㉒ ㉓		X		Medicine ball, wall
Standing Scoop Pass	⑨ ⑪ ⑫ ⑭ ⑮ ⑰ ㉑ ㉒ ㉓		X		Medicine ball, wall
Medicine Ball Chop Slam Progression 1: Half-Kneeling	⑨ ⑪ ⑫ ⑭ ⑮ ⑰ ㉑ ㉒ ㉓		X		Medicine ball, wall
Medicine Ball Chop Slam Progression 2: Tall Kneeling	⑨ ⑪ ⑫ ⑭ ⑮ ⑰ ㉑ ㉒ ㉓		X		Medicine ball, wall
Medicine Ball Chop Slam Progression 3: Standing	⑨ ⑪ ⑫ ⑭ ⑮ ⑰ ㉑ ㉒ ㉓		X		Medicine ball, wall
Medicine Ball Chop Slam Progression 4: Staggered Stance	⑨ ⑪ ⑫ ⑭ ⑮ ⑰ ㉑ ㉒ ㉓			X	Medicine ball, wall
Medicine Ball Chop Slam, Progression 5: Lunge Stance	⑨ ⑪ ⑫ ⑭ ⑮ ⑰ ㉑ ㉒ ㉓			X	Medicine ball, wall
Medicine Ball Side Throw Progression 1: Half-Kneeling	⑨ ⑪ ⑫ ⑭ ⑮ ⑰ ㉑ ㉒ ㉓		X		Medicine ball, wall
Medicine Ball Side Throw Progression 2: Tall Kneeling	⑨ ⑪ ⑫ ⑭ ⑮ ⑰ ㉑ ㉒ ㉓		X		Medicine ball, wall
Medicine Ball Side Throw Progression 3: Standing	⑨ ⑪ ⑫ ⑭ ⑮ ⑰ ㉑ ㉒ ㉓		X		Medicine ball, wall
Medicine Ball Side Throw Progression 4: Staggered Stance	⑨ ⑪ ⑫ ⑭ ⑮ ⑰ ㉑ ㉒ ㉓			X	Medicine ball, wall
Medicine Ball Side Throw Progression 5: Lunge Stance	⑨ ⑪ ⑫ ⑭ ⑮ ⑰ ㉑ ㉒ ㉓			X	Medicine ball, wall

Exercise Name	Specific Benefits (see chapter 5)	Difficulty Level			Equipment
		Easy	Medium	Hard	
Medicine Ball Parallel Throw Progression 1: Half-Kneeling	⑨ ⑪ ⑫ ⑭ ⑮ ⑰ ㉑ ㉒ ㉓		X		Medicine ball, wall
Medicine Ball Parallel Throw Progression 2: Tall Kneeling	⑨ ⑪ ⑫ ⑭ ⑮ ⑰ ㉑ ㉒ ㉓		X		Medicine ball, wall
Medicine Ball Parallel Throw Progression 3: Standing	⑨ ⑪ ⑫ ⑭ ⑮ ⑰ ㉑ ㉒ ㉓		X		Medicine ball, wall
Medicine Ball Parallel Throw Progression 4: Staggered Stance	⑨ ⑪ ⑫ ⑭ ⑮ ⑰ ㉑ ㉒ ㉓			X	Medicine ball, wall
Medicine Ball Parallel Throw Progression 5: Lunge Stance	⑨ ⑪ ⑫ ⑭ ⑮ ⑰ ㉑ ㉒ ㉓			X	Medicine ball, wall
Overhead Medicine Ball Slam Rotation Progression 1: Half-Kneeling	⑨ ⑫ ⑭ ⑮ ⑰ ㉑ ㉒ ㉓		X		Medicine ball
Overhead Medicine Ball Slam Rotation Progression 2: Staggered Stance	⑨ ⑫ ⑭ ⑮ ⑰ ㉑ ㉒ ㉓			X	Medicine ball
Overhead Medicine Ball Slam Rotation Progression 3: Lunge Stance	⑨ ⑫ ⑭ ⑮ ⑰ ㉑ ㉒ ㉓			X	Medicine ball
Tornado Ball Twist	⑨ ⑫ ⑭ ⑮ ⑰ ㉑ ㉒ ㉓			X	Medicine ball on rope, wall

MOVEMENTS

1. Stand upright with the feet parallel and slightly wider than shoulder width. Flex the knees and hips to an athletic stance.

2. With two hands, firmly grasp a medicine ball, bumper plate, dumbbell, or sandbag (one hand on either side). The weight is positioned directly in front of the face; the elbows point to the floor.

3. Brace the core and "trace" the sandbag around the head. The bag remains very close but never touches the head.

4. The bag makes a full revolution (360 degrees) and ends directly in front of the face, elbows pointing to the floor.

5. Immediately repeat in the opposite direction.

6. Clockwise then counter-clockwise equals one complete repetition. Perform a predetermined number of repetitions.

CONSIDERATIONS

1. A common mistake is for the ball or weight to complete a full orbit of the head, but the arms (specifically the elbows) don't fully return to start position. In other words, athletes leave a lazy elbow up before returning in the opposite direction.

2. To add variety and possibly make the exercise more challenging, try these alternatives:
   - Stand with feet together.
   - Stand on a single leg.
   - Stand with both feet on an unstable surface (see photo).
   - Stand with a single leg on an unstable surface.
   - Perform the drill with eyes closed. But be careful! Never take the weight above the head, and use a spotter.

SPECIFIC BENEFITS

 12 **17**

If you incorporate any of the variations or challenges, many more benefits will be realized.

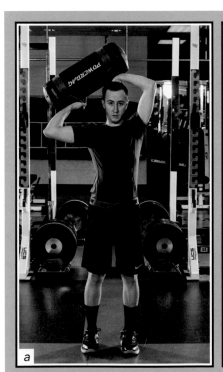
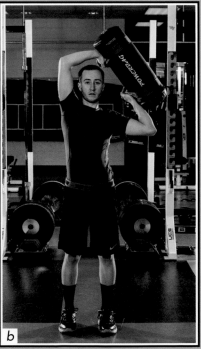
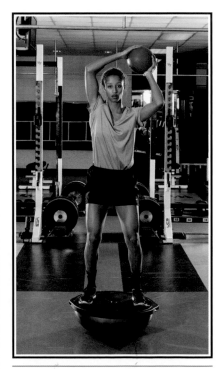

Around the World variation with both feet on an unstable surface.

Modifications

Follow the steps for Around the World except for the following:

1. To begin, the arms are extended. Current levels of strength and balance determine extension distance.

2. During the orbit, maintain a greater degree of separation between the weight and the head. In other words, trace a bigger circle around the head.

3. Clockwise then counter-clockwise equals one complete repetition.

Specific Benefits ⑫ ⑰

If you incorporate any of the variations or challenges noted in Around the World, many more benefits will be realized.

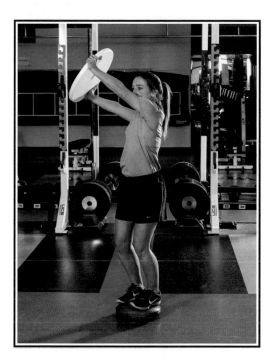

MOVEMENTS

1. Kneel on a gym mat or foam pad, facing a wall.
2. Tighten the glutes; brace the abdomen. Throughout the exercise, maintain a completely straight line in the body (ears, shoulders, hips, and knees are in alignment).
3. Hold a rubber medicine ball over the left shoulder with the arms extended above the head and slightly behind the body (elbows are *not* locked). Forcefully toss the ball against the wall. The toss should be angled so the rebound can be caught over the right (opposite) shoulder.
4. Holding the ball over the right shoulder, repeat the action.
5. Left shoulder, right shoulder equals one repetition. Perform a predetermined number of repetitions.

CONSIDERATIONS

1. Distance from the wall depends on the athlete's current levels of strength and skill and on the resiliency (bounciness) of the medicine ball.
2. The wall should be solid (concrete, cinderblock, brick, solid wood, etc.).
3. The height of the toss depends on current level of strength and on the resiliency (bounciness) of the medicine ball.
4. Avoid undue hip and knee flexion.
5. Benefit 23, gravity load, is a bit of a misnomer for this particular drill and the following progression. In actuality, the rubber medicine ball and its resiliency and therefore the responsive energy stored in the rubber and subsequent horizontal energy released upon contact with the wall act in much the same fashion as vertical gravity load.

SPECIFIC BENEFITS

9 **12** **14** **15** **17** **20** **21** **22** **23** **24**

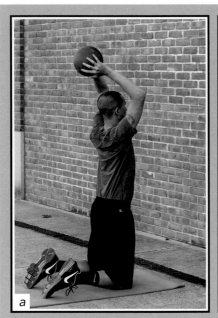
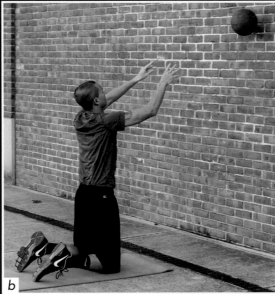
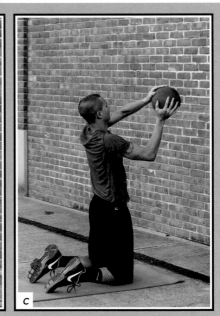

▪ SEATED ANGLE TOSS ▪

Movements

1. To begin, sit facing a solid wall. The knees are flexed and the feet are flat on the ground.
2. The throwing action is the same as for Kneeling Angle Toss. The toss should be angled so the rebound can be caught over the right (opposite) shoulder.
3. On catching the rebound, in a controlled manner, drop and tap the ball to the floor over the shoulder on the side the ball was caught.
4. Immediately counter the rotational forces to return to the start position while simultaneously releasing the ball toward the wall. In effect, the ball is thrown with the core, minimizing the actual throwing motion of the arms. Release the ball from behind the head (or as near as possible).

Specific Benefits ❾ ⑫ ⑭ ⑮ ⑰ ⑳ ㉑ ㉒ ㉓ ㉔

Note Try these variations:

- Sit with the feet off the ground (or mat) and the knees flexed to 90 degrees.
- Sit on an unstable surface with the feet off the ground (or mat) and the knees flexed to 90 degrees.
- Toss using the same-side shoulder for the entire set; then repeat with opposite shoulder.

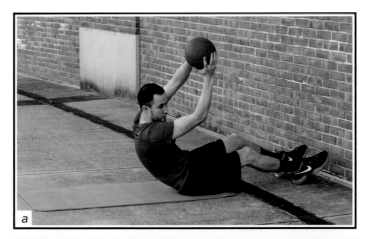

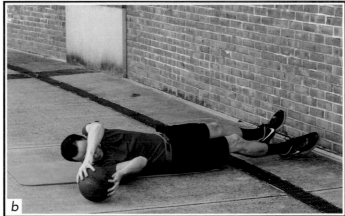

KNEELING REVERSE HALF-ROTATION

MOVEMENTS

1. Kneel on a mat or pad facing away from a wall.
2. Tighten the glutes; brace the abdomen. Throughout the exercise, maintain a completely straight line in the body (ears, shoulders, hips, and knees are in alignment).
3. Hold a rubber medicine ball in the hands and extend the arms forward directly in front of the body (elbows are slightly flexed, arms parallel to the ground).
4. Forcefully rotate the core left and toss the ball against the wall. The toss should be directly back to the wall so the rebound can be caught as close to the release point (on the left side) as possible.
5. Allow the momentum of the ball to rotate the body back toward the right (toward the start position).
6. *Now here is the whole point of the drill!* As soon as the hips and ball cross the midline of the body, snap the hips back to the same (left) side. This snap is against momentum, eliciting a stretch-shortening response.
7. Continue to the left side for a predetermined number of repetitions, then repeat on the right side.

CONSIDERATIONS

1. Distance from the wall depends on the athlete's current levels of strength and skill and on the resiliency (bounciness) of the medicine ball.
2. The wall should be solid (concrete, cinderblock, brick, solid wood, etc.).
3. The height of the toss depends on current level of strength and on the resiliency (bounciness) of the medicine ball.
4. Avoid undue hip and knee flexion.
5. Benefit 23, gravity load, is a bit of a misnomer for this particular drill and the following progressions. In actuality, the rubber medicine ball and its resiliency and therefore the responsive energy stored in the rubber and subsequent horizontal energy released upon contact with the wall act in much the same fashion as vertical gravity load.

SPECIFIC BENEFITS

9 12 14 15 17 20 21 22 23

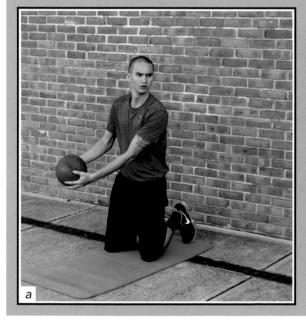

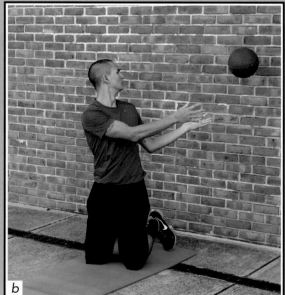

■ STANDING REVERSE HALF-ROTATION ■

Modifications

1. The setup and action are identical to Kneeling Reverse Half-Rotation except stand upright with the feet parallel and slightly wider than shoulder width. Flex the knees and hips to a be in an athletic stance.

2. Continue to the left side for a set number of repetitions. Then repeat on the right side.

Specific Benefits ❾ ⓬ ⓮ ⓯ ⓱ ⓴ ㉑ ㉒ ㉓

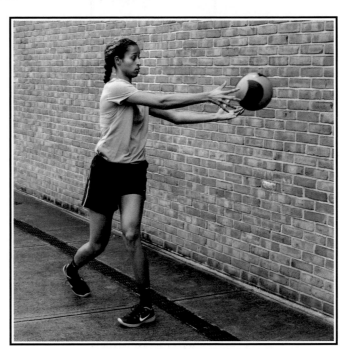

▪ KNEELING REVERSE FULL ROTATION

Modifications

1. The setup and initial action are identical to Kneeling Reverse Half-Rotation.

2. Forcefully rotate the core to the left and toss the ball against the wall. The toss should be directly back to the wall so the rebound can be caught as close to the release point (on the left side) as possible.

3. Allow the momentum of the ball to rotate the body back toward the right. Contract the core rotators and continue to accelerate the ball completely around to the right.

4. Release the ball on the right side; catch the rebound on the right side and repeat to the left. There should be no stopping at any point in the action for the duration of the exercise.

5. Over and back (right side, left side) equals one repetition. Perform for a predetermined number of repetitions or length of time.

Specific Benefits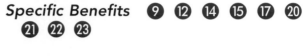

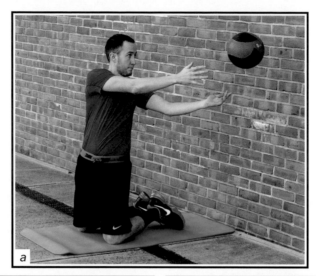

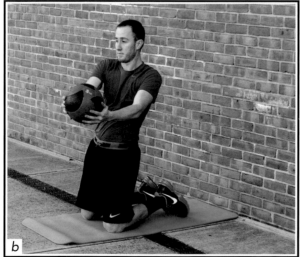

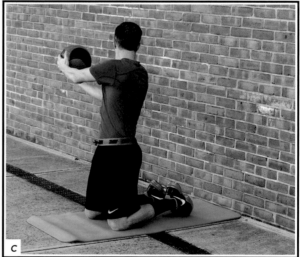

▪ STANDING REVERSE FULL ROTATION ▪

Modifications

1. The setup and action are identical to Kneeling Reverse Full Rotation except stand upright with the feet parallel and slightly wider than shoulder width. Flex the knees and hips to a be in an athletic stance.

2. Over and back (right side, left side) equals one repetition. Perform for a predetermined number of repetitions or length of time.

Specific Benefits ⑨ ⑫ ⑭ ⑮ ⑰ ⑳ ㉑ ㉒ ㉓

KNEELING SCOOP PASS

MOVEMENTS

1. Kneel on a mat facing a wall (both knees down).
2. Tighten the glutes; brace the abdomen. Throughout the exercise, maintain a completely straight line in the body (ears, shoulders, hips, and knees are in alignment).
3. Hold a rubber medicine ball in the hands next to the right hip.
4. Initiate the action with a forceful right hip thrust.
5. Release the ball at an angle toward the wall so the ball makes contact at about the midline of the body (directly in front of the body).
6. Catch the rebound on the opposite (left) hip, allowing the rebound momentum of the medicine ball to take the ball back behind the left hip slightly.
7. Over and back (right side, left side) equals one repetition. Perform for a predetermined number of repetitions or length of time.

CONSIDERATIONS

1. Distance from the wall depends on the athlete's current levels of strength and skill and on the resiliency (bounciness) of the medicine ball.
2. The wall should be solid (concrete, cinderblock, brick, solid wood, etc.).
3. The height of the toss depends on current level of strength and on the resiliency (bounciness) of the medicine ball.
4. Although some arm and shoulder action will occur, the ball should be "thrown" by the hip thrust, not the arms.
5. Benefit 23, gravity load, is a bit of a misnomer for this particular drill and the following progression. In actuality, the rubber medicine ball and its resiliency and therefore the responsive energy stored in the rubber and subsequent horizontal energy released upon contact with the wall act in much the same fashion as vertical gravity load.

SPECIFIC BENEFITS

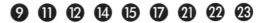

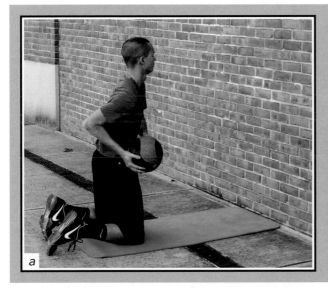 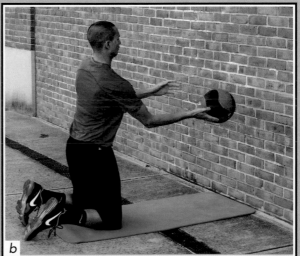

■ STANDING SCOOP PASS ■

Modifications

1. The setup and action are identical to Kneeling Scoop Pass except stand upright with the feet parallel and slightly wider than shoulder width. Flex the knees and hips to a be in an athletic stance.

2. Over and back (right side, left side) equals one repetition.

Specific Benefits **9 11 12 14 15 17 21 22 23**

MOVEMENTS

1. Select a medicine ball light enough to be thrown hard but heavy enough to provide resistance.

2. Kneel on a gym mat or foam pad perpendicular to a wall. The left knee is bent and flat on the mat; the right knee is also bent with the foot flat on the floor. The right leg is in front of the left leg.

3. Tighten the glutes; brace the abdomen. Throughout the exercise, maintain a completely straight line in the body (ears, shoulders, hips, and knees are in alignment).

4. Hold the medicine ball by the midsection with both hands.

5. Raise the ball up to the right side of head. Ensure the side is the same as the up leg.

6. Slam the ball down at an angle from right to left toward the wall, away from the down leg.

7. Maintain good posture throughout; do not break form. Do not rotate the torso.

8. Perform a set number of repetitions; repeat on the opposite side.

CONSIDERATIONS

1. Brace the core throughout the exercise.

2. Maintain good posture with the shoulder blades pulled down and retracted.

3. Benefit 23, gravity load, is a bit of a misnomer for this particular drill and the following progressions. In actuality, the rubber medicine ball and its resiliency and therefore the responsive energy stored in the rubber and subsequent horizontal energy released upon contact with the wall act in much the same fashion as vertical gravity load.

SPECIFIC BENEFITS

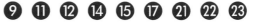

9 11 12 14 15 17 21 22 23

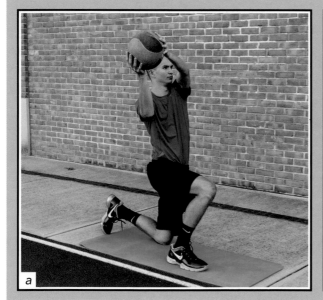 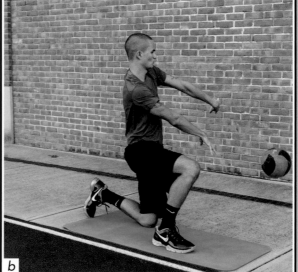

■ MEDICINE BALL CHOP SLAM ■
PROGRESSION 2: TALL KNEELING

Modifications

1. The setup and action are identical to the Medicine Ball Chop Slam Progression 1, except both knees are bent and on the ground.

Specific Benefits ⑨ ⑪ ⑫ ⑭ ⑮ ⑰ ㉑ ㉒ ㉓

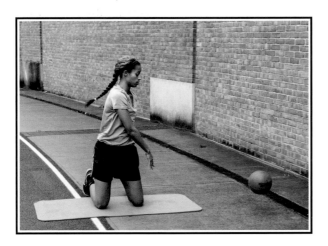

■ MEDICINE BALL CHOP SLAM ■
PROGRESSION 3: STANDING

Modifications

1. Stand upright with the feet parallel and slightly wider than shoulder width. Set up with the ball at the midsection and both hips and knees flexed.
2. The action is identical to the Medicine Ball Chop Slam Progression 1.

Specific Benefits ⑨ ⑪ ⑫ ⑭ ⑮ ⑰ ㉑ ㉒ ㉓

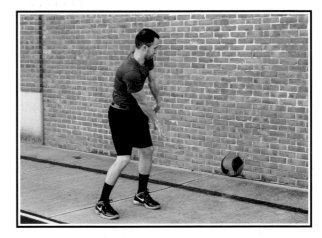

■ MEDICINE BALL CHOP SLAM ■
PROGRESSION 4: STAGGERED STANCE

Modifications

1. Set up with the medicine ball at the midsection and the feet split staggered one in front of the other.
2. The action is identical to the Medicine Ball Chop Slap Progression 1.

Specific Benefits ⑨ ⑪ ⑫ ⑭ ⑮ ⑰ ㉑ ㉒ ㉓

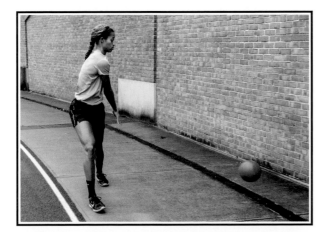

■ MEDICINE BALL CHOP SLAM ■
PROGRESSION 5: LUNGE STANCE

Modifications

1. Set up with the medicine ball at the midsection and feet split staggered one in front of the other. Brace the core; bend both knees to 90 degrees and come up onto the ball of the back foot.
2. The action is identical to the Medicine Ball Chop Slam Progression 1.

Specific Benefits ⑨ ⑪ ⑫ ⑭ ⑮ ⑰ ㉑ ㉒ ㉓

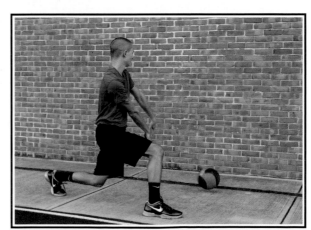

MEDICINE BALL SIDE THROW

PROGRESSION 1: HALF-KNEELING

MOVEMENTS

1. Select a medicine ball light enough to be thrown hard but heavy enough to provide resistance.
2. Kneel on a gym mat or foam pad perpendicular to a wall. The right knee is bent and flat on the mat; the left knee is also bent with the foot flat on the floor. The left leg is in front of the right leg.
3. Tighten the glutes; brace the abdomen. Throughout the exercise, maintain a completely straight line in the body (ears, shoulders, hips, and knees are in alignment).
4. Hold the medicine ball by the midsection with both hands.
5. Rotating through the shoulders (not the lower back) toward the up leg, throw the ball as hard as possible in a baseball-swing fashion.
6. Maintain good posture throughout; do not break form.
7. Control the rebound; perform a predetermined number of repetitions.
8. Repeat on the opposite side.

CONSIDERATIONS

1. Brace the core throughout the exercise.
2. Maintain good posture with the shoulder blades pulled down and retracted.
3. Benefit 23, gravity load, is a bit of a misnomer for this particular drill and the following progressions. In actuality, the rubber medicine ball and its resiliency and therefore the responsive energy stored in the rubber and subsequent horizontal energy released upon contact with the wall act in much the same fashion as vertical gravity load.

SPECIFIC BENEFITS

9 11 12 14 15 17 21 22 23

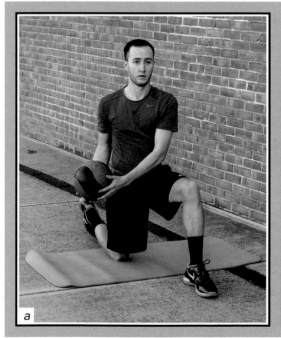

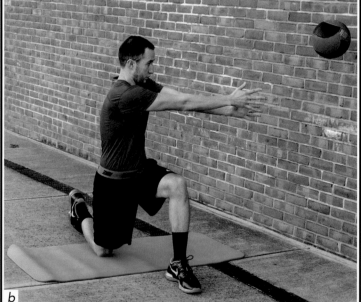

■ MEDICINE BALL SIDE THROW ■
PROGRESSION 2: TALL KNEELING

Modifications

1. The setup and action are identical to the Medicine Ball Side Throw Progression 1, except both knees are bent and on the floor.

Specific Benefits ❾ ⑪ ⑫ ⑭ ⑮ ⑰ ㉑ ㉒ ㉓

■ MEDICINE BALL SIDE THROW ■
PROGRESSION 3: STANDING

Modifications

1. Stand upright with the feet parallel and slightly wider than shoulder width. Set up with the ball at the midsection and both hips and knees flexed.

2. The action is identical to the Medicine Ball Side Throw Progression 1.

Specific Benefits ❾ ⑪ ⑫ ⑭ ⑮ ⑰ ㉑ ㉒ ㉓

■ MEDICINE BALL SIDE THROW ■
PROGRESSION 4: STAGGERED STANCE

Modifications

1. Set up with the medicine ball at the midsection and the feet split staggered one in front of the other.

2. The action is identical to the Medicine Ball Side Throw Progression 1.

Specific Benefits ❾ ⑪ ⑫ ⑭ ⑮ ⑰ ㉑ ㉒ ㉓

■ MEDICINE BALL SIDE THROW ■
PROGRESSION 5: LUNGE STANCE

Modifications

1. Set up with the medicine ball at the midsection and the feet split staggered one in front of the other. Brace the core, bend both knees to 90 degrees, and come up onto the ball of the back foot.

2. The action is identical to the Medicine Ball Side Throw Progression 1.

Specific Benefits ❾ ⑪ ⑫ ⑭ ⑮ ⑰ ㉑ ㉒ ㉓

MEDICINE BALL PARALLEL THROW

PROGRESSION 1: HALF-KNEELING

MOVEMENTS

1. Kneel on a gym mat or foam pad, facing a wall. The right knee is bent and flat on the mat; the left knee is also bent with the foot flat on the floor. The left leg is in front of the right leg.
2. Tighten the glutes; brace the abdomen. Throughout the exercise, maintain a completely straight line in the body (ears, shoulders, hips, and knees are in alignment).
3. Hold the medicine ball in both hands by the right hip. Rotating through the shoulders (not the lower back), throw the ball as hard as possible in a tennis-backhand fashion.
4. Control the rebound.
5. Continue the action for a predetermined number of repetitions, then switch legs and repeat on the opposite side.

CONSIDERATIONS

1. Distance from the wall depends on the athlete's current levels of strength and skill and on the resiliency (bounciness) of the medicine ball.
2. The wall should be solid (concrete, cinderblock, brick, solid wood, etc.).
3. The height of the toss depends on current level of strength and on the resiliency (bounciness) of the medicine ball.
4. Brace the core throughout the exercise.
5. Maintain good posture throughout with shoulder blades pulled down and retracted. Do not break form.
6. Benefit 23, gravity load, is a bit of a misnomer for this particular drill and the following progressions. In actuality, the rubber medicine ball and its resiliency and therefore the responsive energy stored in the rubber and subsequent horizontal energy released upon contact with the wall act in much the same fashion as vertical gravity load.

SPECIFIC BENEFITS

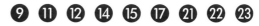

9 11 12 14 15 17 21 22 23

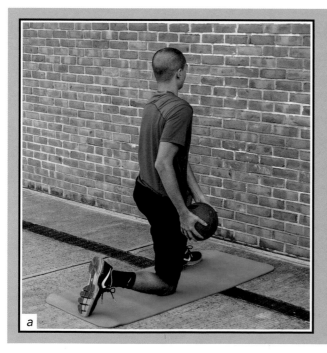

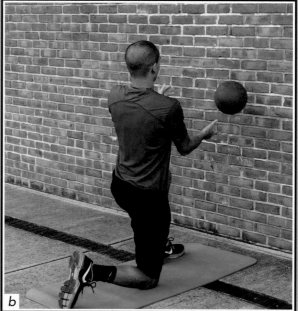

■ MEDICINE BALL PARALLEL THROW ■
PROGRESSION 2: TALL KNEELING

Modifications

1. The setup and action are identical to the Medicine Ball Parallel Throw Progression 1, except both knees are bent and on the floor.

Specific Benefits ❾ ⓫ ⓬ ⓮ ⓯ ⓱ ㉑ ㉒ ㉓

■ MEDICINE BALL PARALLEL THROW ■
PROGRESSION 3: STANDING

Modifications

1. Stand upright with the feet parallel and slightly wider than shoulder width. Set up with the ball at the right hip and both hips and knees flexed.

2. The action is identical to the Medicine Ball Parallel Throw Progression 1.

Specific Benefits ❾ ⓫ ⓬ ⓮ ⓯ ⓱ ㉑ ㉒ ㉓

■ MEDICINE BALL PARALLEL THROW ■
PROGRESSION 4: STAGGERED STANCE

Modifications

1. Set up with the medicine ball at the right hip and the feet staggered one in front of the other.

2. The action is identical to the Medicine Ball Parallel Throw Progression 1.

Specific Benefits ❾ ⓫ ⓬ ⓮ ⓯ ⓱ ㉑ ㉒ ㉓

■ MEDICINE BALL PARALLEL THROW ■
PROGRESSION 5: LUNGE STANCE

Modifications

1. Set up with the medicine ball at the right hip and the feet staggered one in front of the other. Brace the core, bend both knees to 90 degrees, and come up onto the ball of the back foot.

2. The action is identical to the Medicine Ball Parallel Throw Progression 1.

Specific Benefits ❾ ⓫ ⓬ ⓮ ⓯ ⓱ ㉑ ㉒ ㉓

MOVEMENTS

1. Select a medicine ball light enough to be thrown hard but heavy enough to provide resistance.
2. One knee is bent and flat on the floor; the other knee is also bent with the foot flat on the floor.
3. Hold the ball by the midsection with both hands.
4. Keep the hips pointing forward and, rotating through the shoulders, rotate to the down-leg side.
5. Raise the ball overhead and slam it down into the open space.
6. Control the speed of the recoil; catch the ball at about chest height.
7. Rotate back to start position.
8. Perform a predetermined number of repetitions, then repeat to the opposite side.

CONSIDERATIONS

1. Brace the core throughout the exercise
2. Maintain good posture throughout with shoulder blades pulled down and retracted. Do not break form.
3. Benefit 23, gravity load, is a bit of a misnomer for this particular drill and the following progressions. In actuality, the rubber medicine ball and its resiliency and therefore the responsive energy stored in the rubber and subsequent horizontal energy released upon contact with the wall act in much the same fashion as vertical gravity load.

SPECIFIC BENEFITS

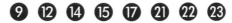

9 · 12 · 14 · 15 · 17 · 21 · 22 · 23

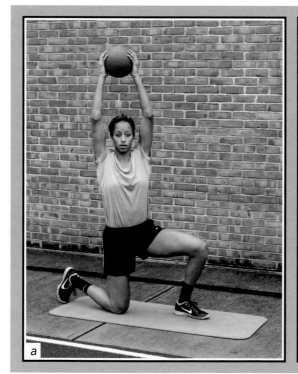

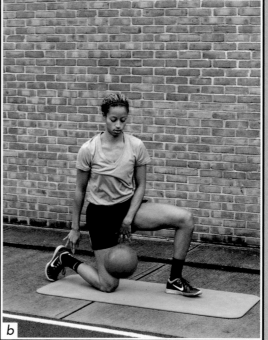

■ OVERHEAD MEDICINE BALL SLAM ROTATION ■
PROGRESSION 2: STAGGERED STANCE

Modifications

1. Set up with the medicine ball at the midsection and the feet staggered one in front of the other.

2. The action is identical to the Overhead Medicine Ball Slam Rotation Progression 1.

Specific Benefits (9) (12) (14) (15) (17) (21) (22) (23)

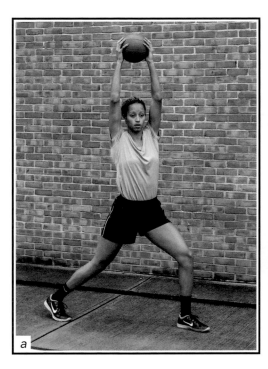

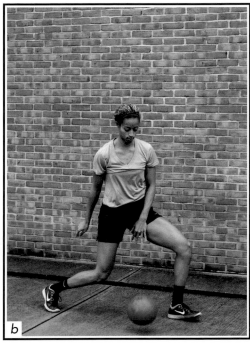

■ OVERHEAD MEDICINE BALL SLAM ROTATION ■
PROGRESSION 3: LUNGE STANCE

Modifications

1. Set up with the medicine ball at the midsection and the feet staggered one in front of the other. Brace the core, bend both knees to 90 degrees, and come up onto the ball of the back foot.

2. The action is identical to the Overhead Medicine Ball Slam Rotation Progression 1.

Specific Benefits (9) (12) (14) (15) (17) (21) (22) (23)

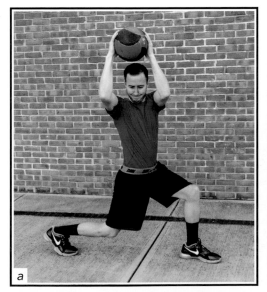

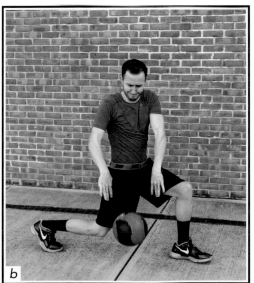

MOVEMENTS

1. Select a medicine ball (on a rope) light enough to be thrown hard but heavy enough to provide resistance.
2. Stand facing away from a wall about a foot (.3 m) from touching. Both the hips and knees are flexed. The feet are parallel and pointing straight. Hold the rope tightly in both hands.
3. Rotating through the shoulders (not the lower back), slam the ball against the wall on one side. Sit back into the movement so the force of the recoil does not pull you off balance.
4. Control the rebound and then slam the ball against the wall on the opposite side.
5. Repeat in strong, rhythmic fashion for a predetermined number of repetitions.

CONSIDERATIONS

1. Brace the core.
2. Maintain good posture throughout with shoulder blades pulled down and retracted. Do not break form.
3. Benefit 23, gravity load, is a bit of a misnomer for this particular drill and the following progressions. In actuality, the rubber medicine ball and its resiliency and therefore the responsive energy stored in the rubber and subsequent horizontal energy released upon contact with the wall act in much the same fashion as vertical gravity load.

SPECIFIC BENEFITS

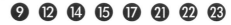

9 12 14 15 17 21 22 23

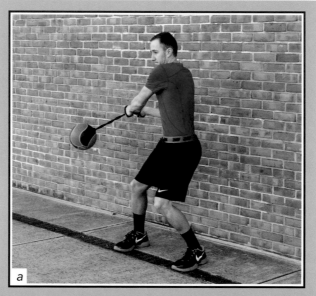

a

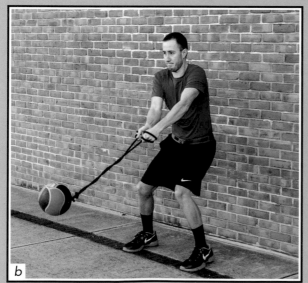

b

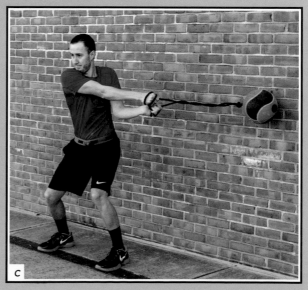

c

Lumbo-Pelvic Hip Exercises

We have espoused the many incredible benefits of training the lumbo-pelvic hip complex (LPHC) throughout this book, particularly in chapters 9 and 13. It is now time to turn our attention to the be-all and end-all of sports... power! An explosive LPHC is a weapon you can't do without and one that will change the nature of your athletic output. How do you get this? Through well-thought out plyometric strategies. This chapter is a snapshot into the world of plyometrics that will lead you in the right direction with form, exercise selection, and placement.

You can think of plyometrics as fundamental movement patterns on steroids. Plyometric exercises involve hopping, skipping, jumping, and bounding on a flat surface, up and down hills and stairs, over barriers, and onto and off of boxes with the upper and lower body alike, all within a multiplicity of plane combinations. Sandwiched between primitive and postural reflexes and the rudimentary movement stages on one side, and years before the onset of the sport skill application stage on the opposite side, are the above mentioned fundamental movement patterns—the third stage in the motor development continuum—which are critical for the further expansion of athletic development.

But fear not—regardless of the age of the athlete, new movements *can* be learned. However, with advancing age comes the intensified importance of cognitive involvement. In other words, a compulsory thought process on the part of the athlete is essential for comprehensive development and successful application of any new learned movement pattern (a pattern new to that athlete). So tell that therapist to remove his text-messaging elbows from your glute medius, get up off the table, and get out on the field and actually do some hard work toward developing that new motor skill. Knowingly comprehend the movement that you want to acquire, and you will take your game to the next level.

The exercises in this chapter will effectually apply fundamental movement patterns in a controlled and explosive sport skill application. The drills should also serve as an impetuous in developing your own movement patterns specific to your needs. The surface area for the exercises in this chapter should be semiresilient, clean, and clear of obstructions. In other words, avoid cluttered, hard, and unforgiving surfaces.

The following exercise finder lists the benefits, difficulty level, and equipment needed for every exercise that appears in this chapter. Primary exercises are highlighted in beige with their progressions in green. The primary exercises are also noted in the text with a green title bar.

Lumbo-Pelvic Hip Power Exercise Finder

Exercise Name	Specific Benefits (see chapter 5)	Difficulty Level			Equipment
		Easy	Medium	Hard	
Bound	④ ⑧ ⑨ ⑪ ⑫ ⑭ ㉒ ㉓ ㉔			X	
Ice Skater	④ ⑧ ⑨ ⑪ ⑫ ⑭ ㉒ ㉓		X		
Box Hop Up	④ ⑧ ⑨ ⑪ ㉒ ㉓		X		Raised platform*
Box Hop Down	④ ⑧ ⑨ ⑪ ㉒ ㉓		X		Raised platform
Medial Box Hop Up	④ ⑧ ⑨ ⑪ ㉒ ㉓		X		Raised platform
Medial Box Hop Down	④ ⑧ ⑨ ⑪ ㉒ ㉓		X		Raised platform
Single-Leg Power Step-Up	④ ⑧ ⑨ ⑪ ⑫ ㉒ ㉓		X		Raised platform
Alternating Leg Power Step-Up	④ ⑧ ⑨ ⑪ ⑫ ㉒ ㉓		X		Raised platform

* Many options are available for the raised platform, including a box, bench, stair, or step.

MOVEMENTS

1. Stand on the right leg. The left leg is up with the knee slightly forward (*a*).

2. With a quick drop action, flex the hip, knee, and ankle of the right leg and bound forward as far as comfortably possible to land on the left leg (*b*). Use proper deceleration mechanics: Land with a shock absorption action where the ankle, knee, and hip execute a natural flexion to reduce the abruptness of the landing. Correct posture remains intact throughout.

3. On landing, body weight is distributed directly over the base of support. Hold this position (stabilization component) for a second or two.

4. Maintaining postural control, stand a little more erect just prior to a rapid "drop" (prestretch) and then bound backward to the start position, landing on the right leg.

5. Laterally bound to the left (*c*), again landing on the left leg with the above mentioned proper decelerative action. Maintaining postural control, bound laterally back to the start position.

6. Now comes the tricky part. Adhering to the same mechanics as described (prestretch and countermovement action), simultaneously bound while rotating the body counterclockwise (right leg takeoff, left leg landing) to land *behind* the start position (*d-e*). You need not turn a full 180 degrees. Rotate only as far as comfortably possible without compromising body awareness, balance, or control. This drill is risky, so proceed with care. Attempt to land on a solid base of support (left foot). When landing, the body should no longer be turning counter-clockwise. This will greatly lessen the torsion forces at the ankle, hip, and particularly the knee. If pain or discomfort is felt then discontinue this portion of the drill or the entire drill.

7. After a split-second of stabilization, jump and rotate back to the start position (jump clockwise: left leg to right leg). The same care must be taken during the return jump. Anytime pain or discomfort is felt then discontinue this portion of the drill or the entire drill. Bound back under control.

8. Forward, lateral, and transverse (backward) equals one repetition. Perform a predetermined number of repetitions on the same leg or alternate legs. Regardless, repeat with an equal number of repetitions on each leg.

CONSIDERATIONS

1. Brace the core throughout the exercise.

2. Maintain good posture; depress and retract the scapulae.

3. The distance of the bound depends on the athlete's current levels of strength and coordination. Never sacrifice technique for greater distance.

4. Of critical importance is the ability to comfortably stick the landing prior to a subsequent action. Complete control of the body requires a synchronous effort throughout the kinetic chain. Drills such as this one, which requires controlled deceleration, balance, and body precision, are absolutely specific to the physical demands of sport participation. These drills require a shock-absorbing (or sticking) component that greatly enhances proprioceptive awareness.

5. Maintain a knee position directly above the base of the support foot.

SPECIFIC BENEFITS

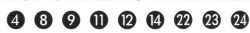

(continued)

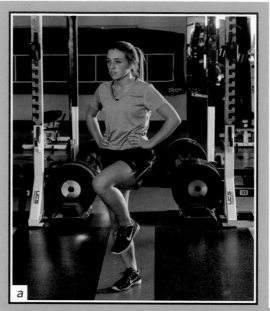

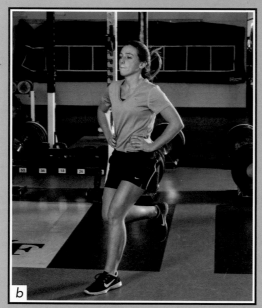

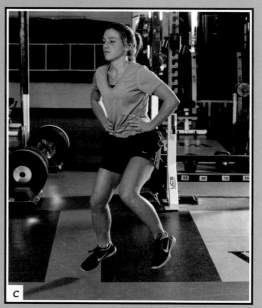

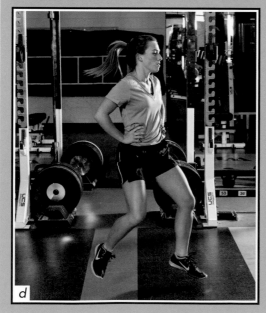

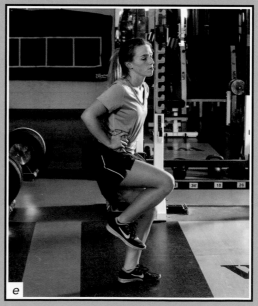

■ ICE SKATER ■

Modifications

1. Stand on the right leg. The left leg is up with the knee slightly forward.
2. Bound powerfully to the left side (lateral bound). Land on the left leg and execute good deceleration mechanics by flexing the hip, knee, and ankle on landing.
3. Bound back to the start position.
4. The bound to the left and back equals one repetition. Continue bounding in a rhythmic fashion for a predetermined number of repetitions.

Specific Benefits ④ ⑧ ⑨ ⑪ ⑫ ⑭ ㉒ ㉓

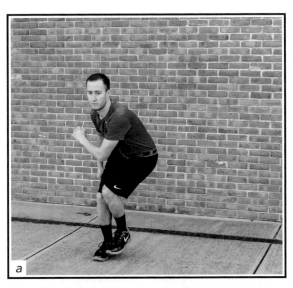

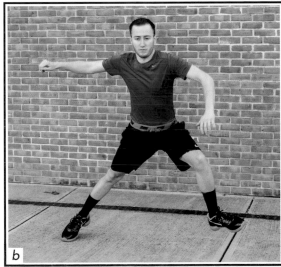

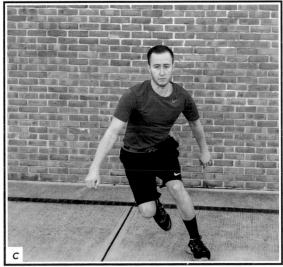

MOVEMENTS

1. Stand on the left leg in front of a box or other raised platform that is tall enough for a quality jump but short enough for a comfortable landing.
2. Push hard (drive) against the ground and hop up onto the box.
3. Land on the left leg; execute proper deceleration mechanics by flexing the hip, knee, and ankle on landing.
4. Maintain good posture throughout; do not break form or allow the knee to drift to the left or right as you land.

5. Step down from the box and reset.
6. Perform a predetermined number of repetitions with the same leg. Repeat on the opposite leg.

CONSIDERATIONS

1. Brace the core throughout the exercise.
2. Maintain good posture; depress and retract the scapulae.

SPECIFIC BENEFITS

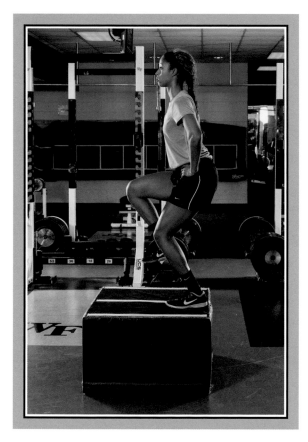

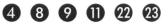

■ BOX HOP DOWN ■

Modifications

1. Stand on the right leg on top and near the edge of a box or raised platform that is between 3 inches to no taller than 15 to 20 inches (38-50 cm).
2. Hop down. Land on the right leg and execute proper deceleration mechanics by flexing the hip, knee, and ankle on landing. Do not break form or allow the knee to drift to the left or right as you land.

3. Step back onto the box and reset. Perform a predetermined number of repetitions on the same leg or alternate legs. Regardless, repeat with an equal number of repetitions on each leg.

Specific Benefits

▪ MEDIAL BOX HOP UP ▪

Modifications

1. Stand next to a box or raised platform that is tall enough for a quality jump but short enough for a comfortable landing. Stand on the right leg with the raised platform next to the lifted left leg.
2. Push hard (drive) against the ground and hop lateral to the left, up onto the box. Do not break form or allow the knee to drift to the left or right as you land.

3. Land on the right leg and execute proper deceleration mechanics by flexing the hip, knee, and ankle on landing.
4. Step down from the box and reset.

Specific Benefits

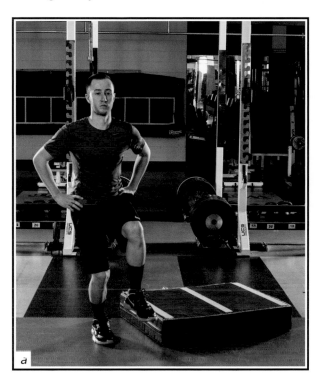

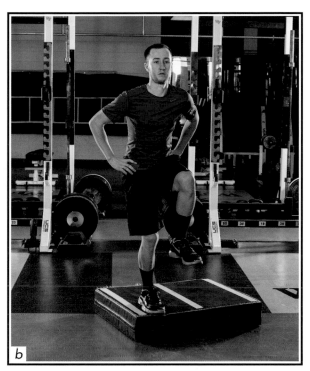

▪ MEDIAL BOX HOP DOWN ▪

Modifications

1. Stand on the right leg on top and near the edge of a box or raised platform.
2. Hop down lateral to the left.
3. Land on the right leg and execute proper deceleration mechanics by flexing the hip, knee, and ankle on landing. Do not break form or allow the knee to drift to the left or right as you land—the most important part of the drill!

4. Step back onto the box and reset. Continue with the same leg for a predetermined number of repetitions. Repeat with the opposite leg.

Specific Benefits

■ SINGLE-LEG POWER STEP-UP ■

Modifications

1. Stand facing a bench (or box) with the left foot on the bench and the right foot on the floor. The height of the box will be dictated by the athlete's strength and comfort level. Our recommendation is to never exceed a 90 degree angle at the knee when the foot is on the box. To begin, the athlete may start with a 3-inch box and progress from there as strength and comfort levels improve.

2. Push (drive) hard onto the bench, using the left leg to accelerate the body upward. The right leg knee drive and dual arm action combine to transfer energy through your solid core to the left foot on the box. The right leg will also help to facilitate landing.

3. Land back on the box with the left leg; execute proper deceleration mechanics by flexing the hip, knee, and ankle and controlling the lowering of the right leg and foot.

4. After landing, immediately reset your posture, and continue with the same leg for a predetermined number of repetitions. Repeat with the opposite leg.

Specific Benefits

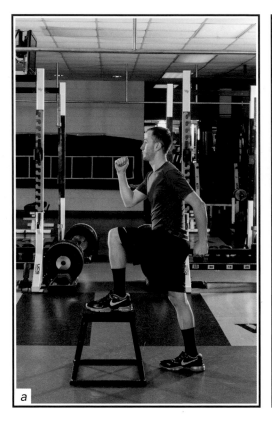 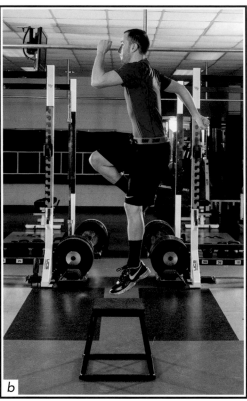

■ ALTERNATING-LEG POWER STEP-UP ■

Modifications

1. The setup is identical to the Single-Leg Power Step-Up

2. Push hard into the bench, using only the left leg to jump upward. The right leg and knee will drive hard to the ceiling.

3. In the air, change legs and land with the right leg on the bench, executing proper deceleration mechanics by flexing the hip, knee, and ankle and controlling the lowering of the left leg and foot.

4. After landing, immediately reset your posture in a split second, and continue alternating legs for a predetermined number of repetitions.

Specific Benefits

CORE TESTING AND PROGRAM DESIGN

To this point we have provided a great deal of information about the core from a historical, anatomical, functional, and contemporary perspective. In the final part of this book we pull everything together and address questions about program design and layout.

BEGINNING THE PROGRAM

The great majority of people will abandon a training program within the first three months of starting it. The reasons for quitting are as varied as the participants. Lifestyle change must be understood and accepted; otherwise you too will become another statistical exercise fugitive. Once you start an exercise program and start burning those additional calories daily, you will have to make other adjustments in your life to accommodate the changes that your body is experiencing . For example, you will certainly need more sleep. Fatigue is one of the primary culprits of attrition, and lack of sleep will greatly impact the grinding down or slow destruction of your body. Additionally, you must also focus on your dietary needs. Your body will certainly require more high-quality macronutrients (proteins, fats, and carbs) to create the energy you need to exercise at a high intensity.

Other areas of comprehensive training must be diligently attended to as well. Having a sound core is of strategic importance to the complete athletic body. However transference of power is only productive if overall power can be created through diligent full-body strength work. Movement inefficiencies need to be corrected through mobility and flexibility exercises and so on. Each training brush stroke fills in the full athletic painting to create what we hope will be your own personal masterpiece. This book is designed to give you a heightened awareness of the core and an organized and efficient training plan, but as we mentioned before it should be an important part of a more complete workout.

Be patient. You might see rapid improvements in fitness, followed by plateaus that seem to last forever. It is during these lulls that many novice fitness enthusiasts lose enthusiasm and quit the program. If progress levels off, try mixing things up a bit. Change your routine. We hope the hundreds of exercises in this book give you plenty of variety. Do not get discouraged. You might have to adjust your goals and thus adjust your training. Just be sure to *adjust* your goals and not eliminate them. Goals are important to making progress.

Goal setting can be tricky. Success in achieving goals is often a product of intrinsic motivation of the goal setter. For example, high achievement–oriented individuals respond best to goals that provide task-specific standards with a performance focus. In contrast, low achievement–oriented individuals respond best to mastery-focused goals. Always determine your own goals. Trainers or coaches can give you realistic feedback about goal complexity and being able to physiologically achieve your goals, but you know yourself better than anyone. You know what best motivates you, which is ultimately what goal achievement depends on.

Goal setting is an evolving, dynamic process. A couple of issues related to goal setting are limiting yourself to a single goal or selecting a goal that is too easily attainable. Once you achieve the goal, you simply drop off and fall back to old habits. Goals should be achievable and incrementally organized to keep your training on track toward further development. As each goal is achieved, aggressively move to the next goal, which should be progressively more challenging than the previous one.

So, exactly what type of core training is appropriate and for whom? Utilizing the tests in chapter 18 will help to answer this question, and the information gathered will provide the basis for determining your specific goals. More daunting than setting a goal is establishing a starting place, particularly for those who do not have a long exercise history. Understand that you must determine your current level of core functionality before developing a plan for where you need to go. Use chapter 18 as your guide. These tests will establish your current level of core physical fitness, osteoarticular stabilization, and dynamic functionality. Established baseline test results give you insights to help you plan your first steps into our system.

Periodic retesting allows you to monitor your progress and identify your current levels of conditioning. Retesting keeps you on the right track toward achieving your physical potential in each area of concentration. Subsequent testing is also beneficial for times when you cannot train because of injury, personal problems, or other life circumstances. For whatever reason that training was interrupted, test data will expose performance decrements. When compared to previous test scores or even the initial baseline data, the most recent test results will become an obvious consideration for determining how and where to start back up again.

Do not be capricious with your training. Do not jump in and out of programs, and do not just pick the new "cool" exercise that you saw online. Develop a plan, get to know your body, and work toward a goal.

WORKING WITHIN THE PROGRAM

Once you have established a starting point, a broad understanding of our training concepts in their entirety is critical to success. Chapters 19 and 20 present the infrastructure of the plan. You will learn to maneuver within the philosophy and program design with ease. As of this writing, most core-training protocols are one dimensional or fad driven. Understand that training is not only a never-ending process, but a process that develops cyclically, with peaks and valleys. Our intent is to present guidelines and examples that put you in the driver's seat when making critical training decisions. Always base decisions on a sound understanding of purpose and procedure, with an eye on your fitness and performance goals.

We live in a world of hyper-competitiveness in which we are all looking to gain an advantage over opponents. This being the case, in chapter 21 we include core-training protocols for several popular sports. Our intent here is to provide blueprints from which to build an appreciation of what sport specificity is all about and how to train for it.

Train your core as it was developed, allow it to express itself appropriately, and reap the many benefits of its abilities. The time for half measures and misinformation is over. You must take control of your training and be accountable to yourself. We have given you all the information you need. Knowledge is power, and the informed always come out on top.

Core Assessment Tools

Before you can design a core-training plan, be it for yourself or for an athlete you are working with, you must determine a starting point. Every type of workout should be constructed through direct, individualized physiological feedback from the athlete in question (or *you*, if you are the athlete). Anything less relies on guesswork and assumption, which is an inadequate way of approaching training. These simple tests can be administered with minimal time and equipment, but the information garnered is extremely valuable in highlighting the athlete's strengths and weaknesses. Test data will assist in evaluating the effectiveness of the training program, support goal setting, help identify health status, and establish a preinjury baseline that we hope will never be necessary to revisit.

ESTABLISHING YOUR BASELINE

Your baseline is your present level of strength and fitness. On beginning a training program, you must know where you are from a robustness standpoint. By establishing your baseline, you can then use quantifiable information to better adjust important variables such as quantity, intensity, frequency, duration, and the effectual training modality of your program design. The adaptation associated with that program might be unexpectedly substantial, or it might be slow and incremental, but it is progress nonetheless. Regardless, without baseline evidence you cannot accurately evaluate the effectiveness of your program. Likewise, if for some reason a stoppage occurs in your training (caused by injury, travel, game schedule, etc.), there will be associated decrements in your conditioning. An understanding of your baseline will demonstrate how much you have lost and how far you must go to get back to the starting point.

In this chapter we present a series of simple tests to help you establish this starting point. You can then begin to tap your athletic potential. Your skill level in a previous core-training plan does not allow you to skip this step—the methodology and principles we use here are likely to be quite different from what you have used before.

An overriding physiological principle to note is that your body will be only as powerful as your foundation allows. Stability is the foundation from which all athletic action emanates. In other words, an overused but useful analogy is that "You can't fire a cannon from a canoe." This is true as it relates to the human body, conceptually falling in line with our stability before strength and strength before power methodology. With this in mind, and regardless of prior training experience, no one should start a core regimen using the more advanced and dynamic movements such as those associated with power training.

If test results indicate that you have an effectively stable core, you can bypass the stability stage and proceed directly to the strength-oriented drills. However, the precondition necessary to integrate power-training drills will have to be earned, and in doing so, you must demonstrate full readiness to participate in those activities. Another determining factor is your ability to demonstrate proper mechanics in the execution of the drills. Progressing on to higher reps, additional sets, or added load or resistance of more difficult drills should never occur at the expense of sacrificing technique. Furthermore, just because your test results indicate you are fully capable of performing the strength and power drills, incorporating stability drills is nonetheless important. The best athletes in the world continue to reinforce their stabilization foundation by performing stability drills on a daily basis.

We recommend devoting at least four to six weeks to each phase (stability, strength, and power) before progressing to the next. As you progress with your core training, you will continually reevaluate yourself using the same tests. That said, randomly testing yourself from time to time is also appropriate to get on-the-spot feedback. The test–retest approach is critically important to systematically evaluate fluctuations in your training and to both empirically and quantifiably measure your progress. Assessments such as these are subject to many variables that might affect outcome. Thus when replicating a test, try to limit as many of the unique variables as possible. Variables that might affect the outcome of repeated testing include but aren't limited to the following:

- Environment (surface, equipment, temperature, etc.)
- Various testers
- Hydration
- Energy level
- Time of day
- Athlete stress level

Make every attempt to note all variables prior to testing and to replicate them on subsequent assessments. Ensuring that the retest conditions are as close to the original conditions as possible is extremely important from a validity standpoint. The assessments we recommend have been chosen because they are specific to the objectives of the program. It makes little sense to run a mile time trial when our intent is to measure lumbar stability. All testing must be objective. In other words, the outcome should be reliable regardless of who administers the test. If you are performing the test on yourself repeatedly, then you can be pretty well assured that consistency will prevail—especially with practice.

It would be irresponsible to suggest that you can accurately predict the incidence, timing, or severity of a future injury. That said, it is possible to examine some of the markers that relate directly to injury potential. Three of the most important indicators are these:

- Level of motor control
- Injury history
- Bilateral asymmetries

The tests are an excellent way to gain a better understanding of your body's current performance potential and how it functionally relates to these variables. For example, if during the anti-rotation testing you feel strong or more stable on one side, or if during the lumbo-pelvic hip complex unilateral bridge test you are stronger on one leg, you have a noticeable asymmetry that if ignored could become problematic. Briefly, if an asymmetry is discovered, you must perform at least a two-to-one bilateral work ratio to address the deficit and restore symmetry (e.g., two sets on the affected leg to one set on the good leg).

Described below are two integrated tests for each of the core areas emphasized. The first is a simple stability test to determine your core's essential strength. The second set of tests adds a light load to establish how your core responds to additional stimulus. Our guidelines suggest that in order to advance from the stability level to the strength level of the core-training regimen, you must successfully pass both tests. If you pass the first but fail the second, you must remain at the stability level. There is nothing wrong with that. The stability level exercises will still kick your butt.

You might discover differing levels of stability or strength throughout the core region. If this is the case, your training focus will be on eliminating those weaknesses prior to additional training of your strengths. For example, if your test data indicates that you are strong in the anti-extension movements but weak in the anti-rotation movements, the entire core must be trained at the stability level until better balance is achieved. The core works at its most optimal when synergy prevails throughout, which can occur only when limitations are identified and corrected.

For all of the tests that follow, if at any point during the test you experience pain, stop testing immediately.

ANTI-EXTENSION TESTING

Anti-extension is a fairly simple premise, the basis of which incorporates the core system to actively counter the forces intended to arch backward. A basic example is the elbow plank, a primary structural body alignment activity that can be made progressively more difficult by increasing load, adding time, and challenging balance through base of support manipulation or perturbation techniques. Ultimately, the longer someone can hold this joint-aligned plank position without slipping into extension, the stronger that person is within this capacity of anti-extension.

ANTI-EXTENSION TEST 1: ELBOW PLANK, 20 SECONDS

Lie prone on the floor with the feet dorsiflexed (toes toward the shins) and the elbows and forearms under the chest area. Position a broomstick along your spine to confirm symmetrical orientation.

1. To begin, lift the body off the floor so that the only points of contact are the forearms, balls of the feet, and flexed toes. After lifting up, the body will shift slightly to a position in which the upper arms are perpendicular to the floor, with the elbows directly under the shoulders and the forearms angled slightly to a position in which the hands are under the face.

2. Brace the core, stabilize the scapulae, lock the knees, and tighten the glutes.

3. Start the clock only when you have successfully aligned the shoulders, hips, knees and ankles (straight body alignment). Maintain this solid posture for 20 seconds.

Fail

The test is interpreted as a failure if at some point during the 20 seconds any part of the torso sags away from the broomstick or substantial shaking (joint instability) throughout the body ensues. In this case, the training program begins at the **anti-extension stability level**.

Pass

If the torso remains fully in contact with the broomstick for a minimum of 20 seconds with no noticeable quivering (figure 18.1), this test has been passed. Progress to anti-extension test 2.

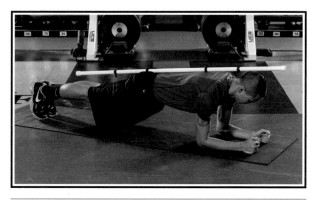

Figure 18.1 Anti-extension test 1: Elbow plank, 20 seconds.

ANTI-EXTENSION TEST 2: ELBOW PLANK, 60 SECONDS

The additional load in this test comes simply from increasing the test duration. With an increase in duration to 60 seconds, the overall time under tension intensifies, challenging the body to work harder against slipping into a negative posture identified as an undesirable extension.

Again, lie prone on the floor with the feet dorsiflexed (toes toward the shins) and the elbows and forearms under the chest area. Position a broomstick along your spine to confirm symmetrical orientation.

1. To begin, lift the body off the floor so that the only points of contact are the forearms, balls of the feet, and flexed toes. After lifting up, the body will shift slightly to a position in which the upper arms are perpendicular to the floor, with the elbows directly under the shoulders and the forearms angled slightly to a position in which the hands are under the face.

2. Brace the core, stabilize the scapulae, lock the knees, and tighten the glutes.

3. Start the clock only when you have successfully aligned the shoulders, hips, knees and ankles (straight body alignment). Maintain this solid posture for 60 seconds.

Fail

The test is interpreted as a failure if at some point during the 60 seconds any part of the torso sags away from the broomstick or substantial shaking (joint instability) throughout the body ensues. In this case, the training program begins at the **anti-extension stability level**.

Pass

If the torso remains fully in contact with the broomstick for a minimum of 60 seconds with no noticeable quivering (see figure 18.1), this test has been passed. Begin the training program at the **anti-extension strength level**.

ANTI-ROTATION TESTING

Anti-rotation control is one of the most important qualities in effective sports performance. More often than not, athletes perform activities on a single leg and in spiral patterns (for example, executing a right-handed layup while jumping off the left leg). Additionally, movement in the transverse plane, which is a biomechanical inevitability and is inherent to just about all sport movement, all too frequently exposes bilateral asymmetries, especially when the athlete is forced into rotational movement patterns. Alarmingly, many injuries, particularly noncontact injuries, occur during these rotational type movements. Control over this critical area pays dividends in both the possibility of injury reduction as well as increased performance.

ANTI-ROTATION TEST 1: BIRD-DOG

In a kneeling position with hands on the floor, place a broomstick on the back, in line with the spine.

1. To begin, raise the left arm up and extend it parallel to the floor.
2. Simultaneously, raise the right leg up and extend it backward, also parallel to the floor.
3. Draw both limbs back under the body and touch the left elbow to the right knee.
4. Return to the fully extended position and repeat.
5. Continue touching the left elbow to the right knee for six repetitions; then repeat on the opposite side (i.e., right arm and left leg extended, right elbow to left knee).

Fail

The test is interpreted as a failure if at any point during the test the torso sags away from the broomstick, the broomstick rolls off the back, or balance is lost. If any of these occur, training begins and remains at the **anti-rotation stability level** until successful completion of both tests.

Pass

If the torso remains in complete contact with the broomstick, and body control and balance are maintained throughout the test (figure 18.2), this test has been deemed a success Progress to anti-rotation test 2.

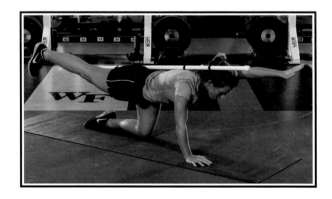

Figure 18.2 Anti-rotation test 1: Bird-dog.

ANTI-ROTATION TEST 2: ROTARY STABILITY

The additional load and balance required in this test come via extending the lever length of the body. This is an intensive contralateral co-contraction activity that requires strength, stability, body control, and, above all, concentration. Remember that this is anti-rotation. Focus on avoiding twisting or tipping.

Begin in a push-up position with the feet roughly hip-width apart and the hands directly under the shoulders. The arms are locked, and the head is up slightly with the eyes focused on the floor about 3 to 5 feet (or about .9 to 1.5 meters) forward. The body should be in a straight line (i.e., ears, shoulders, hips, knees, and ankles are lined up, with no sagging or piking). Place a broomstick on the back, in line with the spine.

1. When ready, keep the feet still but raise one arm up to parallel, and then lower it back down again.
2. Do six repetitions on each side.

Fail

If the body twists, hips sag, hips pike, or shoulders drop, any of which causes the broomstick to fall, the test is deemed a failure. Also, if the hips roll back and forth, causing the broomstick to roll or fall, or if balance is lost at any point or a foot is raised off the floor to counterbalance, the test has been failed. Training begins and remains at the **anti-rotary stability level** until both have been passed.

Pass

If the torso remains in full contact with the broomstick, with no hip rolling or loss of balance (figure 18.3), this test has been passed. Begin training at the **anti-rotation strength level.**

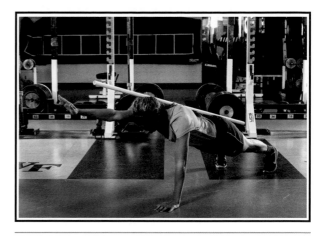

Figure 18.3   Anti-rotation test 2: Rotary stability.

SCAPULOTHORACIC MUSCULATURE TESTING

The intricate web of interwoven muscle and fascia, together with the structural support of the skeletal system, provide a framework that facilitates the production of force, the reduction of force, and the stabilization of the kinetic chain during all functional movements. Without this integrated synergism, functional upright posture would be impossible.

Unfortunately, although the muscles that cover the scapula and thoracic regions are incredibly complex and a vitally important structural element, they are consistently undertrained, which means the scapulothoracic musculature is constantly losing the battle against gravity because of this lack of focus in program design and application. Biomechanically, this region has major implications relating to postural control, breathing function, rotator cuff stability, glenohumeral joint positioning, and force transfer from lower to upper limbs, to name but a few. With this in mind, assessment is critically important because of the uniqueness of this region's integrated functional performance implications.

Because of its visibly obscure location, the athlete rarely can see the adaptive fruits of his labor. In other words, these are not a "mirror" group requiring extensive training for beach season. But from a stability, strength, and power standpoint, the scapulothoracic musculature is a critically important component of the body's musculoskeletal system. Functional assessment of this region helps determine an ability to control scapular retraction and depression (sometimes called a packed shoulder) and maintain that position when standing statically as well as when forces are applied through movement.

SCAPULOTHORACIC MUSCULATURE TEST 1: THUMBS UP

Begin in an upright standing position. Stand up straight with the arms against the sides.

1. Close your eyes, take a deep breath, and release. Do not change the position of the wrists or hands.
2. Extend both thumbs into a thumbs-up position.
3. Open your eyes and look at your hands.

Fail

If the thumbs are pointing at the hips or at each other, the test has been failed. Begin training at the **scapulothoracic musculature stability level**.

Pass

If the thumbs are pointing straight forward (figure 18.4), this test has been passed. Progress to scapulothoracic musculature test 2.

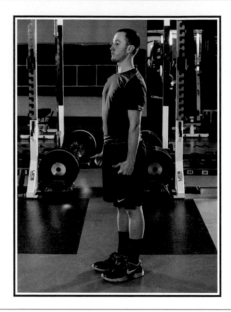

Figure 18.4 Scapulothoracic musculature test 1: Thumbs up.

SCAPULOTHORACIC MUSCULATURE TEST 2: OVERHEAD ARM DROP

Begin in an upright standing position with the arms at the sides.

1. Rotate the arms backward in a large cyclical motion until they are straight overhead. (At this point, the shoulders will be pulled back and down in optimal posture.)
2. When ready, let the arms drop forward quickly back to the starting point. Note the position of the shoulders.

Fail

If after the arms drop, the shoulders remain rolled forward and do not retain any posterior translation, the test has been failed. Begin training at the **scapulothoracic musculature stability level.**

Pass

If after the arms drop, the shoulders remain back in a solid postural position (figure 18.5), this test has been passed. Begin training at the **scapulothoracic musculature strength level.**

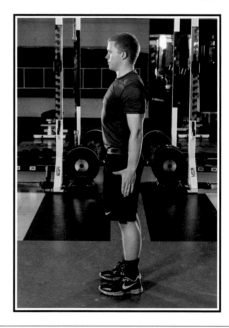

Figure 18.5 Scapulothoracic musculature test 2: Overhead arm drop.

LUMBO-PELVIC HIP COMPLEX TESTING

As stated in earlier chapters, the lumbo-pelvic hip complex (LPHC) is a major structural factor within the body. As the vertebral foundation with ligamentous attachments that impact femoral control, this complex controls and supports everything above and below it. It is the driving force for acceleration and change of direction and also affects posture.

The importance of a strong core as it relates to neuromuscular efficiency is critically important for dynamically stabilizing the LPHC. All mechanical functioning originates and is stabilized by LPHC musculature (global and local alike). The following tests determine interdependent functioning and neuromuscular efficiency of the lumbo-pelvic hip complex from a stability and strength perspective throughout the kinetic chain.

LUMBO-PELVIC HIP COMPLEX TEST 1: TWO-FOOT BRIDGE

Lay supine on the floor with the knees flexed to 90 degrees. The feet are flat on the floor, parallel to each other and positioned hip-width apart. Place the hands on the floor at the sides and relax the head and neck.

1. To begin, brace the core, contract the glutes, and smoothly lift upward until the hips are fully extended. The up position is attained when there is a straight line from the knees to the hips to the shoulders (which are on the floor). Avoid lifting up onto the head and neck. The load of the body should be held by the shoulders and upper back, not the head and neck.

2. Hold the up position for 10 seconds.

3. Slowly lower to the start position and immediately repeat three times.

Fail

If any adverse stress is felt through the lower back or if the contraction is felt entirely in the hamstrings musculature while the hips are in the up position, the test is a decided failure. Training

begins and remains at the **lumbo-pelvic hip complex stability level** until a successful completion of both tests is achieved.

Pass

If during each of the three 10-second sets, only a consistent tightening of the glutes is felt (figure 18.6), this test has been passed. Proceed to the lumbo-pelvic hip complex test 2.

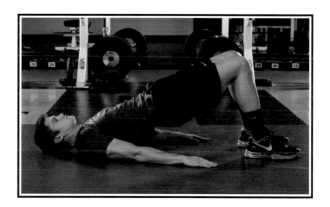

Figure 18.6 Lumbo-pelvic hip complex test 1: Two-foot bridge.

LUMBO-PELVIC HIP COMPLEX TEST 2: UNILATERAL BRIDGE

Lay supine on the floor with the knees flexed to 90 degrees. The feet are flat on the floor, parallel to each other and positioned hip-width apart. Place the hands on the floor at the sides and relax the head and neck.

1. To begin, pull one knee up tight to the chest. To ensure quality of movement, place a tennis ball (or similar object) near

the bottom of the rib cage and hold it in place with the thigh of the up leg.

2. Dorsiflex the foot on the floor by lifting the toes upward to the ceiling, brace the core, and extend the hips fully by driving down into the heel that is on the floor. The up position is attained when there is a straight line from the knee of the down leg

(continued)

to the hips to the shoulders (which are on the floor). Avoid lifting up onto the head and neck. The load of the body should be held by the shoulders and upper back, not the head and neck.

3. Hold the up position for 10 seconds.
4. Slowly lower to the start position and immediately repeat three times.
5. Perform the test with the opposite leg.

Fail

If at any point the tennis ball falls out of position, the test has been failed. Also, if any adverse stress is felt through the lower back or if the contraction is felt entirely in the hamstring musculature, the test is a failure. Training begins and remains at the **lumbo-pelvic hip complex stability level** until both tests have been passed.

Pass

If during each of the three 10-second sets with each leg, the ball stays in place throughout (figure 18.7), and if a consistent tightening of only the glutes is felt, this test has been passed. Begin training at the **lumbo-pelvic hip complex strength level**.

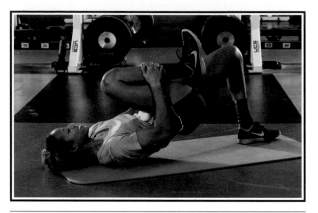

Figure 18.7   Lumbo-pelvic hip complex test 2: Unilateral bridge.

TESTING CHECKLIST

For a quick and concise test battery, use the provided checklist in table 18.1 for each test and each region. Document all your checklists. Over time, these data will provide you with a chronologically sequential record of your progress. This information provides both context and validation as you pursue your ever-expanding objectives.

By now you have determined your starting points for each of the core areas. Now go back into the book and pick an exercise that corresponds to your results. Each exercise follows a systematic progression. The exercise selection must mirror your current level and also work within the constraints of equipment availability and your comfort level. Do not attempt the most impressive looking stability or strength exercise unless you know you can master it. Remember that we want all facets of the core to be working optimally, so if some areas fail the given tests and require stability training, then pass or fail, *all* areas need stability training.

Note that when you have tested to a higher starting point, that doesn't necessarily mean that the drills from the stability or strength levels are any less important. Including these drills in your training will reinforce stability and strength and add variety to your program design. The body adapts specific to the stress imposed, so the more varietal angles that you attack within your training, the more complete the adaptive qualities.

Table 18.1 Testing Checklist

Focus	Test	Pass	Fail	Diagram
Anti-extension testing	1: Elbow plank, 20 seconds			
	2: Elbow plank, 60 seconds			
Anti-rotation testing	1: Bird-dog			
	2: Rotary stability			
Scapulothoracic musculature testing	1: Thumbs up			
	2: Overhead arm drop			

(continued)

Table 18.1 Testing Checklist *(continued)*

Focus	Test	Pass	Fail	Diagram
Lumbo-pelvic hip complex testing	1: Two-foot bridge			
	2: Unilateral bridge			

Complete Core Program

A stable, strong, and powerful core lasts a lifetime. Core efficiency is not a passing fad or something that needs to be trained only while actively involved in sport. Core efficiency is an essential part of a weekly routine that will enhance your daily quality of life for years to come. With this in mind, we have developed a core program that is functionally cyclical—and without a conclusion. After establishing a starting point through the assessment protocols in chapter 18, the workouts begin at a predetermined point, but as you move steadily through each phase, you will never reach an end point. In fact, given the space limitations, hundreds of possible core exercises have been intentionally omitted from this text. Not to worry: Even if you burn through all of the drills presented in the previous chapters, the concepts and guidelines described in these following pages will certainly apply to your program design regardless of the source of the exercises you choose to incorporate. Exercise selection, load, reps, sets, temporal considerations, intensity, duration, and frequency can all be manipulated in a progressively challenging system—forever.

A CYCLICAL PROGRAM

The concept of a cyclical program might seem strange and is perhaps unfamiliar or uncomfortable for some. The truth is, you will never really be able to fully exhaust your ability or variable options during each phase. As you move through the stability phase and become more efficient at controlling your body, you will see improvements both physically and posturally, and also from a performance perspective. After four to six weeks and a successful follow-up retest, you will begin the strength portion of the training regimen. Although some stability-based components appear in these exercises, they are designed primarily to improve the overall strength of the musculoskeletal system. As you progress through the four to six weeks of this strength-focused phase, you will recognize improvement in several areas. Next, you move on to the power phase, in which the focus is almost entirely based on developing, commanding, and using speed.

Upon completion of these initial three phases, you will then cycle back to a stability phase. Since the training focus over the past two to three months shifted in each of the successive phases, returning to stabilization will ensure continued maintenance of this critically important dynamic functional quality. As you start to organize your second round through all of the phases (beginning with stability-based training), it is important to add variety with regard to the above-mentioned variables (exercise selection, reps, sets, intensity, etc.). This will ensure progressive adaptation. An example might be shifting from straightforward, ground-based elbow plank activities, which you will have mastered during your first stability sequence, to progressively more challenging exercises such as a stability ball elbow plank or other unstable and asymmetrical stabilization choices. Remember, this same conceptual protocol will be applied through the strength and power phases as well. Pay close attention when selecting exercises. For example, if you were overly challenged with a simple ground-based elbow plank, it would not be prudent to select a highly challenging unstable drill for the second go-around. As you become more and more familiar with the exercises in the book you will become adept at choosing those drills with a similar intensity. Not only does the body adapt more readily to drill variety, but it will also avert boredom.

In each of the exercise chapters (6 through 17), there are logical progressions in addition to judicious regressions to aid you in this adaptive process. You can choose to follow the exercises as outlined in this book, or as your understanding of the program concepts and confidence with the methodology expands, you can select additional exercises, including some we have not presented in this book.

UNDERSTANDING THE PROGRAM PHASES

View the phases that follow as a spectrum of progressiveness: proximal to distal, slow to fast, stable to unstable, load absent to load present. In other words, move from low classification to highly concentrated intensities. The program phases will be systematic and developmentally efficient. Variables that will be manipulated include exercise selection, body positioning, load considerations, planes of movement, intensity, frequency, and duration. Progression will be predicated on previous successes (primarily with exercise performance accuracy) and periodic testing. Finally, the phases follow a global functioning perspective with regard to the entire muscle contraction continuum (force reduction, isometric and force production). Regardless of the exercise selection, unloaded or loaded, stable or unstable, or any other variable you add, always retain proper fundamental mechanics.

The foundation is the least aesthetically appealing aspect of a house, but the structure above would not be functionally achievable without the substructure's sturdiness. Likewise, because of the less than dynamic nature of the majority of the activities, stability training is sometimes viewed as the least exciting of the three program phases. Most athletes find it more stimulating and innately fulfilling to do exercises that require movement, increasing loads, or the slamming of a medicine ball onto the ground. This is why even fitness enthusiasts and seasoned professionals alike tend to neglect training for stability and opt instead for the more sexy movement-oriented drills. Many people, especially those just starting a core program, plunge directly into the strength phase of their training—directed by any combination of individual comfort level, irrational misinformation from ill-intentioned physiotherapists, or nefarious product promises that ultimately do not live up to their claims. As we have stated repeatedly, working strength before stability is reckless and often leads to developmental setbacks and heightened injury potential.

Interestingly, many individuals never advance to the power-training phase, choosing instead to work only strength. It is true that power training should not be taken lightly, and that the body must be well prepared before attempting it. But the hard work involved in the previous phases, stability and strength, will sufficiently lay the groundwork for progressing to power. Do not let the explosive nature of the power drills deter you. Instead, view them as a necessary and essential piece of the complete core puzzle. As we age, our power levels diminish, and as we move into our later years, the deficiency of explosive vigor can detrimentally affect our quality of life. Power is relative to the individual, and can have far-different motivations—compare three-time Olympic and world champion weightlifter Pyrros Dimas, who wants to dominate his competition, with an elderly person who, when necessary, wants to get out of the way of an oncoming bus. Although it should be respected and earned, power training can be fun, and it is essential for success in the athletic world.

So that you clearly understand their purposes within the program philosophy and why each component is synergistically essential to the successful outcome of the total design, we will now review all three phases—stability, strength, and power—with additional detail. The level of importance for each phase is moment specific. You have undoubtedly heard the adage, "Live in the moment." For our purposes, the importance of the moment is the demarcated progression of advancing from stability to strength and from strength to power, and then repeating the cycle as development dictates.

The most important phase is always the one you are presently in. Progressing through the program is dependent upon mastery of the exercises at the previous phase. If you maintain a singular focus on one specific phase, or for that matter, one specific exercise, to the exclusion of the others, the probable results will be inefficient movement patterns and methodological deficiencies. Thus the crucial aspect of the program is the collective completion of each phase in its entirety. Along the way, and as you cycle through the phases again and again, you will always freshly appreciate your improved athleticism on the court, on the field, or in the backyard.

Stability Phase

Stability is one of the most important yet sadly misunderstood elements necessary for both heightened athletic performance and maintaining a healthy lifestyle. Most of us have heard the statistics from the massive quantities of research on the topic: 80 percent of us will suffer debilitating back pain at some point during our adult lives. Some 16 million adults—8 percent of all adults—experience persistent or chronic back pain, and as a result are limited in certain everyday activities.

As we have emphasized though, the back is often the most neglected part of the core-training continuum. Stability training is an essential foundation for every other part of athletic success. It is inaccurately burdened with the identity of static positions sustained for extended periods of time, which, while indeed an element of stability, does not fully represent its dynamic functionality within a comprehensive athletic context. Prominent physical therapist Charlie Weingroff provides us with an insightful perspective of stability, defining it as "the ability of a joint system to maintain position in the presence of change." With this acumen strongly influencing our philosophy, the following program will both statically and actively challenge the deep stabilizers typically associated with osteoarticular equilibrium to maintain postural alignment and dynamic postural efficiency during functional movement patterns. If we can accomplish this challenging task and then link it to strength and power, we will have laid the groundwork for a championship contender.

Take a look at the corresponding stability guidelines. As with the other program phases, stability training covers a four- to six-week cycle. The core musculature generally tends to be slow-twitch, which dictates the suggested repetition range. In addition, some movements are classified as total-body or complex exercises. Thus there might be as many as six or seven movement variations within the same exercise. We will identify these exercises on a drill-by-drill basis with a suggested repetition range specific to that particular complex. To keep the training session progressing smoothly and to maintain athlete productivity and focus, the various core regions should be executed in a circuit procedure. This system of training is sometimes called *supersetting*, in which one drill moves directly into the next with no rest interval. The prescribed rest interval will follow each cycle. However, if you ever need to rest in order to ensure proper technique with subsequent exercises, then by all means, *rest*. Never sacrifice mechanics for any reason; if a brief rest is necessary to maintain accuracy, then rest is warranted.

Stability Phase Guidelines

- **Phase duration:** 4 to 6 weeks
- **Session frequency per week:** Minimum of 3 (not to exceed 6)
- **Repetition range:** 10 to 20 reps
- **Timed exercise duration (if applicable):** 15 seconds to 3 minutes
- **Circuit repetition:** 3 or 4 cycles, with 30-second rest between cycles

Note: Drill selection can remain constant or can vary from session to session or even set to set.

For a sample stability circuit, see table 19.1. Remember, these are just examples. Your exercise selection, sets, and time or rep intervals will vary.

Table 19.1 Stability Phase

Region	Exercise	Sets	Time or reps
Anti-extension	Elbow Plank	3	35 seconds
Anti-rotation	Rolling Pattern I Soft Roll, Upper Body	3	12 reps, 6 each side
Scapulothoracic	Prone Scapular Retraction and Depression (A), Incline Bench	3	12 reps
Lumbo-pelvic hip complex	Unilateral Bridge	3	12 reps each side

Strength Phase

As we discussed in chapter 18, on completion of the stability phase, there will be a retest before the strength phase begins. Once you pass the testing you are now ready to move into the strength phase.

We can increase the level of difficulty of an exercise in many ways. Simply increasing the proprioceptive requirement by using a multisensory environment makes a relatively simple drill more complicated. Shifting the drill from stable to unstable, adding perturbation techniques, tossing a ball to the athlete while in a challenging posture, or any other type of multimodal manipulation is often more substantially valuable than increasing external load. Thus, in this phase, the progressive distinction of increasing intensity might range from discreetly manipulating the weight of the body or as demanding as moving against an external load such as a cable weight stack column.

Refer to the corresponding strength guidelines. The repetition range will be lower than in the stability phase, whereas the time for isometric-based (static) exercises will again be predicated on individual capability, as screened through the tests in chapter 18. When selecting appropriate load, use good critical judgment; additional weight should challenge the exercise but not impair overall form. In other words, never sacrifice technique or postural control for additional reps, sets, or supplemental load. As with the other two phases, the strength phase is performed in circuit fashion of three to four rotations with minimal breaks between each. Safety considerations regarding precise technique always apply.

Within the strength exercises, you will find a group labeled "total core." These complex exercises aggressively challenge each of the areas outlined throughout the text. Although all our exercises are globally focused, some will suggest an anatomical emphasis. These exercises will be apparent and are necessary for establishing a global foundation and, ultimately, performance efficiency. The total-core exercises are far more inclusive in nature. Outside of their physical impact, doing these exercises is useful for many reasons; for the more advanced athlete, they can be included in a typical circuit.

Because of its large blood supply in the region, the core repairs rapidly, lending to quick recovery. Thus when you have suitably prepared yourself through training in the stability phase and have passed the retests, advancing into the strength phases with a focus on higher volume training (from either sets, reps, or duration or a combination or all three) is warranted. Also, in some cases you can pair a total-core exercise with

Strength Phase Guidelines

- **Phase duration:** 4 to 6 weeks
- **Session frequency per week:** Minimum of 3 (not to exceed 6)
- **Repetition range:** 10 to 15 reps
- **Timed exercise duration (if applicable):** 15 seconds to 1 minute
- **Circuit repetition:** 3 or 4 cycles, with 30-second rest between cycles

Note: Drill selection can remain constant or can vary from session to session or even set to set.

Table 19.2   Strength Phase

Region	Exercise	Sets	Time or reps
Anti-extension	Plank on Stability Ball: Stir the Pot	4	10 reps, 5 each side
Anti-rotation	Pallof Press Progression 1: Half-Kneeling Isometric	4	10 reps, 5 each side
Scapulothoracic	Band Pull Apart	4	10 reps
Lumbo-pelvic hip complex	Hip Lift, Shoulders Elevated	4	10 reps each side
Total core	Bilateral Waiter's Walk	4	10 steps

an anatomical region that might need emphasis. An example would be pairing the Turkish Get-Up (see chapter 14) with Prone YTA movement (chapter 12).

Many people are short on time. When necessary (while not ideal), you can use one or more total-core exercises for an entire core workout. If you do this, you will need to do multiple sets. Doing three or four sets of one total-core exercise is not enough to effect positive adaptive change. Upward of six sets would certainly be apt.

For a sample strength circuit (including total core), see table 19.2. Remember, these are just examples. Your exercise selection, sets, and time or rep intervals will vary.

Power Phase

The power phase will begin after successfully testing to determine readiness. The important element in this phase is speed of movement, so the weight you select must reflect your ability to control the load quickly. Too heavy will equal too slow a movement and will provide minimal benefit. Of course the weight you select should never control *you*.

Refer to the corresponding power guidelines. Adhering to the previous guideline parameters, the rep range for the power phase is again lower than in the stability and strength phases. No exercises outlined in the power section involve static movement isometrics, so programming

time will not be an issue. The entire power set moves in a circuit of three or four cycles, with 60-second breaks.

Note that at this stage there are no prescribed scapulothoracic exercises. Explosively drawing back your shoulder blades in an isolated fashion is generally not a good idea, primarily because it puts many of the supporting structures of the shoulder girdle at risk. Additionally, during many of the power exercises, the scapulothoracic musculature plays a key role in an integrated fashion and thus requires no additional stress.

For a sample power circuit, see table 19.3. Remember, these are just examples. Your exercise selection, sets, and time or rep intervals will vary.

Power Phase Guidelines

- **Phase duration:** 4 to 6 weeks
- **Session frequency per week:** Minimum of 3 (not to exceed 4)
- **Repetition range:** 5 to 10 reps
- **Set recovery:** 90 seconds between sets
- **Circuit repetition:** 3 or 4 cycles, with 60-second rest between cycles

Note: Drill selection can remain constant or can vary from session to session or even set to set.

Table 19.3 Power Phase

Region	Exercise	Sets	Time or reps
Anti-extension	Overhead Medicine Ball Slam	4	8 reps
Anti-rotation	Tornado Ball Twist	4	8 reps
Lumbo-pelvic hip complex	Power Step-Up	4	16 reps, 8 each leg

BASIC PROGRAM TENETS

For ease of understanding and to help identify the important tenets of our core program, use the following list as a quick-check reference guide:

- The program is functionally cyclical and constantly rotates through each phase.
- Testing establishes an appropriate starting point.
- Each phase lasts between four and six weeks.
- Exercise selection should vary throughout the entire phase. Variety might be as simple as changing the exercise from session to session or as complex as changing the exercise from set to set within the session. One recommendation, however: If you have less than perfect technique in the attempted drill, stick with that drill until mastery dictates the selection of another drill.
- Exercises follow a circuit format.
- A 30-second break is taken between each of the stability- and strength-phase circuits; a 90-second break is taken during the power-phase circuits.
- Successful completion of the preceding test is required before advancing into that specific phase
- Stability rep range is 10 to 20; strength rep range is 10 to 15; power rep range is 5 to 10.
- Isometric-focused exercises have a minimum duration time of 15 seconds and a maximum length of 3 minutes.
- Circuit set range is 3 or 4.
- Technique or postural control is never sacrificed for additional reps, sets, duration, supplemental load, or shortened rest interval.

In chapter 20 we present more advanced sample programs for you to get a feel for the training system and better understand the effective flow of the phases. Ultimately, you are looking to be appropriately challenged throughout, never accepting the status quo and always pursuing excellence.

Advanced Core Programs

In this chapter we provide a number of sample workouts. Our intent is to establish a format and to represent a variety of scenarios that allows for a broad spectrum of training possibilities. Note that these are *sample* workouts. Your program will absolutely vary. Be creative! There are a lot of exercises in the book to choose from.

BASIC TEMPLATE

The model shown in tables 20.1 to 20.3 illustrates the rhythm and flow of a complete core system throughout three cycles (a 12- to 18-week period).

The initial stability phase (table 20.1) is concise yet critical. Do not overlook its value just because it seems less than demanding at times. Stabilization qualities are necessary to optimize dynamic postural control and ultimately maximize functional efficiency throughout the kinetic chain. At the conclusion of the four to six weeks, you will be required to retest to ensure you possess adequate strength development and the mechanical precision necessary to advance safely to the strength phase (table 20.2). The strength phase is more progressively challenging than the stability phase. A point of safety bears repeating: Never progress to more advanced exercises at the sacrifice of technique. Proper mechanics are paramount. We cannot emphasize this enough. Added reps, sets, stability challenges, velocity, accelerative or decelerative properties, rest intervals (or lack thereof), or any other challenge to make the drill more difficult must never be implemented without mastering the previous level of difficulty beforehand. Remember that periodic testing is necessary for assessment before advancing from stability to strength or strength to power (table 20.3). Use the tests presented in chapter 18.

Table 20.1 Stability Phase 1 (4 to 6 Weeks): Basic Template

Region	Exercise	Sets	Time or reps
Anti-extension	Elbow Plank	3	15-30 sec
Anti-rotation	Lateral Elbow Plank, Feet Elevated	3	15-25 sec each side
Scapulothoracic	Prone Scapular Retraction and Depression (A), Floor	3	15 reps
Lumbo-pelvic hip complex	Bridge on Floor With Resistance Band	3	15 reps

Table 20.2 Strength Phase 1 (4 to 6 Weeks): Basic Template

Region	Exercise	Sets	Time or reps
Anti-extension	Plank on Stability Ball: Rock the Cradle	3	12
Anti-rotation	Cable Chop Progression 1: Half-Kneeling	3	12 each side
Scapulothoracic	Prone Loaded Scapular Retraction and Depression (A), Incline Bench	3	12
Lumbo-pelvic hip complex	Hip Lift, Shoulders Elevated	3	12

Table 20.3 Power Phase 1 (4 to 6 Weeks): Basic Template

Region	Exercise	Sets	Time or reps
Anti-extension	Overhead Medicine Ball Slam Progression 1: Tall Kneeling	3	10
Anti-rotation	Medicine Ball Chop Slam Progression 1: Half-Kneeling	3	10 each side
Lumbo-pelvic hip complex	Box Hop Up	3	10 each leg

After progressing through the workouts in tables 20.1 through 20.3, you have completed 12 to 18 weeks of training, which is a fantastic accomplishment. Now for a bit of a conjectural shift. Our experience has shown that to avoid the possibility of languishing on a training plateau or, worse yet, experiencing a performance regression as a result of stagnation, you must cycle back through each phase, but at an increasingly demanding intensity (tables 20.4 to 20.6). In addition to increased intensity, make sure you continue to alter the exercise selection, which will further help to challenge the body's adaptive qualities (from a physiologic and movement diversity standpoint). The body modifies more readily to a program that includes an array of unique challenges rather than the same drill performed time and again. For example, once you've mastered the elbow plank, it is superfluous to continue the same exercise for the next two months. Increasing the intensity, adding load, or incorporating instability will further challenge the functional system. Or simply change the exercise.

The body is capable of an infinite number of movement combinations, so it is not prudent to train only one. Therefore, be creative with your exercise selection. Remember, as long as you follow the aforementioned guidelines—*stability before strength, strength before power,* and include the necessary *regions* within the structured template format—you have complete control over the exercises to include within a phase, within a session, and within the sets. In other words, you can pick an exercise and perform it for the entirety of the 4 to 6 week phase (not the best option). Or you could pick an exercise and perform the prescribed number of sets for that session and then change the exercise for the next session (solid option). Or you could perform a different exercise for each of the sets within the session (requires some planning, but this is our favorite option). However, never rehearse a bad habit! After a couple of sessions, if you are still unable to perform the exercise that you have chosen with good mechanics, then rethink including that particular exercise until you have sufficient strength and body control to allow for enhanced performance.

By the end of the second round of phases, you will have experienced a profound functional adaptation to your core. The results should be visible, but more importantly, you should begin to recognize a noticeable improvement in the efficiency and functionality of movement patterns and additionally measured athletic performance variables. At the end of this second cycle, you will have completed 24 to 36 weeks of training. As you begin your third cycle through the phases (tables 20.7 to 20.9), your selection of exercises should follow the same increasing intensity and varietal flow as the previous two cycles but be more demanding.

Table 20.4 Stability Phase 2 (4 to 6 Weeks): Basic Template

Region	Exercise	Sets	Time or reps
Anti-extension	Elbow Plank, Unstable Lower, Feet Elevated	4	20-30 sec
Anti-rotation	Lateral Elbow Plank, Unstable Upper, Feet Elevated	4	15-20 sec each side
Scapulothoracic	Prone Scaption (Y), Floor	4	12
Lumbo-pelvic hip complex	Unilateral Bridge	4	12 each leg

Table 20.5 Strength Phase 2 (4 to 6 Weeks): Basic Template

Region	Exercise	Sets	Time or reps
Anti-extension	Rollout: Dolly	4	12
Anti-rotation	Cable Chop Progression 2: Tall Kneeling	4	12 each side
Scapulothoracic	Prone Loaded Scaption (Y), Incline Bench	4	12
Lumbo-pelvic hip complex	Hip Lift With Resistance Band, Shoulders Elevated	4	12

Table 20.6 Power Phase 2 (4 to 6 Weeks): Basic Template

Region	Exercise	Sets	Time or reps
Anti-extension	Overhead Medicine Ball Slam Progression 2: Standing	4	10
Anti-rotation	Medicine Ball Chop Slam Progression 2: Tall Kneeling	4	10 each side
Lumbo-pelvic hip complex	Ice Skater	4	10 each side

Table 20.7 Stability Phase 3 (4 to 6 Weeks): Basic Template

Region	Exercise	Sets	Time or reps
Anti-extension	Plank, Suspended Upper	4	20-30 sec
Anti-rotation	Lateral Elbow Plank, Unstable Upper, Arm and Leg Abduction, Feet Elevated	4	15-20 sec each side
Scapulothoracic	Prone Scapulothoracic Combination (YTA), Floor	4	12
Lumbo-pelvic hip complex	Single-Leg Bridge on Stability Ball	4	12 each leg

Table 20.8 Strength Phase 3 (4 to 6 Weeks): Basic Template

Region	Exercise	Sets	Time or reps
Anti-extension	Rollout: Ab Wheel	4	12
Anti-rotation	Cable Chop Progression 3: Standing	4	12 each side
Scapulothoracic	Prone Loaded Scapulothoracic Combination (YTA), Incline Bench	4	12
Lumbo-pelvic hip complex	Hip Lift, Shoulders Elevated, Single Leg	4	12 each leg

Table 20.9 Power Phase 3 (4 to 6 Weeks): Basic Template

Region	Exercise	Sets	Time or reps
Anti-extension	Overhead Medicine Ball Slam Progression 4: Standing With Wind-Up	4	10 each side
Anti-rotation	Medicine Ball Chop Slam Progression 3: Standing	4	10 each side
Lumbo-pelvic hip complex	Medial Box Hop Up	4	10 each side

The previous workout plan provides an efficient, integrated template to move you closer to achieving your goals. However, realistically speaking, it is unlikely that the initial stages of this or any program will be entirely regular. Nothing ever goes exactly as planned. In the remainder of this chapter we present workouts and guidelines for dealing with unpredictable situations and peculiarities that will undoubtedly arise.

BEGINNER: MINIMAL TRAINING EXPERIENCE

Do not be disappointed if the tests in chapter 18 indicate starting at the beginner level with stability training. Honestly, this is where most core neophytes begin. Likewise, do not be alarmed if you find yourself back in this category if you do not pass the retest and are required to do a second four to six weeks of stability training. Additional stabilization is not to your eternal detriment—it is simply your body letting you know that your foundation is not quite yet established to advance on. Proper development of your core musculature promotes the subsequent and more rapid adaptation of the core complex and its resultant involvement in athletic performance. A lifetime of evolving workouts is ahead of you, so give your body a chance to adapt to the stress that will be imposed.

The following template (tables 20.10 to 20.16) is an example of an athlete who completed the initial stability phase, failed the retest, and was required to do a second four to six weeks of stability training before moving to the strength phase. If it wasn't done the first time through, this individual should manipulate the variables of exercise selection, intensity, and proprioceptive challenges. While the testing is important to assess progress as measured against a baseline of performance, it will not fully disclose global core development. Therefore, to reiterate, a variety of training will accelerate adaptation, and improvements should be disclosed with subsequent testing.

Test: FAIL

Table 20.10 Stability Phase 1(4 to 6 Weeks): Beginner

Region	Exercise	Sets	Time or reps
Anti-extension	Elbow Plank	3	20-30 sec
Anti-rotation	Rolling Pattern 1	3	12 each side
Scapulothoracic	Prone Shoulder Abduction (T), Floor	3	12
Lumbo-pelvic hip complex	Bridge on Floor	3	12

Retest: FAIL

Table 20.11 Stability Phase 2 (4 to 6 Weeks): Beginner

Region	Exercise	Sets	Time or reps
Anti-extension	Elbow plank, Feet Elevated	4	20-30 sec
Anti-rotation	Rolling Pattern 1: Soft Roll, Upper Body	4	12 each side
Scapulothoracic	Prone Shoulder Abduction (T), Incline Bench	4	12
Lumbo-pelvic hip complex	Bridge on Floor With Resistance Band	4	12

Retest: PASS

Table 20.12   Strength Phase 1 (4 to 6 Weeks): Beginner

Region	Exercise	Sets	Time or reps
Anti-extension	Rollout: Stability Ball, Kneeling	3	12
Anti-rotation	Pallof Isometric Press Progression 1: Half-Kneeling	3	15-20 sec each side
Scapulothoracic	Prone Loaded Shoulder Abduction (T), Incline Bench	3	12
Lumbo-pelvic hip complex	Hip Lift, Shoulders Elevated	3	12

Table 20.13   Power Phase 1 (4 to 6 Weeks): Beginner

Region	Exercise	Sets	Time or reps
Anti-extension	Overhead Medicine Ball Slam Progression 1: Tall Kneeling	3	10
Anti-rotation	Medicine Ball Side Throw Progression 1: Half-Kneeling	3	10 each side
Lumbo-pelvic hip complex	Box Hop Down	3	10 each leg

Table 20.14   Stability Phase 3 (4 to 6 Weeks): Beginner

Region	Exercise	Sets	Time or reps
Anti-extension	Elbow Plank, Unstable Lower, Feet Elevated	4	20-30 sec
Anti-rotation	Rolling Pattern 2	4	12 each side
Scapulothoracic	Prone Shoulder Abduction (T), Stability Ball	4	12
Lumbo-pelvic hip complex	Bridge on Stability Ball	4	12

Table 20.15   Strength Phase 2 (4 to 6 Weeks): Beginner

Region	Exercise	Sets	Time or reps
Anti-extension	Rollout: Dolly	4	12
Anti-rotation	Pallof Isometric Press Progression 2: Tall Kneeling	4	15-20 sec each side
Scapulothoracic	Band Pull Apart	4	12
Lumbo-pelvic hip complex	Hip Lift With Resistance Band, Shoulders Elevated	4	12

Table 20.16   Power Phase 2 (4 to 6 Weeks): Beginner

Region	Exercise	Sets	Time or reps
Anti-extension	Overhead Medicine Ball Slam Progression 2: Standing	4	8
Anti-rotation	Medicine Ball Side Throw Progression 2: Tall Kneeling	4	8 each side
Lumbo-pelvic hip complex	Single-Leg Power Step-Up	4	8 each leg

INTERMEDIATE: MODERATE TRAINING EXPERIENCE

If your chapter 18 test results indicate that you can begin your program with the strength phase, follow the template outlined in tables 20.17 to 20.25. Do not be afraid to challenge yourself; always keep in mind that proper form is crucial, but be prepared to push the envelope. Remember, be creative. Include a variety of drills and challenges.

Test: PASS

Table 20.17 Strength Phase 1 (4 to 6 Weeks): Intermediate

Region	Exercise	Sets	Time or reps
Anti-extension	Slideboard Feet: Elbow Bodysaw	3	10
Anti-rotation	Landmine Rotation	3	5 each side
Scapulothoracic	Band Pull Apart	3	10
Lumbo-pelvic hip complex	Overhead Squat Series Progression 1: Prisoner Squat With Resistance Band	3	10

Table 20.18 Power Phase 1 (4 to 6 Weeks): Intermediate

Region	Exercise	Sets	Time or reps
Anti-extension	Overhead Medicine Ball Slam Progression 1: Tall Kneeling	3	10
Anti-rotation	Medicine Ball Parallel Throw Progression 1: Half-Kneeling	3	10 each side
Lumbo-pelvic hip complex	Box Hop Up	3	10 each leg

Table 20.19 Stability Phase 1 (4 to 6 Weeks): Intermediate

Region	Exercise	Sets	Time or reps
Anti-extension	Straight-Arm Plank, Single-Leg Hip Abduction	3	15-20 sec each leg
Anti-rotation	Prone Rotary Stability Progression 1: Single-Leg Hip Extension	3	12 each leg
Scapulothoracic	Prone Scapulothoracic Combination (YTA), Floor	3	12
Lumbo-pelvic hip complex	Foundational Core Squat Series Progression 1: Prisoner Squat	3	12

Table 20.20 Strength Phase 2 (4 to 6 Weeks): Intermediate

Region	Exercise	Sets	Time or reps
Anti-extension	Slideboard Feet: Straight-Arm Bodysaw	4	10
Anti-rotation	Landmine Rotation With Handle	4	5 each side
Scapulothoracic	Prone Loaded Scapulothoracic Combination (YTA), Incline Bench	4	10
Lumbo-pelvic hip complex	Overhead Squat Series Progression 3: Weighted Overhead Squat	4	10

Table 20.21 Power Phase 2 (4 to 6 Weeks): Intermediate

Region	Exercise	Sets	Time or reps
Anti-extension	Overhead Medicine Ball Slam Progression 2: Standing	4	10
Anti-rotation	Medicine Ball Parallel Throw Progression 2: Tall Kneeling	4	10 each side
Lumbo-pelvic hip complex	Box Hop Down	4	10 each leg

Table 20.22 Stability Phase 2 (4 to 6 Weeks): Intermediate

Region	Exercise	Sets	Time or reps
Anti-extension	Straight-Arm Plank, Single-Leg Hip Abduction, Feet Elevated	4	15-20 sec each leg
Anti-rotation	Prone Rotary Stability Progression 2: Single-Leg Full Flexion	4	12 each leg
Scapulothoracic	Prone Scapulothoracic Combination (YTA), Incline Bench	4	12
Lumbo-pelvic hip complex	Single-Leg Balance	4	20-30 sec each leg

Table 20.23 Strength Phase 3 (4 to 6 Weeks): Intermediate

Region	Exercise	Sets	Time or reps
Anti-extension	Dolly Walks	4	10 steps
Anti-rotation	Landmine Rotation With Handle and Load	4	5 each side
Scapulothoracic	Prone Loaded Scapulothoracic Combination (YTA), Stability Ball	4	10
Lumbo-pelvic hip complex	Overhead Squat Series Progression 5: Single-Arm Weighted Overhead Squat	4	10 reps

Table 20.24 Power Phase 3 (4 to 6 Weeks): Intermediate

Region	Exercise	Sets	Time or reps
Anti-extension	Overhead Medicine Ball Slam With Rotation, Progression III: Lunge Position	4	8 each side
Anti-rotation	Medicine Ball Parallel Throw Progression 3: Standing	4	8 each side
Lumbo-pelvic hip complex	Medial Box Hop Down	4	8 each leg

Table 20.25 Stability Phase 3 (4 to 6 Weeks): Intermediate

Region	Exercise	Sets	Time or reps
Anti-extension	Straight-Arm Plank, Unstable Upper, Single-Leg Hip Abduction	4	15-20 sec each leg
Anti-rotation	Prone Rotary Stability Progression 3: Single-Leg Hip Internal Rotation and Tap	4	12 each side
Scapulothoracic	Prone Scapulothoracic Combination (YTA), Stability Ball	4	12
Lumbo-pelvic hip complex	Single-Leg Balance and Reach	4	12 each leg

ADVANCED: HIGH TRAINING EXPERIENCE

If you have made it this far, congratulations! You have demonstrated that you are at an advanced level of core development. Your foundation is evidently considerable, but the program that follows (tables 20.26 to 20.34) should further challenge both the inner and outer mobilizers. Remember that your body must be well prepared for the explosive activities of the power phase. Err on the side of caution. With osteoarticular control, you can now more fully develop your strength, power, proprioceptive awareness, and neuromuscular control essential for enhanced sports performance.

Test: PASS

Table 20.26   Strength Phase 1 (4 to 6 Weeks): Advanced

Region	Exercise	Sets	Time or reps
Anti-extension	Rollout: Ab Wheel	4	12
Anti-rotation	Landmine Rotation	4	6 each side
Scapulothoracic	Prone Loaded Scapulothoracic Combination (YTA), Incline Bench	4	12
Lumbo-pelvic hip complex	Lateral Band Slide	4	12 steps each side

Table 20.27   Power Phase 1 (4 to 6 Weeks): Advanced

Region	Exercise	Sets	Time or reps
Anti-extension	Overhead Medicine Ball Slam Progression 1: Tall Kneeling	4	10 each side
Anti-rotation	Medicine Ball Parallel Throw Progression 1: Half-Kneeling	4	10 each side
Lumbo-pelvic hip complex	Ice Skater	4	10 each leg

Table 20.28   Stability Phase 1 (4 to 6 Weeks): Advanced

Region	Exercise	Sets	Time or reps
Anti-extension	Elbow Plank Stationary Walk Out and Back	4	12 steps
Anti-rotation	Lateral Elbow Plank, Arm Abduction, Foot Taps	4	12 each side
Scapulothoracic	Prone Scaption (Y), Incline Bench	4	12
Lumbo-pelvic hip complex	Foundational Core Squat Series Progression 2: Overhead Squat	4	12

Table 20.29   Strength Phase 2 (4 to 6 Weeks): Advanced

Region	Exercise	Sets	Time or reps
Anti-extension	Mountain Climber: Slideboard, Unstable Upper	4	6 each leg
Anti-rotation	Landmine Rotation With Handle	4	6 each side
Scapulothoracic	Prone Loaded Scapulothoracic Combination (YTA), Incline Bench	4	12
Lumbo-pelvic hip complex	X-Band Walk	4	12 steps each side

Table 20.30   Power Phase 2 (4 to 6 Weeks): Advanced

Region	Exercise	Sets	Time or reps
Anti-extension	Overhead Medicine Ball Slam Progression 2: Standing	4	5 each side
Anti-rotation	Medicine Ball Parallel Throw Progression 2: Tall Kneeling	4	10 each side
Lumbo-pelvic hip complex	Single-Leg Power Step-Up	4	10 each leg

Table 20.31   Stability Phase 2 (4 to 6 Weeks): Advanced

Region	Exercise	Sets	Time or reps
Anti-extension	Straight-Arm Plank Stationary Walk Out and Back	4	12 steps
Anti-rotation	Lateral Straight-Arm Plank, Arm Abduction, Foot Taps	4	12 each side
Scapulothoracic	Prone Shoulder Abduction (T), Incline Bench	4	12
Lumbo-pelvic hip complex	Single-Leg Balance	4	20-30 sec each leg

Table 20.32   Strength Phase 3 (4 to 6 Weeks): Advanced

Region	Exercise	Sets	Time or reps
Anti-extension	Mountain Climber: Stability Ball, Elastic Band Resistance	4	6 each leg
Anti-rotation	Landmine Rotation With Handle and Load	4	6 each side
Scapulothoracic	Prone Loaded Scapulothoracic Combination (YTA), Stability Ball	4	12
Lumbo-pelvic hip complex	Lateral Band Slide, Straight Legs	4	12 steps each

Table 20.33   Power Phase 3 (4 to 6 Weeks): Advanced

Region	Exercise	Sets	Time or reps
Anti-extension	Overhead Medicine Ball Slam Progression 3: Tall Kneeling With Wind-Up	4	8 each side
Anti-rotation	Medicine Ball Parallel Throw Progression 3: Standing	4	8 each side
Lumbo-pelvic hip complex	Alternating Leg Power Step-Up	4	8 each leg

Table 20.34   Stability Phase 3 (4 to 6 Weeks): Advanced

Region	Exercise	Sets	Time or reps
Anti-extension	Elbow to Straight-Arm Plank Box Walk Up	4	12 steps
Anti-rotation	Lateral Elbow Plank, Arm Abduction, Knee Drive to Chest	4	12 each leg
Scapulothoracic	Prone Scapular Retraction and Depression (A), Incline Bench	4	12
Lumbo-pelvic hip complex	Single-Leg Balance and Reach	4	12 each leg

ADVANCING WITHIN FOUR TO SIX WEEKS

We hope that this protocol format allows you a level of comfort so that you will not require multiple cycles to advance from one level to the next. An exciting goal is for you to develop a kind of symbiotic relationship with the phases and exercise progressions. This inevitably leads to a desire to experiment within the phases. We encourage this type of thinking and believe you should continuously challenge yourself whenever possible. That said, you must stay within the constructed framework.

As an example, we will now reexamine what we presented earlier for the intermediate trainee with a mind to advance within each four- to six-week phase. In the following examples (tables 20.35 to 20.46), each of the first tables outlines a workout for two to four weeks, and each of the second an additional same-phase workout for three to six weeks. This shows you how to subtly change your workout by selecting harder exercises from the same group to push yourself within a given phase. If after two to four weeks you need to increase the exercise difficulty level, simply adjust as you go along and retest as needed.

During the initial phases of training, you will develop a good sense for exercise purpose and procedure. Core adaptation in the form of high-quality mechanics and precision in performance for each new exercise will also occur. You might find it necessary to advance progressively at a slower pace in order to better identify the key muscles and how they facilitate a specific function. As with any type of strength and conditioning protocol, accurate muscle influence must be specific to the desired outcome. Thus a greater intrinsic control of the core unit is necessary before advancing to progressively more difficult phases. Trust the system. Your improvement is built on a subsequent progression in which successive exercise endeavors and their intensities are based on preceding achievements. Proceed at a comfortable pace, and never advance to more difficult exercises without mastering the rudimentary exercises in the progression. Everyone advances at a different pace. Progression might be as subtle as marginally influencing body position through leg abduction or as significant as adding an external load such as a sandbag. Any progressive increase in balance, body control, neuromuscular efficiency, force generation, or the speed of that generation will result in better performance. Additionally, variety in your drill selection will assure that progress will be consistently progressive.

First and foremost, on securing superior levels of dynamic spinal stabilization, you must turn your core focus toward managing an external load (tables 20.35 and 20.36). In the weight room this can be done using plates and dumbbells, bands and cables, sandbags and medicine balls, and much more. Be smart with your exercise selection, but don't be reserved with your choice of equipment.

The importance of speed in the power equation, and ultimately to power performance, is significant to say the least. With this in mind, as exercise difficulty intensifies (tables 20.37 and 20.38) through any combination of challenges—such as including balance modalities, changing body position, or increasing load—it cannot be at the detriment of velocity.

Test: PASS

Table 20.35	Advancing Within Strength Phase 1 (2 to 4 Weeks)		
Region	Exercise	Sets	Time or reps
Anti-extension	Hanging L Series: Straight Legs to L and Return	3	10
Anti-rotation	Pull and Press Progression 1: Half-Kneeling	3	5 each side
Scapulothoracic	Band Pull-Apart	3	10
Lumbo-pelvic hip complex	Overhead Squat Series Progression 1: Prisoner Squat With Resistance Band	3	10

Table 20.36 Advancing Within Strength Phase 1 (3 to 6 Weeks)

Region	Exercise	Sets	Time or reps
Anti-extension	Hanging L Series: Alternating Straight Leg to L	3	10 each leg
Advancing the anti-extension exercise is simple initially by changing from a bilateral leg movement to a unilateral one.			
Anti-rotation	Pull and Press Progression 2: Tall Kneeling	3	5 each side
In the case of the anti-rotary exercise, instead of adding weight or increasing repetitions, it is appropriate to change lower body positioning from a half-kneeling position to a tall-kneeling position, entirely removing any assistance from the legs and thus increasing overall difficulty.			
Scapulothoracic	Band Pull-Apart	3	10
The Band Pull-Apart can be advanced in one of two ways: either by increasing the tension of the band by using a slightly thicker band (they are often colored-coded to represent tension) or by holding the band a little closer to the center on both sides.			
Lumbo-pelvic hip complex	Overhead Squat Series Progression 1: Prisoner Squat With Resistance Band	3	10
To advance the Prisoner Squat With Resistance Band, use a band with greater tension to increase the load requirement targeting the lateral hip musculature or, in the case of this example, add a further component of difficulty by performing an overhead squat. The act of stretching the arms overhead alters the dynamic effect on the entire core system (principally the back musculature) and also dramatically impacts the overall lumbo-pelvic hip complex.			

Table 20.37 Advancing Within Power Phase 1 (2 to 4 Weeks)

Region	Exercise	Sets	Time or reps
Anti-extension	Overhead Medicine Ball Slam Progression 1: Tall Kneeling	3	8
Anti-rotation	Medicine Ball Parallel Throw Progression 1: Half-Kneeling	3	8 each side
Lumbo-pelvic hip complex	Box Hop Up	3	8 each leg

Table 20.38 Advancing Within Power Phase 1 (3 to 6 Weeks)

Region	Exercise	Sets	Time or reps
Anti-extension	Overhead Medicine Ball Slam Progression 1: Tall Kneeling	3	8
For the entirety of this 3- to 6-week phase, you will remain in the tall kneeling position, but as strength improves, use progressively heavier medicine balls.			
Anti-rotation	Medicine Ball Parallel Throw Progression 1: Half-Kneeling	3	8 each side
Again, the appropriate progression for this exercise would be an increase in the weight of the medicine ball.			
Lumbo-pelvic hip complex	Box Hop Up	3	8 each leg
Depending on the height of the box chosen, during your first time through the power phase consider increasing the height to maximize the effort required to jump, land, and stabilize. However, be aware that jumping requires your body to handle four to six times the force of your body weight; prudent selection of box height is critical.			

The development of the greatest levels of neuromuscular control and stabilization helps provide an improved biomechanical position and a balanced muscular functioning of the entire kinetic chain. The extent of your neuromuscular control along with core stabilization factors will significantly affect postural control throughout the kinetic chain, thus facilitating efficient movement and heightened athletic performance. Compensation factors such as asymmetrical domination patterns, arthrokinetic inhibition, and variable postural control issues can be the result of this lack of dynamic control. All of this can in turn stress the musculoskeletal system and possibly initiate the pain–injury cycle.

The stability phase is predisposed to be inherently less demanding on the central nervous system. Thus progressions must be more challenging in complexity to ensure adaptation and continued neuromuscular control. Regardless of which level of stability training you are presently performing, maintaining proper dynamic control of your posture will certainly facilitate a positive influence toward preventing chronic postural alterations that can lead to injury. Although certainly an option, it is not always necessary to add external load to make drills progressive. Introducing instability variables, maneuvering the body, and including perturbation techniques will add challenges without adding load (tables 20.39 and 20.40).

Table 20.39　Advancing Within Stability Phase 1 (2 to 4 Weeks)

Region	Exercise	Sets	Time or reps
Anti-extension	Straight-Arm Plank, Single-Leg Hip Abduction	3	15-20 sec each leg
Anti-rotation	Prone Rotary Stability Progression 1: Single-Leg Hip Extension	3	12 each leg
Scapulothoracic	Prone Scapulothoracic Combination (YTA), Floor	3	12
Lumbo-pelvic hip complex	Foundational Core Squat Series Progression 1: Prisoner Squat	3	12

Table 20.40　Advancing Within Stability Phase 1 (3 to 6 Weeks)

Region	Exercise	Sets	Time or reps
Anti-extension	Straight-Arm Plank, Single-Leg Hip Extension, Feet Elevated	3	15-20 sec each leg
Make this exercise more difficult by raising the legs up. Extend one leg up slightly (not to the side in an adducted fashion), allowing the load to remain on only one leg.			
Anti-rotation	Prone Rotary Stability Progression 2: Single-Leg Full Flexion	3	12 each leg
This progression is as simple as switching from lifting the legs in an extension pattern to rotating through the hip with the leg flexed.			
Scapulothoracic	Prone Scapulothoracic Combination (YTA), Incline Bench	3	12
This is the same movement with the same concepts as the prone floor YTA but adds a bench to facilitate a more forward movement of the arms.			
Lumbo-pelvic hip complex	Foundational Core Squat Series Progression 2: Overhead Squat	3	6 each side
To advance the overhead squat, move from an evenly distributed two hands overhead to an asymmetrically loaded one hand overhead. This unilateral mechanic creates a new challenge for the core section to deal with and causes the ipsilateral hip musculature and contralateral adductor complex to work harder.			

Adaptation to stress imposed is directly proportional to the intensity of the imposition. As such, if you continuously train within your comfort zone, little, if any, adaptation will occur. Regular increases in intensity are necessary to ensure continued development. Thus as you initiate your second time through this phase, challenging yourself a little more and experimenting with your limits will both keep you motivated and create more of an overall effect (tables 20.41 to 20.46).

Table 20.41 Advancing Within Strength Phase 2 (2 to 4 Weeks)

Region	Exercise	Sets	Time or reps
Anti-extension	Mountain Climber: Slideboard	4	6 each leg
Anti-rotation	Landmine Rotation With Handle	4	6 each side
Scapulothoracic	Prone Loaded Scapulothoracic Combination (YTA), Incline Bench	4	12
Lumbo-pelvic hip complex	Overhead Squat Series Progression 3: Weighted Overhead Squat	4	12

Table 20.42 Advancing Within Strength Phase 2 (3 to 6 Weeks)

Region	Exercise	Sets	Time or reps
Anti-extension	Mountain Climber: Slideboard, Unstable Upper	4	12
To increase the difficulty of the mountain climber exercise, place the forearms on an additional piece of unstable apparatus.			
Anti-rotation	Landmine Rotation With Handle and Load	4	6 each side
As the name suggests, adding weight to make the exercise more challenging will increase the difficulty level without getting too far ahead of yourself.			
Scapulothoracic	Prone Loaded Scapulothoracic Combination (YTA), Stability Ball	4	12
In general, the prone bench YTA is a challenging exercise, so any additional changes should be well thought out, and proper form should always be retained. That said, if by the latter part of this phase of training you feel ready to add weight, you can do so.			
Lumbo-pelvic hip complex	Overhead Squat Series Progression 4: Weighted Overhead Squat With Resistance Band	4	12
Once the overhead component of the lift is mastered, adding a load to the lateral aspect of the hips is a simple but effective way of comfortably progressing without dramatically changing the nature of the lift.			

Table 20.43 Advancing Within Power Phase 2 (2 to 4 Weeks)

Region	Exercise	Sets	Time or reps
Anti-extension	Overhead Medicine Ball Slam Progression 2: Standing	4	10
Anti-rotation	Medicine Ball Parallel Throw Progression 2: Tall Kneeling	4	10 each side
Lumbo-pelvic hip complex	Box Hop Down	4	10 each leg

Table 20.44 Advancing Within Power Phase 2 (3 to 6 Weeks)

Region	Exercise	Sets	Time or reps
Anti-extension	Overhead Medicine Ball Slam Progression 4: Standing With Wind-Up	4	8 each side
The addition of the sledgehammer-type wind-up on each side will reduce momentum and create a different effect within the core, making this exercise slightly more challenging.			
Anti-rotation	Medicine Ball Parallel Throw Progression 2: Tall Kneeling	4	8 each side
Maintain the tall-kneeling position, but as with the first time through, begin to throw a heavier medicine ball.			
Lumbo-pelvic hip complex	Box Hop Down	4	10 each leg
When performing hopping or jumping activities, the act of landing requires dealing with force equal to five or six times your body weight, which comes back up from the ground through your body. In this activity, increasing the height of the box is a good way to increase the difficulty of the exercise, but this must be done carefully to allow your body to adapt to the increased level of gravitational stress.			

Table 20.45 Advancing Within Stability Phase 2 (2 to 4 Weeks)

Region	Exercise	Sets	Time or reps
Anti-extension	Straight-Arm Plank, Single-Leg Hip Abduction, Feet Elevated	4	15-20 sec each leg
Anti-rotation	Prone Rotary Stability Progression 2: Single-Leg Full Flexion	4	12 each arm
Scapulothoracic	Prone Scapulothoracic Combination (YTA), Incline Bench	4	12
Lumbo-pelvic hip complex	Single-Leg Balance	4	20-30 sec each leg

Table 20.46 Advancing Within Stability Phase 2 (3 to 6 Weeks)

Region	Exercise	Sets	Time or reps
Anti-extension	Straight-Arm Plank, Unstable Upper, Single-Leg Hip Extension, Feet Elevated	4	15-20 sec each leg
The challenge in this advancement comes from resting your arms on an unstable device such as a BOSU or stability ball. The exercise is challenging already, and adding greater instability creates additional demands.			
Anti-rotation	Prone Rotary Stability Progression 3: Single-Leg Hip Internal Rotation and Tap	4	12
Moving from progression 2 to 3 is an excellent way to advance here. In this exercise, you have gone from rotating a flexed leg outward to crossing the midline of the body and tapping the floor under the opposite hip.			
Scapulothoracic	Prone Scapulothoracic Combination (YTA), Stability Ball	4	12
As with the anti-extension exercise from this group, adding instability guarantees a positive physiological response to the task (as long as good form is maintained).			
Lumbo-pelvic hip complex	Single-Leg Balance and Reach	4	12 each leg
After you master statically holding a position on one leg, add movement. Reaching out gently in different directions with your free leg involves engaging many of the body's proprioceptive receptors and provides rapid neural feedback, forcing your body to remain stable while reaching out. This increases the difficulty simply and effectively.			

As always, focusing on what is warranted from each phase is important, but as your comfort level rises, so too will your ability and desire to extend yourself.

As the cycles progress, more and more variations are possible. Experiment, challenge yourself, and appreciate the specific adaptive process. The results will be worth it.

IN-SEASON ATHLETES

The serious athlete is always confronted with the important issue of how to organize a training schedule within a competitive season. An otherwise meticulously organized plan will more than likely be altered, expanded, or possibly altogether scrapped. As such, a structurally detailed training program has to evolve with the individual distinctiveness of the competitive season. Professional and scholarship athletes alike often find it problematic to organize their training phases in precise four- to six- week cycles, as is optimal in a periodization design. High-level athletes are often at the mercy of their game, practice, and travel schedules, so sticking to a proportionately organized program is sometimes impossible.

For our purposes, we will assume that these athletes have worked hard and followed the off-season core program as outlined in this book. We now want to provide a plan of action should they find themselves unable to adhere to the typical four- to six-week periodization phase.

We will use two examples from our own experience: the New York Knicks and the Siena College women's tennis team. The expectations of both teams are clear. During their off-seasons, or downtime, these athletes should steadfastly adhere to a total athletic development regime that places a strong emphasis on functional core development; however, once their competitive seasons begin, program scheduling becomes a challenge. For the Knicks, this period of time begins around training camp in October and can run through to the finals in June. The Siena women's tennis team's season is traditionally split from September through October, and then picks back up again from February until April, often with a week or two between matches.

To further explain our thought process on core training for in-season athletes, let's first examine the early portion of the Knicks' schedule from the 2010-2011 season (table 20.47). Remember, this table reflects the Knicks *core training* schedule, not other variables, such as regeneration,

conditioning, preventative techniques, total body strength and power, movement mechanics, or basketball-specific skill development. The schedule is a guide and should be individually adjusted.

While spending two decades in the NBA, I learned that no two seasons have ever had an identical or even similar game schedule, so in-season personal training schedules must be adjusted from year to year. Liberties will be taken in scheduling to ensure that during nongame days players are not overtraining and thus negatively affecting performance variables. An all too frequent and completely misguided approach to deflect this undesirable inevitability is to simply forego any unnecessary additional training that might result in a player performing less than optimally on game day. Over the years, many of our head coaches and, unfortunately, even some of our colleagues have believed that additional in-season training detracts from performance.

It is an interesting dichotomy. For example, during dynamic fundamental movements that will most certainly occur during a basketball game, players with a weak core will eventually experience chronic compensation injuries throughout the kinetic chain. These injuries could be upper-, lower-, or total-body focused. It is a vicious cycle, and unfortunately for the athlete, too much emphasis on *preservation* as opposed to *development* perpetuates kinetic chain weaknesses and musculoskeletal imbalances, ultimately leading to chronic injury cycles. A comprehensive core strength and stabilization program can reduce the occurrence and severity of injury and likely decrease the incidence of an incredible 85 percent of athletes who will experience low-back pain at some point in their career.

As mentioned, we both believe that when a training program is intelligently implemented, positive physiological adaptation can occur *during* the season—even in a season as hectic as the NBA's. Thus, manipulating frequency, intensity, and duration is paramount to ensure continued progress while minimizing the potential deleterious effects from fatigue. Doing nothing at all to maintain fresh legs and to keep players sharp will amount to detraining as the season grinds along. All of the benefits of the hard work during the off-season and preseason will vanish possibly when the team needs them the most—when heading into the playoffs. The worst possible scenario is one in which a team has a strong showing during the initial stages of the season, then chronic

Intensity Levels per Training Session

Level	Focus	Volume
High	Explosive power, strength, stability	Low to high, depending on focus
Moderate	Strength, stability	Moderate to high
Low	Stability	High (typically)
Off	N/A	N/A

Table 20.47   New York Knicks 2010-2011 Schedule, October and November

OCTOBER

Sunday	Monday	Tuesday	Wednesday	Thursday	Friday	Saturday
					1	2
3	4	5	6	7	8	9
10	11	12	13	14	15	16
17	18	19	20	21	22	23
24	25	26	27 Game @ Toronto	28	29 Game @ Boston	30 Game vs. Portland
31						

NOVEMBER

Sunday	Monday	Tuesday	Wednesday	Thursday	Friday	Saturday
	1	2 Game @ Orlando	3	4 Game @ Chicago	5 Game vs. Washington	6
7 Game vs. Philadelphia	8	9 Game @ Milwaukee	10 Game vs. Golden State	11	12 Game @ Minnesota	13
14 Game vs. Houston	15	16 Game @ Denver	17 Game @ Sacramento	18	19 Game @ Golden State	20 Game @ Los Angeles
21	22	23 Game vs. Charlotte	24 Game @ Charlotte	25	26	27 Game vs. Atlanta
28 Game @ Detroit	29	30 Game vs. New Jersey				

injuries start to rear their ugly head and keep key players off the court. Ultimately the team, which was considered a championship contender early on, barely makes the playoffs and is eliminated in the second round, ending in far worse shape in May, during the playoffs, than they were at tip-off during opening night in October. The teams that win championships are strong at the end of the season and keep their best players on the court.

The actual training calendar shown in table 20.47 is unique to the 2010-2011 season and will not be used during subsequent seasons. Modifications are required based on a team's unique situation and schedule. Circumstances that might interfere with a prescheduled training session cannot be foreseen, so adjustments will certainly be required. A double-overtime game, plane delays, community appearances, and interviews can take their toll on athletes' recovery processes. What they need most, in some cases, is sleep. There will always be another day for a high-intensity core workout. Sometimes recovery far outweighs any possible adaptation than can be gained from a single core-training session. The physical and mental fatigue of the athletes must always be considered before implementing any additional training, core training included. In short, be willing to adapt to the situation.

NBA basketball is a grueling schedule of games, practice, and travel that extends through an eight-month time span in cities all over the country. At the other end of the sporting spectrum, the Siena's women's tennis team for the most part plays at a regional level over a split season with fairly extensive noncompetitive gaps between matches. Their spring schedule from 2012 looks vastly different from the Knicks' with regard to options for core implementation (table 20.48). Considering these greater opportunities, the women's tennis program design would reflect more of a conventional periodization process with specific work–rest intervals and consistent intensity, frequency, and duration variables.

Early February is the end of the break between fall and spring seasons, so we put a lot of strength- and power-based work into the schedule. Once the matches start up, they are relatively sparse, so we can strategically place strength and power days around them. Conceptually, the matches themselves are power based, so during a heavy competitive period, such as in April, it makes sense for athletes not to focus on power in the weight room. At this point in the school year, the tennis players also tend to become fatigued, which affects thought process and recovery, suppresses the immune system, causes tissue breakdown, and alters eating and sleeping habits. Focusing on less taxing movements that aim to increase reaction, response, precision, ambidexterity, whole-brain thinking, and total body control is a great way to keep players fresh and motivated, while keeping injury rates low.

Table 20.48 Siena Women's Tennis Team 2011-2012 Schedule With Core Training Plan, February to April

FEBRUARY

Sunday	Monday	Tuesday	Wednesday	Thursday	Friday	Saturday
		1	2 Power	3	4 Power	5
6	7 Power	8	9 Power	10	11 Power	12
13	14 Strength	15	16 Strength	17	18 Stability	19 Home match
20	21 Strength	22	23 Strength	24	25 Strength	26
27 Away match	28 Stability					

(continued)

Table 20.48   (continued)

MARCH

Sunday	Monday	Tuesday	Wednesday	Thursday	Friday	Saturday
		1	2 Stability	3	4 Stability	5 Away match
6	7 Strength	8	9 Strength	10	11 Stability	12 Home match
13	14 Strength	15	16 Strength	17	18 Strength	19
20	21 Power	22.	23 Power	24	25 Power	26
27	28 Power	29	30 Power	31		

APRIL

Sunday	Monday	Tuesday	Wednesday	Thursday	Friday	Saturday
					1 Stability	2 Home match
3 Away match	4 Stability	5	6 Stability	7	8 Home match	9
10 Home match	11	12 Away match	13 Stability	14	15 Stability	16 Home match
17 Away match	18 Stability	19	20 Stability	21	22 MAAC*	23 MAAC*
24 MAAC*	25	26	27	28	29	30

*Metro Atlantic Athletic Conference Championships

The style of the stability workouts, for example, would be challenging but not drastically taxing (see table 20.49). The strength workouts in February and March would be a great time to use the complex focused total-body core exercises, particularly the Turkish get-up because of its shoulder stability component (table 20.50). The power exercises during these same months are focused and succinct, with carryover to the movement requirements of match play, such as standing throws (table 20.51).

Table 20.49   Stability Phase: February, March, and April

Region	Exercise	Sets	Time or reps
Anti-extension	Straight-Arm Plank, Suspended Upper	3	20-30 sec
Anti-rotation	Lateral Elbow Plank, Arm and Leg Abduction	3	15-20 sec each side
Scapulothoracic	Prone Scaption (Y), Incline Bench	3	12
Lumbo-pelvic hip complex	Single-Leg Hip Lift on Stability Ball	3	12 each leg

Table 20.50   Strength Phase: February and March

Region	Exercise	Sets	Time or reps
Total core	Turkish Get-Up	5	10 each side

Table 20.51   Power Phase: February and March

Region	Exercise	Sets	Time or reps
Anti-extension	Overhead Medicine Ball Slam Progression 3: Tall Kneeling With Wind-Up	3	8
Anti-rotation	Medicine Ball Parallel Throw Progression 3: Standing	3	8 each side
Lumbo-pelvic hip complex	Ice Skater	3	8 each leg

A great thing about this core program is that although parameters must be met for each phase, the program is flexible enough to be used by anyone at any time during any stage of the season. Challenge the core, and enjoy the results.

Sport-Specific Core Programs

Sport specificity is an interesting concept that has been taken too far by some members of the strength and conditioning community. Sport-specific training has little to do with mimicking actual sporting movements and much to do with appropriate athletic preparation and an individualized approach to training. The confusion often comes from the individuals involved who are not looking at the bigger physiological picture. For example, if increasing bat speed in baseball were as simple as picking up a heavier bat and swinging away wildly, baseball strength and conditioning coaches would be out of a job. The same is true for those who are seeking a faster jab in boxing and thus train by throwing punches with light dumbbells in their hands. The mistake here is that when holding a weight that is not going to be released (unlike a medicine ball), the body is actually working on braking and slowing down the movement. As the weighted punch extends outward, all the protective mechanisms throughout the shoulder and arm musculature engage to stop the shoulder from coming out of the socket or creating trauma in the elbow region. Thus this poorly selected exercise ends up slowing down jab speed instead of speeding it up.

In fact, sport-specific training can be any action specific to the movement patterns, energy systems, or strength and power requirements of a selected activity, including a given athlete's sport. If an athlete wants to train for her sport, she should not bowl to improve her free-throw shooting. However, she could execute sets of triceps extensions, perform three-ball juggling drills, or throw darts at a target to improve strength, coordination, and accuracy, respectively. This newly discovered athleticism can then be applied to the sport-specific task of shooting free throws. The focus on sport-specific training is not so much on a definitive action with some additional overload feature, but rather on training within the realm of physiological and biomechanical similarities. The emphasis of sport-specific training is more on muscle balance and kinesthetic awareness necessary to ensure proper functioning of the kinetic chain. Thus a scientifically based mechanical and physiological program that contains skill-specific components is essential to optimizing performance and preventing injury.

This type of thinking also applies to core training. Across the sporting landscape, athletes should be training their torso and hip regions in a cylindrical fashion with a stability to strength to power methodology. This should not change no matter the activity because force propagation and transmission between upper and lower limbs are present in all sports—even sports such as rowing, in which the transfer is not as obvious. For this reason, the layout and exercise selection for core programming can be similar from sport to sport. Volleyball and badminton are far-different activities, but both employ leg-driving motions combined with explosive overhead movements, so exercise programming for the two sports would have similarities. Following this line of thinking, Chauncey Billups and Chris Bosh are both exceptional NBA basketball players, but they have unique, individualized needs relating to their core functionality.

When designing a core-development program, the important thing to consider is not necessarily the athletic activity but the specifics of core functionality that must be highlighted because of the inherent nature of the sport, along with any individualized deficiencies unique to each athlete. To give you a better feel for how we want you to view sport-specific core training, we will outline two series of phases for some popular sports and some specific positions within those sports. For each of these sports, we will highlight areas of concern that would almost certainly be exposed by the tests in chapter 18 and how to go about attacking them. Note that these are sample workouts: Your program will absolutely vary. Be creative! There are a lot of drills in the book to choose from.

AMERICAN FOOTBALL, OFFENSIVE LINEMAN

An offensive lineman's typical anthropometry is a large frame carrying a substantial amount of body mass. His primary position responsibilities are protecting his quarterback from a charging defensive onslaught and creating openings to initiate an offensive attack. In doing so, his initial setup position is a three-point stance: on the balls of his feet, knees and hips flexed, and one hand on the ground at the line of scrimmage. The instant the ball is snapped, he explodes into action and, using his strong upper body supported by massive legs, pushes and shoves the opposing defensive lineman in a sort of Sumo style, trying to prevent him from breaking through to rush the quarterback or tackle the ball carrier.

The best of the best do their job amazingly well, but they do so at the cost of a tightened anterior hip girdle musculature (caused by their bent-over position), which, through reciprocal inhibition, reduces conveyance through the neural pathways and restricts gluteal complex action. Also, and perhaps more devastating to these athletes, being firmly planted while being powerfully pushed in the upper body leads to increased extension forces in the lumbar spine, causing disc and vertebral issues in their later years. With regard to areas of highlighted focus for core programming, we see a direct need for hip extension work and torso-based anti-extension exercises, particularly ones that incorporate movement of the upper body (tables 21.1 to 21.6).

Test: PASS

Table 21.1   Stability Phase 2 (4 to 6 Weeks): Football Offensive Lineman

Region	Exercise	Sets	Time or reps
Anti-extension	Straight-Arm Plank, Feet Elevated	4	60 sec
Anti-rotation	Prone Rotary Stability Progression 2: Single-Leg Full Flexion	4	12
Scapulothoracic	Prone Scapular Retraction and Depression (A), Incline Bench	4	12
Lumbo-pelvic hip complex	Unilateral Bridge	4	12 each leg

Test: PASS

Table 21.2   Strength Phase 1 (4 to 6 Weeks): Football Offensive Lineman

Region	Exercise	Sets	Time or reps
Anti-extension	Push-Up With Box, Skewed	4	6 each arm
Anti-rotation	Pallof Press Progression 1: Half-Kneeling Horizontal Press	4	20 sec each side
Scapulothoracic	Prone Loaded Scapular Retraction and Depression (A), Incline Bench	4	12
Lumbo-pelvic hip complex	Hip Lift With Resistance Band, Shoulders Elevated	4	12

Test: PASS

Table 21.3 Power Phase 1 (4 to 6 Weeks): Football Offensive Lineman			
Region	**Exercise**	**Sets**	**Time or reps**
Anti-extension	Overhead Medicine Ball Slam Progression 1: Tall Kneeling	4	8
Anti-rotation	Medicine Ball Parallel Throw Progression 1: Half-Kneeling	4	8 each side
Lumbo-pelvic hip complex	Single-Leg Power Step-Up	4	8 each leg

Test: PASS

Table 21.4 Stability Phase 3 (4 to 6 Weeks): Football Offensive Lineman			
Region	**Exercise**	**Sets**	**Time or reps**
Anti-extension	Straight-Arm Plank, Single-Leg Hip Extension	4	25 sec each leg
Anti-rotation	Prone Rotary Stability Progression 3: Single-Leg Hip Internal Rotation and Tap	4	12
Scapulothoracic	Prone Scapular Retraction and Depression (A), Stability Ball	4	12
Lumbo-pelvic hip complex	Bridge on Stability Ball	4	12

Test: PASS

Table 21.5 Strength Phase 2 (4 to 6 Weeks): Football Offensive Lineman			
Region	**Exercise**	**Sets**	**Time or reps**
Anti-extension	Push-Up, Unstable Upper With Asymmetrical Medicine Ball	4	6 each arm
Anti-rotation	Pallof Press Progression 2: Tall Kneeling Horizontal Press	4	20 sec each side
Scapulothoracic	Prone Loaded Scaption (Y), Incline Bench	4	12
Lumbo-pelvic hip complex	Hip Lift, Shoulders Elevated, Single Leg	4	12 each leg

Test: PASS

Table 21.6 Power Phase 2 (4 to 6 Weeks): Football Offensive Lineman			
Region	**Exercise**	**Sets**	**Time or reps**
Anti-extension	Overhead Medicine Ball Slam Progression 2: Standing	4	8
Anti-rotation	Medicine Ball Parallel Throw Progression 2: Tall Kneeling	4	8
Lumbo-pelvic hip complex	Power Step-Up	4	8

BASEBALL, PITCHER

Pitchers in all sports are a fascinating set of athletes. They have an incredible ability to manipulate their bodies in such a way as to produce 100 miles an hour of velocity. They come in all shapes and sizes with differing techniques and pitch specialties. When slowed down, their pitching action looks incredibly painful, but through the naked eye it is often a thing of fluid beauty.

What makes pitching so complicated is that the biomechanical manipulation leaves the body riddled with asymmetries. You can never predict an injury, but two of the three indicators of potential *reinjury* are asymmetries and former injury. Considering that research has shown that high percentages of asymptomatic professional baseball pitchers have abnormal labrum features and rotator cuff damage, this clearly leads to the assumption that the potential for *reinjury* is elevated. Because of these ever-present issues, baseball pitchers are at a higher risk for injury than athletes whose sporting events do not lead to such irregularities throughout their physiological systems. Unfortunately, all of this frequently leads to a hands-off approach in training these athletes; some consider pitchers to be regular athletes who

have a dominant skill and believe they should be left alone with the occasional ice bag! This could not be more mistaken, as we have discussed in part I of this book. Improving their overall athleticism, streamlining their core strength, and working with and around their asymmetrical issues will create pitchers who throw harder with more consistent accuracy and have a higher level of resiliency.

The tests in chapter 18 were not designed to show asymmetries, but you will nevertheless feel and see them, and they should be noted and dealt with using the two-to-one ratio of work described in chapter 18. This will likely be displayed in scapular retraction and depression strength from side to side, as well as a discrepancy in anti-rotary strength. Scapulothoracic strength and stability are critical to ensure a healthy shoulder, so this must be a major focus, along with improving the strength of the nonthrowing anti-rotators. Large differences will also be prevalent between the lead and pushoff legs. On the mound, pitchers are required to do one thing well, using one side of the body for many, many repetitions. As strength and conditioning professionals, it is our job to unwind the damage caused by this imbalance and make both sides function adequately. Tables 21.7 to 21.12 show sample core programming for pitchers.

Test: PASS

Table 21.7   Stability Phase 2 (4 to 6 Weeks): Baseball Pitcher

Region	Exercise	Sets	Time or reps
Anti-extension	Straight-Arm Plank, Suspended Upper	4	40 sec
Anti-rotation	Lateral Elbow Plank, Arm and Leg Abduction	4	20 sec each side
Scapulothoracic	Prone Scaption (Y), Floor	4	12
Lumbo-pelvic hip complex	Foundational Core Squat Series Progression 1: Prisoner Squat	4	12

Test: PASS

Table 21.8   Strength Phase 1 (4 to 6 Weeks): Baseball Pitcher

Region	Exercise	Sets	Time or reps
Anti-extension	Rollout: Dolly	4	12
Anti-rotation	Lateral Elbow Plank Cable Row, Feet Elevated	4	12 each arm
Scapulothoracic	Prone Loaded Scaption (Y), Incline Bench	4	12
Lumbo-pelvic hip complex	Overhead Squat Series Progression 2: Overhead Squat With Resistance Band	4	12

Test: PASS

Table 21.9 Power Phase 1 (4 to 6 Weeks): Baseball Pitcher

Region	Exercise	Sets	Time or reps
Anti-extension	Overhead Medicine Ball Slam Progression 3: Tall Kneeling With Wind-Up	4	8
Anti-rotation	Medicine Ball Chop Slam Progression 1: Half-Kneeling	4	8 each side
Lumbo-pelvic hip complex	Medial Box Hop Down	4	8 each leg

Test: PASS

Table 21.10 Stability Phase 3 (4 to 6 Weeks): Baseball Pitcher

Region	Exercise	Sets	Time or reps
Anti-extension	Straight-Arm Plank, Suspended Upper, Feet Elevated	4	30 sec
Anti-rotation	Lateral Elbow Plank, Unstable Upper	4	20 sec each side
Scapulothoracic	Prone Scapulothoracic Combination (YTA), Floor	4	12
Lumbo-pelvic hip complex	Foundational Core Squat Series Progression 2: Overhead Squat	4	12

Test: PASS

Table 21.11 Strength Phase 2 (4 to 6 Weeks): Baseball Pitcher

Region	Exercise	Sets	Time or reps
Anti-extension	Rollout: Ab Wheel	4	12
Anti-rotation	Lateral Straight-Arm Plank Cable Row, Feet Elevated	4	12 each arm
Scapulothoracic	Prone Loaded Scapulothoracic Combination (YTA), Incline Bench	4	6
Lumbo-pelvic hip complex	Overhead Squat Series Progression 5: ingle-Arm Weighted Overhead Squat	4	6 each arm

Test: PASS

Table 21.12 Power Phase 2 (4 to 6 Weeks): Baseball Pitcher

Region	Exercise	Sets	Time or reps
Anti-extension	Overhead Medicine Ball Slam Progression 4: Standing With Wind-Up	4	8
Anti-rotary	Medicine Ball Chop Slam Progression 2: Tall Kneeling	4	8 each side
Lumbo-pelvic hip complex	Medial Box Hop Up	4	8 each leg

BASKETBALL

Athletes who are most successful in basketball tend to be one of two somatotypes: ectomorph or mesomorph. The ectomorph is long and lean with little overall muscle mass. A true ectomorph has a straight-line appearance with a narrow waist, narrow chest, and narrow shoulders. Think of seven-foot center Marcus Camby of the NBA. A mesomorph, on the other hand, looks more athletic, with broad shoulders and a narrow waist. Athletes possessing this classic V shape include Australian surfer Claire Bevilacqua, LeBron James of the NBA's Miami Heat, and NFL football and MLB baseball great Bo Jackson.

When Dr. William H. Sheldon introduced the concept of body types in the 1940s, doctors, researchers, coaches, and physical therapists began to individualize training and nutritional plans based on an individual's body type. However, it is rare that a person falls strictly into one classification without exhibiting signs of one or both of the others. Most people possess varying combinations of all three somatotypes (including the endomorph, which in the athletic world includes Sumo wrestlers like Asashōryū Akinori.) For the purposes of our discussion here, let's look at a young NBA player and the challenges a strength coach might face given his unique somatotype.

Basketball players tend to be taller than the average population and blessed with long limbs. This extreme length, combined with a very long spine, might create a number of core challenges for trainers and strength coaches, not the least of which is the required vertebral stability and strength, specifically in the thoracic and lumbar regions, central to support extremity functionality. Furthermore, high-top shoes, ankle braces, and taping have reached such a level of ubiquity in this sport that many coaches *require* them to be used, even though they often severely restrict mobility in the talocrural joint of the ankle. This condition can cause a variety of knee issues, and can also move right up the kinetic chain to affect the mechanics of the hip girdle. Combine these complications with the basketball player's freakishly long levers of the spine and extremities, and you are left with an athlete who could be at an excessive disadvantage because of his body's characteristics. However, if trained correctly, this same athlete has the capability of creating immense amounts of positive leverage and gaining a performance advantage over most opponents.

When working with such athletes, the focus of the functional core program should be on correcting kyphotic posture and hip imbalances (see tables 21.13 to 21.18).

Test: FAIL

Table 21.13 Stability Phase 1 (4 to 6 Weeks): Basketball

Region	Exercise	Sets	Time or reps
Anti-extension	Mountain Climber, Incline	4	12
Anti-rotation	Lateral Elbow Plank Ball Toss	4	12 each side
Scapulothoracic	Prone Shoulder Abduction (T), Floor	4	12
Lumbo-pelvic hip complex	Single-Leg Balance	4	30 sec each leg

Test: PASS

Table 21.14 Strength Phase 1 (4 to 6 Weeks): Basketball

Region	Exercise	Sets	Time or reps
Anti-extension	Straight-Arm Plank on Stability Ball: Rock the Cradle	4	12
Anti-rotary	Pallof Horizontal Press Progression 4: Staggered Stance	4	12 each side
Scapulothoracic	Prone Loaded Shoulder Abduction (T), Incline Bench	4	12
Lumbo-pelvic hip complex	X-Band Walk	4	12 steps each way

Test: PASS

Table 21.15	Power Phase 1 (4 to 6 Weeks): Basketball		
Region	**Exercise**	**Sets**	**Time or reps**
Anti-extension	Overhead Medicine Ball Slam Progression 3: Tall Kneeling With Wind-Up	4	8
Anti-rotation	Medicine Ball Side Throw Progression 3: Standing	4	8
Lumbo-pelvic hip complex	Medial Box Hop Up	4	8 each leg

Test: PASS

Table 21.16	Stability Phase 2 (4 to 6 Weeks): Basketball		
Region	**Exercise**	**Sets**	**Time or reps**
Anti-extension	Mountain Climber, Unstable Upper	4	12
Anti-rotation	Lateral Straight-Arm Plank Ball Toss	4	12 each side
Scapulothoracic	Prone Shoulder Abduction (T), Incline Bench	4	12
Lumbo-pelvic hip complex	Single-Leg Balance and Reach	4	12 each direction

Test: PASS

Table 21.17	Strength Phase 2 (4 to 6 Weeks): Basketball		
Region	**Exercise**	**Sets**	**Time or reps**
Anti-extension	Straight-Arm Plank on Stability Ball: Stir the Pot	4	12
Anti-rotation	Pallof Horizontal Press Progression 5: Lunge Stance	4	12 each side
Scapulothoracic	Prone Loaded Shoulder Abduction (T), Stability Ball	4	12
Lumbo-pelvic hip complex	Lateral Band Slide, Skating	4	12

Test: PASS

Table 21.18	Power Phase 2 (4 to 6 Weeks): Basketball		
Region	**Exercise**	**Sets**	**Time or reps**
Anti-extension	Overhead Medicine Ball Slam Progression 4: Standing With Wind-Up	4	8
Anti-rotation	Tornado Ball Twist	4	8
Lumbo-pelvic hip complex	Ice Skater	4	8

SWIMMING

We have mentioned swimming several times in this book because the aqueous challenge of pulling yourself horizontally through high drag forces in the fastest possible time will in fact create a unique set of core challenges. Spending such large amounts of time in a highly unstable environment performing greatly repetitious movements triggers a number of muscular and mechanical compensations. Because of the almost continual requirements on the body's anterior musculature, the posterior chain of muscle becomes underutilized, leading to the common, and feasibly distressful, thoracic kyphosis and unstable scapulae. Considering the vast number of shoulder problems that plague swimmers, such an extreme imbalance can cause an inescapable cycle of chronic shoulder trauma. This upper-crossed syndrome must be addressed and will thus be the focus of all core work for these athletes. Another common area of concern for the swimmer is the gluteal complex, which tends to exhibit a sport-wide underdevelopment (depending on type of swimmer, event, and stroke selection). The glutes play a huge role in the required explosive extension of the hip when coming off the blocks or pool walls, and they are needed for lumbo-pelvic hip stability throughout. Combine with this a propensity for hypermobile joints, and we find that swimmers have a number of problems to address.

All of this must be considered when developing a core program for swimmers. Hypermobile joints tend to respond well to isometric core activities in the short term because the body learns to control itself on stable surfaces. Integrated strength lifts such as the heavy carry walking series (for example, Farmer's Walks and Waiter's Walks) and Turkish Get-Ups can also influence a swimmer's core success because swimmers tend to have large strength deficiencies compared to other athletes. This is often a cultural issue, in which strength and conditioning at the sub-elite levels is either poorly performed or omitted altogether in favor of more pool time. Such insufficiencies can be corrected through total core strength development lifts, which additionally help to train overall body awareness and control. As is true for all athletes, creating higher levels of efficiency is the ultimate objective, but in the case of swimmers, we need to always be mindful of the environment they operate in and the resulting impact on their bodies. Tables 21.19 to 21.24 show examples of core programming for swimmers.

Test: FAIL

Table 21.19 Stability Phase 1 (4 to 6 Weeks): Swimming

Region	Exercise	Sets	Time or reps
Anti-extension	Elbow Plank, Single-Leg Hip Extension	3	20 sec each leg
Anti-rotation	Rolling Pattern 2: Hard Roll With Ball	3	12 each side
Scapulothoracic	Prone Scapulothoracic Combination (YTA), Incline Bench	3	12
Lumbo-pelvic hip complex	Hip Lift on Stability Ball	3	12

Test: PASS

Table 21.20 Strength Phase 1 (4 to 6 Weeks): Swimming

Region	Exercise	Sets	Time or reps
Anti-extension	Rollout: Stability Ball, Kneeling	3	12
Lumbo-pelvic hip complex	Hip Lift, Shoulders Elevated	3	12 each leg
Total core	Waiter's Walk	3	20 feet (6 m)

Test: PASS

Table 21.21	Power Phase 1 (4 to 6 Weeks): Swimming		
Region	**Exercise**	**Sets**	**Time or reps**
Anti-extension	Overhead Medicine Ball Slam Progression 1: Tall Kneeling	3	8
Anti-rotation	Medicine Ball Chop Slam Progression 2: Tall Kneeling	3	8 each side
Lumbo-pelvic hip complex	Single-Leg Power Step-Up	3	8 each leg

Test: PASS

Table 21.22	Stability Phase 2 (4 to 6 Weeks): Swimming		
Region	**Exercise**	**Sets**	**Time or reps**
Anti-extension	Straight-Arm Plank, Single-Leg Hip Extension	4	20 sec each leg
Anti-rotation	Rolling Pattern 2: Hard Roll	4	12 each side
Scapulothoracic	Prone Scapulothoracic Combination (YTA), Stability Ball	4	12
Lumbo-pelvic hip complex	Single-Leg Hip Lift on Stability Ball	4	12 each leg

Test: PASS

Table 21.23	Strength Phase 2 (4 to 6 weeks): Swimming		
Region	**Exercise**	**Sets**	**Time or reps**
Anti-extension	Rollout: Dolly	4	12
Total core	Turkish Get-Up	4	6 each side

Test: PASS

Table 21.24	Power Phase 2 (4 to 6 Weeks): Swimming		
Region	**Exercise**	**Sets**	**Time or reps**
Anti-extension	Overhead Medicine Ball Slam Progression 2: Standing	4	8
Anti-rotation	Medicine Ball Chop Slam Progression 3: Standing	4	8 each side
Lumbo-pelvic hip complex	Power Step-Up	4	8

DISTANCE RUNNING

Of all the sports discussed in this book and across the spectrum of athletic endeavor, running is one that resonates with all of us. It is an activity that requires deep commitment and supreme focus, but it does not require physical mastery over a piece of equipment or an opponent, and it is not restricted to a court or a field. Most people can enjoy running and compete at any level, even if only against themselves.

Like swimming, running requires copious, repetitive motions that lead to a high joint-impact quotient with a number of physiological and mechanical adaptations and exposure to a myriad of overuse injuries. Patello-femoral issues can run rife in runners, as can lower leg and foot issues.

Many of these complications can be reduced and even eliminated by improving stability in the hip and allowing the leg to align more appropriately as we forcefully drive the foot into the ground. Quality hip extension—or, more accurately, *repeated* quality hip extension—is critical for effective running, as is the ability to cross the finish line as quickly as possible. Focusing on our cylinder and aiming to limit unwanted extraneous rotation between torso and hips makes for more efficient running. Core training is no more or less important to running than to any other sport, but the act of terrestrial locomotion is a request to your body to undergo a heavy-duty task, and rewarding the body by preparing it for the rigors and impact of multiple-leg cycles is fundamental to success. Tables 20.25 to 20.30 present sample core programming for distance runners.

Test: FAIL

Table 21.25 Stability Phase 1 (4 to 6 Weeks): Distance Running

Region	Exercise	Sets	Time or reps
Anti-extension	Mountain Climber, Unstable Upper	4	12
Anti-rotation	Lateral Elbow Plank, Unstable Upper, Arm and Leg Abduction	4	20 sec each arm
Scapulothoracic	Prone Shoulder Abduction (T), Floor	4	12
Lumbo-pelvic hip complex	Unilateral Bridge	4	12 each leg

Test: PASS

Table 21.26 Strength Phase 1 (4 to 6 Weeks): Distance Running

Region	Exercise	Sets	Time or reps
Anti-extension	Rollout: Dolly	4	12
Anti-rotary	Landmine Rotation	4	12
Scapulothoracic	Band Pull Apart	4	12
Lumbo-pelvic hip complex	Lateral Band Slide, Straight Legs	4	10 steps each way

Test: PASS

Table 21.27   Power Phase 1 (4 to 6 Weeks): Distance Running

Region	Exercise	Sets	Time or reps
Anti-extension	Overhead Medicine Ball Slam Progression 1: Tall Kneeling	4	8 each side
Anti-rotation	Medicine Ball Side Throw Progression 4: Staggered Stance	4	8 each side
Lumbo-pelvic hip complex	Medial Box Hop Up	4	12

Test: PASS

Table 21.28   Stability Phase 2 (4 to 6 Weeks): Distance Running

Region	Exercise	Sets	Time or reps
Anti-extension	Mountain Climber, Suspended Upper or Lower	4	12
Anti-rotation	Lateral Elbow Plank, Unstable Upper, Arm and Leg Abduction	4	25 sec each side
Scapulothoracic	Prone Shoulder Abduction (T), Incline Bench	4	12
Lumbo-pelvic hip complex	Single-Leg Bridge on Stability Ball	4	12 each leg

Test: PASS

Table 21.29   Strength Phase 2 (4 to 6 Weeks): Distance Running

Region	Exercise	Sets	Time or reps
Anti-extension	Rollout: Ab Wheel	4	12
Anti-rotation	Landmine Rotation With Handle	4	12
Scapulothoracic	Prone Loaded Shoulder Abduction (T), Incline Bench	4	12
Lumbo-pelvic hip complex	X-Band Walk	4	10 steps

Test: PASS

Table 21.30   Power Phase 2 (4 to 6 Weeks): Distance Running

Region	Exercise	Sets	Time or reps
Anti-extension	Overhead Medicine Ball Slam Progression 2: Standing	4	8 each
Anti-rotary	Medicine Ball Side Throw Progression 5: Lunge Stance	4	8 each side
Lumbo-pelvic hip complex	Alternating Leg Power Step-Up	4	12

When organizing a suitable training regimen, a total approach strives to improve the following athletic components:

- strength
- power
- agility
- coordination
- balance and body control
- functionality
- speed
- anaerobic and aerobic conditioning
- flexibility
- body composition
- ambidexterity
- dynamic spine stabilization

The purpose of this chapter project was to demonstrate how to construct the most effective, personalized training program focused on enhancing individual strengths and eliminating performance weaknesses as assessed for each athlete. Only playing your sport void of additional adjunct training will not adequately prepare you for the coming season and top-level performance. The requisite skill necessary to play at a high intensity is determined by the level of your physical base. If this physical base is underdeveloped or for some reason is in decline, performance too will decline. It should be obvious that to maximize your performance potential, you must train the skills of your sport as well as the physical base that supports those skills.

Sport is a microcosm of life; if losing becomes acceptable in sport, what chance will we have at winning in life? With over a half a century in the business of sports and athletics and after training thousands of athletes, there is one prevailing characteristic we both recognize that champions demonstrate: They identify a goal and choose the most direct route toward its successful completion. It is within this straight line that the athlete discovers unreserved strength and dominance. We could have taken the inscrutable approach and written a book with all mystifying bells, enigmatic whistles, arrogant medical terminology, and deceptive promises, but it ultimately comes down to you, the athlete. The teams and individuals we've been fortunate enough to work with, including the game-changing Knicks of the 90s; hall-of-fame football, basketball, and baseball players; number-one world-ranked tennis players; Olympians and world record holders; and now, passionate collegiate athletes, have all discovered an important quality about their growth and development. Any program is only as good as the effort put forth by those who see the big picture and realize that they are in control of their own destiny. No one is going to do the work for you. All of the manual therapy in the world will not take your skills to the next level. Passive, low-intensity muscle isolation training is great for playing chess or throwing darts, but in order to perform at a high intensity you must commit to an intelligent training regimen executed at a higher intensity.

The individuals and teams that we have been privileged to work with could see the big picture and chose to devote the effort necessary to maximize their potential. They understood that training should always be more demanding than the game. In other words, the best athletes trained beyond the expectations of their sport. Focus your efforts, eliminate weaknesses, train smart, and train hard. This is how gold medals, top rankings, gold gloves, NCAA tournament appearances, and conference championships are realized.

Enclosed in these pages is the culmination of over 50 years of experience. We have endeavored to provide you with the most up-to-date core-training knowledge available. That said, this project was never intended to be an all-inclusive tome, nor is it the magnum opus of core training. The essence of this book is to put you on the correct path to core-training success, no matter your goal or background. At this point, you have a good working knowledge of a very successful system—one that has a solid structure but is flexible enough to be adapted by any athlete or individual. As your experience grows, you will be able to identify new core exercises, know immediately if they are appropriate for you and your specific needs, and understand precisely where they fall in your cyclical program. You will also be able to regress or progress the exercise as you need to, thereby encouraging experimentation and keeping your protocol fresh.

Through the writing of this book and many conversations and e-mails, we have determined that core training should not have limitations (other than the basic guidelines we have shared). Moreover, core training should be limitless—the benefits should be available to all, not just the elite. You will undoubtedly return to this book for clarification or guidance, but the testament to its success will be your ability to take everything you need from it and go forth to create your own success. Your core training will last you a lifetime. It has been a pleasure working alongside you and showing you the complete ins and outs of conditioning to the core.

About the Authors

Greg Brittenham served as assistant coach for player development and team conditioning with the New York Knicks for 20 years before taking on the position of director of athletic performance for men's and women's basketball at Wake Forest University before the 2011-12 season. He was also the director of the Center for Athletic Performance at the National Institute for Fitness and Sport. In addition to NBA players, he has advised and trained athletes in the NFL, MLB, several number one and many more top ten tennis players in the world and international champions in gymnastics and cycling and the Olympics.

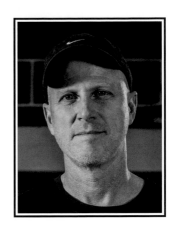

Brittenham's training regimens for improving overall athletic ability have made him a popular speaker and demonstrator at clinics and conferences worldwide. He authored *Complete Conditioning for Basketball* (Human Kinetics, 1995) and coauthored *Stronger Abs and Back* (Human Kinetics, 1997) with his father, Dean Brittenham, a pioneer in the field of strength and conditioning.

Daniel Taylor, MS, PES, CSCS is the head strength and conditioning coach at Siena College and oversees those efforts for all 18 Division I varsity programs at the college, as varied as water polo and lacrosse. He has trained athletes who have advanced to the professional level in soccer, lacrosse, baseball, and basketball. Taylor was part of Siena men's basketball's historic 3 championships in a row (2008-2010) that led to two first round wins in the NCAA tournament (2008 and 2009).

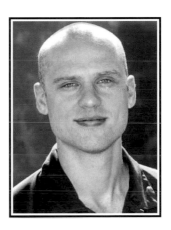

Taylor previously worked with men's and women's basketball at The College of Saint Rose in Albany, New York and with the New York Knicks Training Camps. He has been a speaker at numerous clinics and workshops in the northeast geared to high school through college level athletes. Originally from North Yorkshire, England, he now resides in Scotia, New York

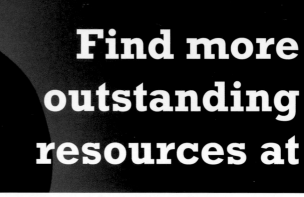
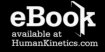
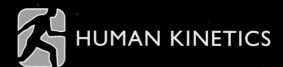